Viral Diseases and One Health in Africa

Juliet Adamma Shenge • Akebe Luther King Abia
Editors

Viral Diseases and One Health in Africa

Springer

Editors
Juliet Adamma Shenge
Virology Research Laboratory
Biological Sciences
Dominican University Ibadan
Ibadan, Nigeria

Akebe Luther King Abia
Total Environment Research (TEN-R) Group
College of Health Sciences
University of KwaZulu-Natal
Durban, South Africa

Environmental Research Foundation
Westville, South Africa

ISBN 978-3-032-09612-8 ISBN 978-3-032-09613-5 (eBook)
https://doi.org/10.1007/978-3-032-09613-5

This Springer imprint is published by the registered company Springer Nature Switzerland AG
The registered company address is: Gewerbestrasse 11, 6330 Cham, Switzerland

Juliet Adamma Shenge
To my father of blessed memory, Fidelis Amajuoyi Nwagwu, my pillar and mentor, who instilled in me the blazing passion for science at an early age.

Akebe Luther King Abia
Dedicated to Guy R. Lanza, whose unwavering belief in me lit the path when the way seemed unclear, and whose mentorship continues to inspire my pursuit of knowledge.

Foreword

Juliet Adamma Shenge and Akebe Luther King Abia

The pain of one is the pain of all. *Swahili proverb*

The recent COVID-19 pandemic challenged health systems worldwide, even in developed countries, prompting the need to develop early warning systems to monitor present pandemics and prevent the emergence of new ones or the re-emergence of once-forgotten ones. However, setting up such surveillance systems requires an in-depth understanding of the disease landscape in any given community. This is particularly important because the impact of COVID-19 and other diseases is not felt equally worldwide.

Africa carries a disproportionately high burden of viral infections such as HIV, hepatitis, Ebola, and emerging zoonoses, making the continent a critical hotspot for both endemic and epidemic diseases. Weak health and surveillance systems, combined with environmental and socioeconomic factors, hinder early detection and timely responses, thereby increasing the risk of outbreaks. Genomic surveillance and a One Health approach are essential for understanding transmission dynamics; guiding diagnostics, vaccines, and therapeutics; and preventing spillover events. Strengthening Africa's capacity to study and respond to viral infections not only improves regional health outcomes but also enhances global pandemic preparedness and health security. Therefore, understanding the dynamics of viral disease emergence in the continent is paramount to protecting the population from future epidemics and pandemics.

Viral Diseases and One Health in Africa comprises 15 chapters featuring, among others, a collection of research on various emerging and re-emerging viral agents emanating from the continent; their presence in the environment, animals, and other hosts and vectors; their resistance to antivirals; existing detection and diagnostic tools; health systems management and mitigation of viral diseases; challenges of implementing early warning systems; surveillance for viral disease outbreaks in Africa; the impact of viral infections on the continent's economy and the psychosocial impacts on its populations; and integrating the one health concept or approach of preventing diseases outbreaks, spillover, and pandemics with emphasis on sustainable participatory strategies to achieving overall human, animal, and environmental health.

Africa has a rich biodiversity and favourable environmental conditions that facilitate increased human-animal interaction, making it an ideal hotspot for the emergence, re-emergence, and transmission of zoonotic diseases. Four chapters in this edited book address viral zoonoses in Africa. Animal Ebola, Marburg, Rift Valley fever, Lassa fever, and Rabies can spread from animals to humans through vectors like mosquitoes or direct contact. As such, one chapter assesses the role of vectors in the transmission of these infections between sectors, while another chapter further examines the public health implications of these zoonotic viral infections on public health in Africa. Some viral infections affect humans indirectly by impacting other sectors, as illustrated by a chapter on the impact of swine flu on food security and another chapter addressing plant viruses and their impact on food security. The environmental dimension of viral diseases is significant within the African context, as many parts, especially in sub-Saharan Africa, still lack provisions for safe sanitary facilities. Thus, two chapters examine environmental reservoirs of viruses generally, while a second chapter focuses on rotaviruses and noroviruses in wastewater. Recognising the environmental presence of viruses, especially in sewage, one chapter proceeds to assess the use of wastewater-based epidemiology as an early warning tool for potential outbreaks in Africa. Although the detection of viruses is complex, at times requiring advanced molecular tools, Africa has made significant strides in this regard, as evidenced by one chapter that sheds light on the use of genomics in viral detection on the continent. Although a health issue, viral infections extend beyond public health to impact the psychological well-being of affected populations, as demonstrated in one chapter. At times, the solutions require political will, as shown in a chapter on the politics of public health, with a specific focus on the ongoing COVID-19 pandemic. Lastly, it is now recognised that a successful fight against infections requires effective and coordinated efforts from all sectors. Hence, two chapters discuss the application of the One Health approach and the associated challenges in tackling viral infections in Africa.

Emerging and re-emerging pathogenic viruses are becoming humanity's worst enemy, especially in an era of rapid globalisation and irrefutable climate change that favours the rapid spread of diseases across borders. However, unlike other disease-causing agents like bacteria, viruses remain the dreadful, yet understudied, enemies. Worse still, there are tremendous disparities in disease burden globally, with low- and middle-income regions, especially in sub-Saharan Africa, bearing the lion's share in terms of the types, numbers, and implications thereof. Combined, the 15 chapters in this edited volume place Africa on the global health map regarding viral infections. Africa undoubtedly has the potential to be on par with the global north, as evidenced by the remarkable achievements made in containing and tracking the recent COVID-19 pandemic. However, achieving this needs more tailored solutions, coupled with political will and effective national and international collaborations. This volume, through its chapters, aims to spur the discourse in this direction to inform measures to combat viral diseases where and whenever they emerge, not only within the continent but across the globe, as it is now clear that viral diseases know little or no boundaries and no one can fight this battle alone.

Preface

Viral diseases continue to be a public health threat, demonstrated by several viral pandemics that have occurred over the years, the most recent being COVID-19, caused by Severe Acute Respiratory Syndrome Coronavirus 2 (SARS-CoV-2). While these pandemics affect humanity globally, low- and middle-income countries are usually the most affected, especially those in Africa. The African continent, especially the sub-Saharan part, represents a unique and complex environmental, economic, health system, and socio-political landscape, which has favoured the emergence, re-emergence, or survival and spread of viral infections.

Although there has been an overall positive outcome of most interventions aimed at fighting viral infections in the continent, most of these countries still contribute to the high global prevalence of viral diseases and their associated impact on society as a whole. This has been fuelled by poor sanitation conditions, the absence of potable water for personal and household hygiene, and weak health systems, usually due to a lack of finances and political will to invest in them. Moreover, social and cultural practices that allow constant interaction between humans, animals, and their environment increase the chances of infection. These factors collectively pose a significant challenge: antiviral resistance, which threatens to reverse the positive strides made so far in the fight against viral infections in Africa.

This 15-chapter volume on viral diseases and One Health in Africa aims to assess the African viral research landscape, examining the prevalence of various viral infections and the associated challenges, while showcasing the successes made and using the lessons learned to address pending challenges, such as antiviral resistance, the environmental dimension of viral infections, and the lack of funding, as well as the socioeconomic and political implications of these infections.

Our firm conviction is that this book will stimulate greater research focus on viral infections in Africa, given that viruses are understudied despite their significant contribution to disease burden on the continent, ensuring that research on the continent uses a one health and multi-dimensional approaches to combat viral diseases where and whenever they emerge on the African continent.

When the disease is on one side, one should not run away to the other. *Ethiopian proverb*

Ibadan, Nigeria
Durban, South Africa

Juliet Adamma Shenge
Akebe Luther King Abia

Contents

Chapter 1
The Concept and Application of One Health in Africa

Juliet Adamma Shenge

1.1 Introduction

The highest burden of infectious diseases in the world occurs in Africa, caused mainly by poor socioeconomic status, inadequate infrastructure, and close human-animal interactions. These include human-livestock, human-wildlife, or human-livestock-wildlife interactions, emanating from the unprofessional management of forest resources, reserves, and agricultural and land use in Africa, but still have a very low capacity for managing risks and the threats of infectious diseases.

The concept of One Health has evolved over centuries, gaining particular importance in recent times due to the increasing environmental changes that correspond to explosive human and animal populations (Evans and Leighton 2014). However, in Africa, several challenges have contributed to the application and practical use of this concept, namely, a lack of collaboration among relevant agencies, limited attention from the government and other stakeholders (Destoumieux-Garzon et al. 2018; Mpundu et al. 2023).

According to the Tripartite (WHO, FAO, and OIE), the One Health approach is defined as an approach employed to tackle disease threats at the human-animal-environment interface across all relevant sectors and disciplines, with the ultimate goal of achieving optimal health outcomes for both people and animals (Bodenham et al. 2021; WHO, FAO and OIE 2019).

A One Health approach to disease prevention and control involves a trans-disciplinary approach to creating a healthy planet for humans, animals and plants, as well as their environment. It reflects the interplay or interconnection between animals and humans in relation to the environment, elicited by several factors, including climate change, globalisation, pathogen adaptation, changing lifestyles

J. A. Shenge (✉)
Virology Research Laboratory, Biological Sciences, Dominican University Ibadan, Ibadan, Nigeria

J. A. Shenge, A. L. K. Abia (eds.), *Viral Diseases and One Health in Africa*,
https://doi.org/10.1007/978-3-032-09613-5_1

and evolving patterns in animal production (Evans and Leighton 2014), with consequent effects such as antimicrobial resistance and environmental degradation. The concept embraces integrated, unifying approaches or team efforts in various fields locally, regionally and globally to sustainably balance and achieve good health for humans, animals and the environment. This means that by protecting one, the other is equally protected (WHO 2024). Numerous health threats significantly affect populations at the human-animal-environment interface, comprising zoonotic diseases, emerging and re-emerging infectious diseases, vector-borne diseases, the menace of antimicrobial resistance, food-borne disease, and unstable or adverse weather conditions, popularly referred to as climate change. Moreover, the surge in infectious diseases triggered by climate change, other environmental factors, and human activities has called for timely collaborative efforts from all stakeholders to prevent future pandemics. In this light, it becomes very necessary to engage all stakeholders with a keen interest in global health to pave the way for a future devoid of infectious diseases using the One Health approach or platform to detect, curb or prevent disease spillover from animals to humans and vice versa.

Africa is a continent endowed with rich natural and human resources. Reflecting on this unique feature, the African continent is poised with the right machinery, if harnessed sustainably, to accomplish all its health needs and stand at par with other continents worldwide. However, conflicts and poor governance have robbed the continent of these strengths. From Central to East, West to South, and Northern Africa, the fragility of the health system on the continent underscores the need for a stable, harmonised and all-encompassing approach to health and development. This was particularly demonstrated by the inability to cope with the outbreak of Ebola between 2014 and 2016, as exhibited by some African countries through their health systems (Mbilo et al. 2020).

Prioritisation, integration and application of the One Health approach to disease prevention and control in the unique environment of the African continent, therefore, becomes necessary with the expectant goal of achieving quality health outcomes for all Africans, as discussed in this chapter with reference to the key tools needed to achieve this goal.

1.2 Disease Surveillance and Intelligence

According to the Centers for Disease Prevention and Control (CDC), disease surveillance and intelligence encompasses all the activities that aim to detect, monitor and respond promptly and adequately to diseases (CDC 2017). The goal of any surveillance system is to strengthen the health system so that it can make proper decisions, policies, and actions that improve the public's health. A strategic, multidisciplinary, trans-disciplinary approach integrated into the One Health concept is needed to achieve this goal. Majorly, these include the detection of early warning signs of diseases, outbreaks in animals and humans, prediction of the risk or actual occurrence of disease in a population, and also evaluation of the effect of critical events such as climate change, antimicrobial resistance, food and water safety (Fasina et al. 2021). These include, but are not limited to, timely data collection, processing, and monitoring of events at local, state, and national levels, which then inform decision-making and policies. There is a need to strengthen public health institutes to raise competent personnel and research teams.

Surveillance data have shown that the burden of diseases among humans, animals and the environment is on the increase with associated costs (Bodenham et al. 2021). Many factors come into play when considering this critical trend in disease surveillance and response. Both communicable and non-communicable human diseases significantly impact the body by altering the physiological and biochemical pathways. Therefore, screening and monitoring human diseases require some unique strategies or approaches. The most important strategy includes assessing disease risks, considering diseases of public health importance, availability and strength of health systems, an inclusive plan of action, actual implementation, monitoring and evaluation of outcomes (WHO 2006).

According to a report by the Institute of Medicine (US) Forum on Emerging Infections (2000), the basic components of disease surveillance include data collection, analysis, dissemination and response, indicating the major steps involved in any disease surveillance. Integrating the One Health approach to every disease surveillance, as stipulated by the International Health Regulations during the COVID-19 pandemic, will facilitate early detection and response to the outbreak by the relevant agencies.

1.3 Food and Water Safety

The Food and Agriculture Organisation of the United Nations (FAO) recognises the importance of food and water safety in human development. Pathogens enter the environment before reaching food and water. Contamination of food and water occurs through various means. The faecal-oral route is particularly significant for the infection of human and animal populations. Water remains the primary vehicle for the transmission of pathogens, with sewage being a significant contributor. This is especially true when sewage enters the environment through the irrigation of crops with partially treated or untreated wastewater used for irrigation or aquaculture. This wastewater that enters the environment may equally contain heavy metals, faeces and greywater, which may harbour more pathogenic microorganisms than other sources of water, such as surface or underground water sources (FAO 2025). Wastewater contains pathogens such as viruses, bacteria, helminths and protozoa. In low-middle-income countries (LMICs), less than 8% of wastewater is treated. Untreated wastewater, when used for crop irrigation, feeding animals and other forms, can transmit infectious diseases and contribute to the spread of antimicrobial resistance. Viruses such as hepatitis A (HAV) and E virus (HEV) have been profiled in wastewater (La Rosa et al. 2014; Rau et al. 2024). Hepatitis A and E infections are neglected tropical diseases that can be transmitted through contaminated water, food and other environmental sources and may result in fulminant hepatitis in infected persons.

Wastewater surveillance and monitoring provide important information for early detection of possible outbreaks and rapid response to public health threats. In most cases, individuals infected with some viruses, such as SARS-CoV-2, respiratory syncytial virus (RSV), and influenza typically transmit these pathogens through human waste, such as faeces and wastewater (CDC 2023). Genomic surveillance in municipal water supplies and other wastewater management sites facilitates the identification of viruses and the tracking of emerging viral variants in communities (CDC 2023). Adopting and applying whole genome sequencing technologies in LMICs will improve surveillance of infectious diseases in humans, animals and the environment.

1.4 Connection Between Human and Animal Health

The One Health approach to detecting and monitoring infectious diseases builds on the understanding that human and animal health are strongly linked. Through the One Health approach, a multidisciplinary outlook is needed to prevent infectious disease transmission in developing nations. Humans not only share the planet with animals but also share several diseases with animals in the environment, where a complex network of interactions goes on, and as such, impact each other in different ways, including the transmission of pathogens (Alves and Policarpo 2018). As people's health is closely connected to that of animals in our shared environment, there is a need to understand early warning signs of diseases in humans and animals and tackle such issues before possible spillover. For instance, the presence of wild birds infected with avian influenza, such as H5N1 or West Nile virus, in a community may lead to the death of the birds as a warning sign of a potential health threat to humans in that environment (CDC 2024).

1.5 Conclusion

Although the One Health approach and its applications remain theoretical in most African nations, there is a pressing need for stakeholders and policymakers to integrate One Health into various sectors. Such activities include emergency preparedness and response to sporadic outbreaks, strengthening laboratory systems for pathogen detection, especially genomic profiling of circulating variants of emerging and re-emerging viruses, upgrading the public health sector and evidence-based research using the One Health approach. These will prevent and control infectious diseases, including those emanating from animal and arthropod vectors, the environment and even humans.

References

Alves RRN, Policarpo IDS (2018) Animals and human health: where do they meet? Ethnozoology 2018:233–259

Bodenham RF, Mtui-Malamsha N, Gatei W, Woldetsadik MA, Cassell CH, Salyer SJ, Halliday JEB, Nonga HE, Swai ES, Makungu S, Mwakapeje E, Bernard J, Bebay C, Makonnen YJ, Fasina FO (2021) Multisectoral cost analysis of a human and livestock anthrax outbreak in Songwe Region, Tanzania (December 2018–January 2019), using a novel Outbreak Costing Tool. One Health 13:100259. https://doi.org/10.1016/j.onehlt.2021.100259

Centers for Disease Control and Prevention (2017) One Health zoonotic disease prioritization for multisectoral engagement in Tanzania

Center for Disease Prevention and Control (2023) National Wastewater sSurveillance System. www.cdc.gov/wastewater

Centers for Disease Control and Prevention (2024) What is One Health?

Destoumieux-Garzon D, Mavingui P, Boetsch G, Boissier J, Darriet F, Duboz P et al (2018) The One Health concept: 10 years old and a long road ahead. Front Vet Sci 5:14

Evans BR, Leighton FA (2014) A history of One Health. Rev Sci Tech 33(2):413–420. https://doi.org/10.20506/rst.33.2.2298

Fasina FO, Fasanmi OG, Makonnem YJ, Bebay C, Beth B, Roesel K (2021) The One Health landscape in Sub-Saharan African countries. One Health 13:100325

Food and Agricultural Organization (2025) FAO land and water and One Health. Innovations and digital technology applications for One Health

Institute of Medicine (US) Forum on Emerging Infections (2000) In: Davis JR, Lederberg J (eds) Public health systems and emerging infections: assessing the capabilities of the public and private sectors: workshop summary. National Academies Press, Washington, DC. 3, Surveillance. Available from: https://www.ncbi.nlm.nih.gov/books/NBK100249/

La Rosa G, Della Libera S, Iaconelli M et al (2014) Surveillance of hepatitis A virus in urban sewage and comparison with cases notified in the course of an outbreak, Italy 2013. BMC Infect Dis 14:419

Mbilo C, Coetzer A, Bonfoh B, Angot A, Bebay C, Cassamá B, De Benedictis P, Ebou MH, Gnanvi C, Kallo V, Lokossou RH, Manjuba C, Mokondjimobe E, Mouillé B, Mounkaila M, Ndour APN, Nel L, Olugasa BO, Pato P, Pyana PP, Rerambyath GA, Roamba RC, Sadeuh-Mba SA, Suluku R, Suu-Ire RD, Tejiokem MC, Tetchi M, Tiembre I, Traoré A, Voupawoe G, Zinsstag J (2020) Dog rabies control in West and Central Africa: a review. Acta Trop 224: 105459. https://doi.org/10.1016/j.actatropica.2020.105459

Mpundu M, Chanda R, Khan S (2023) Antimicrobial stewardship in Africa. In: Abia ALK, Essack SF (eds) Antimicrobial research and One Health in Africa. Springer, Cham, pp 19–29

Rau F, Elsener C, Meister TL, Gomer A, Kallies R, Dittmer U, Steinmann E, Todt D (2024) Monitoring of hepatitis E virus in wastewater can identify clinically relevant variants. Liver Int 44(3):637–643. https://doi.org/10.1111/liv.15842

World Health Organization (2006) Communicable disease surveillance and response systems. Guide to monitoring and evaluating. WHO/CDS/EPR/LYO/2006.2

World Health Organization, Food and Agriculture Organization of the United Nations (2019) World Organisation for Animal Health taking a multisectoral, One Health approach: a tripartite guide to addressing zoonotic diseases in countries

World Health Organization (2024) One Health. https://www.who.int/health-topics/one-health

Chapter 2
Viral Haemorrhagic Fever and Zoonoses in Africa

Juliet Adamma Shenge

2.1 Introduction

In recent years, the world has witnessed a surge in the emergence of infectious zoonotic diseases, which in most cases are seen to be neglected, according to Di Bari et al. (2023). Most viral haemorrhagic fever infections are zoonotic and seriously threaten human and animal health, as they are typically transmitted from animals to humans or vice versa (Di Bari et al. 2023). Recent reports by the World Health Organization (WHO 2020) show an increase in the number of zoonotic diseases, especially those emanating from wildlife, sporadic infections transmitted by domestic and farm animals with the potential to cause outbreaks, spillover and even pandemics. The WHO has warned that zoonotic diseases, including haemorrhagic fever, have jumped 63% compared with transmission a decade ago in Africa (WHO 2020). It has been estimated that about 80% of viruses that infect humans are zoonotic. Most of these viruses are carried in animal reservoirs, including some groups of mammalian, invertebrate vectors, avian, swine or intermediate hosts, and can jump from animals to humans due to mutations in their genome (Shenge and Opayele 2020; Shenge 2023).

African countries, including the Democratic Republic of the Congo (DRC), Sierra-Leon, Uganda, Liberia, Guinea and Nigeria, have experienced outbreaks of haemorrhagic fever of viral origin at different times. Since 2013, pockets of sporadic outbreaks of Ebola have occurred in West and East Africa, particularly. The East African region has particularly experienced a surge in Marburg and Ebola virus outbreaks, while West Africa, including Nigeria, witnessed a rise in Lassa haemorrhagic fever and dengue haemorrhagic fever, two important vector-borne viral diseases, in addition to the existing zoonotic diseases.

J. A. Shenge (✉)
Virology Research Laboratory, Biological Sciences, Dominican University Ibadan, Ibadan, Nigeria

J. A. Shenge, A. L. K. Abia (eds.), *Viral Diseases and One Health in Africa*,
https://doi.org/10.1007/978-3-032-09613-5_2

Nigeria ranks among the top ten countries in the world with the highest burden of infectious zoonotic diseases. Hence, understanding the mechanisms of virus-host interactions, such as viral-host immune evasion, and its role in disease pathogenesis becomes essential in mounting preventive measures against these pathogens (Shenge 2023). The Nigeria Center for Disease Prevention and Control (NCDC) prioritised zoonotic diseases in 2017, and experts from the human-animal-environment health array in Nigeria were engaged using prioritisation tools. From this, 36 of 52 previously selected zoonoses were identified for prioritisation, of which rabies, avian influenza, Ebola virus disease, swine influenza and anthrax were rated most important based on their weighted scores (Ihekweazu et al. 2021). This underscores the importance of one health in addressing the burden of infectious diseases in Africa and the world, irrespective of the origin of the disease. Although infectious diseases such as avian influenza in the past have attracted attention from both local and international bodies due to their pandemic outlook, neglected tropical zoonotic diseases, including monkeypox (mpox), rabies and Lassa, which are endemic yet preventable, should be prioritised to reduce their impact in most rural communities.

2.2 Major Zoonotic Viral Haemorrhagic Fever

2.2.1 Ebola Virus Disease (EBV)

Ebola virus disease (EVD) is caused by the filovirus named Ebola virus (EBOV), an RNA virus that belongs to the family *Filoviridae.* The Zaire species of Ebola virus (ZEBOV) has been the most implicated over the years, with a fatality rate of up to 90%. Bats, known to be the only flying mammals, have been reported to be the presumptive reservoir and natural host of EBOV, especially the Zaire strain (Leroy et al. 2005, 2009; Pigott et al. 2014). Previous outbreaks have shown that a one-time zoonotic transmission of Ebola to an individual can result in a massive Ebola epidemic (Jacob et al. 2020). Symptoms of Ebola virus disease are varied and overlap with many other diseases that are common in West Africa, including malaria, cholera, and Lassa fever (Husseini and Latham 2022). Transmission is typically through direct contact with the bodily fluid of an infected person. As the disease progresses, it presents with severe gastrointestinal manifestations followed by haemorrhage and multiple organ dysfunction or failures (Jacob et al. 2020).

The West African region has experienced an unprecedented, deadliest and most widely spread Ebola virus disease (EVD) in the past, mostly between 2013 and 2020. The outbreaks infected about 29,000 people, with over 11,000 deaths (Husseini and Latham 2022; Husseini and Latham 2022). At different times, the affected countries responded to this public health emergency by imposing restrictions, including closure of national or regional borders resulting in a halt of movement, trade and services, curfews, strict adherence to temperature checks, monitoring of symptoms in health care facilities, schools and business arenas The West African Ebola outbreak and the ongoing outbreaks in Eastern Africa, including outbreak of

Sudan virus strain in Uganda and the DRC have deepened the understanding of Ebola virus disease, its pathogenesis, epidemiology and viral persistence in survivors, which has resulted in improved and advanced strategies for prevention of infection, improvement of clinical management and positive treatment outcomes in patients (Jacob et al. 2020). Different vaccine candidates, including a randomised placebo-controlled trial in children and adults, were used to prevent Ebola (Lee et al. 2024).

2.2.2 Marburg Virus Disease (MVD)

Marburg viral disease (MVD) is another crucial haemorrhagic fever that is threatening the lives of people. The disease is caused by the Marburg virus, an RNA virus that is a member of the *Filoviridae* family. The index case of the Marburg virus (MV) outbreak was first recorded in 1967 in Marburg an der Lahn town in Germany, where poliomyelitis vaccine development and production workers reportedly became sick at three different places in Europe, each having a deadly novel disease connected with grivets (*Chlorocebus aethiops*), which was said to have been imported from Uganda at the time (Ristanović et al. 2020). The disease was tracked to have originated from eastern Africa (Kenya and Uganda), central Africa (DRC), and southern Africa (Angola and Rhodesia [Zimbabwe]). According to Kuhn, up until this day, more than two laboratory-acquired cases have occurred, of which one was fatal in Soviet laboratories (Kuhn 2008).

Similar to Ebola, Marburg causes deadly outbreaks with very high mortality rate and case fatality rate of about 24 to 88%, with an average fatality rate of about 80.6%, associated with most outbreaks (Srivastava et al. 2023; Ristanović et al. 2020). In both humans and non-primates, the disease results in severe haemorrhagic fever, multiple organ failure, and coagulation. The natural hosts of the MV are the Egyptian fruit bat (*Rousettus aegyptiacus*) and some *Chiroptera species* (Srivastava et al. 2023).

Filoviruses, especially Ebola and Marburg viruses, cause deadly zoonotic diseases and exhibit similar structure, pathogenesis, and epidemiology characteristics. The diseases caused by these viral agents progress fast in infected individuals and have been widely dreaded. However, over the years, due to advancements in medical research, there seems to be an improvement, as observed through decreased case fatalities, increased awareness and advanced treatment options. For instance, recently, there was an outbreak of MV in Rwanda, which was effectively contained. The outbreak stopped spreading to neighbouring communities due to the prompt and efficient isolation of positive cases, followed by treatment with monoclonal antibodies and antiviral agents (Butera et al. 2024). It was recorded that throughout the outbreak, the case fatality rate remained at approximately 23% (Butera et al. 2024).

Genomic sequencing of the Marburg genome has deepened our understanding of how the virus evolved. This has helped identify important mutation sites, particularly the VP40 and NP-VP35 proteins at the intergenic regions of the genome, facilitating viral adaptation to new hosts (Wei et al. 2017; Butera et al. 2024). These mutations in the genome enhance the virus's ability to evade an infected person's immune system and cause severe disease (Butera et al. 2024).

2.2.3 Lassa Haemorrhagic Fever

Lassa virus (LASV) is the causative agent of Lassa fever, also known as Lassa haemorrhagic fever (LHF), a severe disease characterised by a high fatality rate. The virus belongs to the family *Arenaviridae*. Rodents, especially *Mastomys natalensis*, are the natural hosts of the virus, which is transmitted to humans when they ingest food or water contaminated with the rodents' droppings, urine or respiratory secretions (Shenge and Opayele 2020). Lassa fever is a zoonotic disease, and infection can occur differently. It can be transmitted by multimammate, peri-domestic rats when they shed their wastes in food through direct contact with infected tissue or blood of the rodents (Agbonlahor et al. 2017). In addition, nosocomial infection can occur in healthcare settings, from patients to healthcare givers or vice versa. Such human-to-human transmission of Lassa fever in hospital settings may result from poor infection prevention and control practices or inadequate infection control infrastructure (Fisher-Hoch et al. 1995; Agbonlahor et al. 2021). Lassa fever can be fatal in infected patients. A study conducted by Fisher-Hoch et al. (1995) among infected patients found that 22 out of 34 infected patients died, giving rise to a 65% fatality rate (Fisher-Hoch et al. 1995).

Lassa fever is endemic in some African countries, such as Sierra Leone and the West African region, including Nigeria, where outbreaks occur repeatedly. As of March 2025, Nigeria had recorded 95 deaths and 509 cases of Lassa fever in 12 states, according to the NCDC. Frequent outbreaks have been attributed to the emergence of novel virus strains due to mutations in the viral genome (Garry 2023). Again, the abundance of *Mastomys* spp. is another possible reason for this repeated infection. Cultural practices, including the consumption of rat meat, can also play a role. Furthermore, another reason is inadequate knowledge about the route of transmission, epidemiology, prevention and control of infection by the public or a total lack of awareness. For instance, some rural and semi-urban communities still spread their food materials for sun-drying along the roads. These rodents emerge from the surrounding bushes, feed, defecate on the food and return to the bush.

Symptoms of infection may vary in individuals, while some infected persons may remain asymptomatic. Initial symptoms may include fever, general body weakness, and malaise. After a few days, sore throat, headache, muscle ache, nausea, vomiting, chest pain, diarrhoea, cough and abdominal pain may follow. However, in severe cases, there may be the accumulation of fluid in the lung, facial swelling, and bleeding (haemorrhage) from all the orifices, including the mouth, nose, vagina and gastrointestinal tract. These may be accompanied by low blood pressure. In about 25% of patients who survive, deafness occurs, while hearing returns after 1–3 months (Africa CDC 2025).

In most cases, about 80% of infected persons may show no sign of infection or present with mild clinical symptoms, while 20% may experience severe disease, which eventually may lead to multiple organ dysfunction or failure and death (Akpede et al. 2019; Agbonlahor et al. 2021). Early diagnosis is vital for disease prognosis and the successful management of the disease. There is no available vaccine for Lassa fever. All efforts are geared toward developing an effective vaccine to prevent Lassa fever in Africa. Eradication of the Lassa virus in Africa can be achieved through collaborative efforts of all stakeholders based on the One Health principle and approach (human-animal-environment), considering the actual rodent-human-environment factors involved in the infection chain.

Efforts to reduce the population of rodent reservoirs and prevent their entrance into new areas, advancements in medical technology to enhance prompt diagnosis, develop vaccines, control infection, and improve patient treatment outcomes are key to tackling the menace of Lassa haemorrhagic fever in Africa and other parts of the world.

2.2.4 *Crimean-Congo Haemorrhagic Fever*

Crimean-Congo haemorrhagic fever (CCHF) is a tick-borne viral infection transmitted by the vector *Hyalomma* tick. The index case of the virus was detected in Soviet soldiers in Crimea in the 1940s; in the 1960s, another virus with similar symptoms to the Crimean virus was detected in the Belgian Congo, the present DRC (Ozdarendeli 2023). It presents with severe illness in infected persons, with a fatality rate of about 30%. The disease has been previously reported in Africa, Asia, the Middle East and Europe (Hawman and Feldmann 2023). The Crimean-Congo haemorrhagic fever virus belongs to the family Bunyaviridae.

According to Temur et al. (2021), a total of 494 cases were reported by 19 countries between 1956 and 2000. Most cases were reported from Mali, Mauritania, Namibia, Nigeria, South Africa, Sudan, and Uganda (Temur et al. 2021). The infection can result in severe symptoms, including haemorrhagic fever, with a mortality rate, which prompted the WHO to classify it as a high-priority pathogen (Ozdarendeli 2023). Although no vaccine is available to prevent infection, technological advancement through animal models has shown promising results for designing effective vaccines (Ozdarendeli 2023).

2.2.5 *Diagnosis of Viral Haemorrhagic Fever*

Due to their highly infectious nature, haemorrhagic fever viruses are typically high-biosafety-level pathogens diagnosed in reference laboratories using biosafety level 4. Highly pathogenic viruses pose a serious threat at every stage of their investigation, including during population screening and laboratory diagnosis. Hence, adequate protection of public health, health workers, and laboratory scientists must be ensured using special personal protective equipment (PPE) and highly secured facilities to store samples.

Rapid diagnosis of VHF is crucial to reduce the further spread of outbreaks (Rasca et al. 2016). Generally, molecular tests are the most frequently used techniques for diagnosing viral haemorrhagic fever, involving nucleic acid extraction (RNA/DNA), amplifying the target genes with polymerase chain reaction (PCR) using specific primers and sequencing of the genes. For Ebola specifically, one commonly used molecular tool is the Real-Star Altona, and this test targets a conserved area of the Ebola L gene. A study by Bettini and colleagues showed that as a very sensitive test, large copies of the viral nucleic acid can be obtained, yielding about 471 copies/mL for Ebola and about 2871 copies/ml for SUDAN virus (Bettini et al. 2023). Several antigen-antibody-based rapid diagnostic tests (RDT) have been developed for Ebola, but none has met the sensitivity level of 99% recommended by the WHO. This implies that RDT-negative results must be confirmed with a molecular test (Bettini et al. 2023).

2.3 Emerging Viral Zoonoses and Role in Pandemics

2.3.1 COVID-19

For five years running, the world has witnessed the ravaging effects of COVID-19, with millions of lives lost. This has placed COVID-19 as one of the deadliest pandemics ever recorded in the history of humans on earth. That notwithstanding, it has not ended this pandemic, as the virus keeps mutating, giving rise to emerging strains that create this lingering pandemic scare, while Long COVID still exists as an aftermath of the COVID-19 pandemic.

Severe acute respiratory syndrome-2 (SARS-CoV-2) is the virus that causes COVID-19, a severe zoonotic respiratory disease that has impacted the world through its pandemic. As it is, understanding the origin of the emergence of SARS-CoV-2 in 2019, especially the zoonotic nature of the outbreak is very important for preventing future outbreaks (Worobey et al. 2024).

Hence, the origin and history of this disease have been a hot debate for the past six years. However, this highly controversial zoonotic origin is beginning to gain some clarity as to the exact origin of the pandemic. Notably, the existence, use and interactive nature of the live-animal market in Wuhan and corroborative evidence emanating from studies conducted on the animals point to the origin of the pandemic, which has formed huge lessons for the future.

According to Michael Worobey et al. (2022), raccoon dogs (*Nyctereutes procyonoides*) have been suspected to be the intermediate hosts or origin of the SARS-CoV-2 virus, passed from bats, that might have spilt over from the animals to humans.

The mounting evidence shows that raccoon dogs are eaten, and their fur serves as raw materials in some countries (Freuling et al. 2020). In 2003, these well-studied animals had passed a related virus that causes severe acute respiratory syndrome (SARS) to civets and raccoon dogs at the live-animal market in Guangdong, China; the same linking axis to Wuhan where SARS-CoV-2 was initially reported (Freuling et al. 2020).

COVID-19 continues to pose a global challenge, with pockets of epidemics still occurring in some locations; now, the question is when the pandemic will be over. As the years run by, there is a need for continuous research on the evolution of the virus and the zoonotic linkages that may shed more light on pandemic trends and inform preparedness for future occurrences.

2.3.2 Mpox Viral Disease

Mpox, formerly known as monkeypox, has existed for ages. However, in recent times, constant outbreaks and severity of infection in affected individuals have increased the scare about a possible pandemic involving the virus. According to Ndembi and colleagues, a total of 45,652 mpox cases were confirmed in 12 African countries between January 1, 2022 and August 18, 2024, with 1492 deaths recorded, resulting in a fatality rate of about 3.3% (Ndembi et al. 2025). There has been a constant increase in mpox cases in different African countries, especially in remote, rural communities, with a global outbreak recorded in 2022 (Ghebreyesus 2025). Mpox clade 1 cases have been reported in other parts of Africa, Europe, North America and Asia, and cases are believed to have been introduced through travel (CDC 2025).

At different times between May 2023 and August 2024, African Centers for Disease Control and Prevention (CDC) declared mpox a public health emergency of continental security (PHECS), with clade 1b of the virus as the predominant strain responsible for the outbreaks in Central and Eastern Africa and clade IIb in West Africa, while that same August 2024, the World Health Organisation declared mpox outbreak in Africa a public health emergency. Altogether, mpox outbreaks have been reported in 17 countries (Ghebreyesus 2025).

The mpox is a viral zoonotic disease caused by the monkeypox virus, which was discovered in Denmark in 1958 in monkeys (reservoirs) and is used mainly for research. The index case was reported in a nine-month-old boy in the DRC around 1970. The mpox virus belongs to the genus *Orthopoxvirus*, Family *Poxviridae*. There are two distinct clades of mpox: clade I, further grouped into subclades Ia and Ib), and clade II, which consists of subclades IIa and IIb (Tomori 2024; WHO 2024).

Monkeypox can be contracted through animal-to-human transmission from infected animals to humans from bites or scratches or during activities such as hunting, skinning, trapping, cooking, playing with carcasses or eating infected animals (WHO 2024). After initial exposure to the virus, signs and symptoms begin within seven days but can start from 1–21 days after exposure. An infected person presents with fever, rash, sore throat, headache, muscle aches, back pain, low energy and swollen lymph nodes. Monkeypox rash often first appears on the face, then spreads to other body parts. Conversely, the rash may also appear on the body at the contact point with an infected individual. Typical monkeypox rash starts as a flat sore but develops rapidly into a blister with accumulated liquid that may be itchy and painful simultaneously (WHO 2024).

The transmission of mpox can sustained in a population through person-to-person contact with an infected person and through sexual contact, fomites such as contaminated clothing or linen, needle-sticks in health care facilities, and body-piercing, such as through tattoos (WHO 2024). It can be transmitted vertically from mother to child during pregnancy and can lead to miscarriage, stillbirth, death of foetus, or even complications for the mother (CDC 2025; WHO 2024). Monkeypox can be equally transmitted through animal bites or scratches from infected animals to humans, contact during hunting, skinning, trapping, cooking, playing with carcasses or consumption of infected animals (WHO 2024).

There is an available vaccine for mpox. Vaccination is highly recommended for people at high risk of infection with mpox, especially in endemic zones or during an outbreak. The vaccine can be administered as a post-exposure prophylaxis for individuals who have been in contact with a mpox-infected person. Typically, those persons should be vaccinated within four days after contact with an infected individual.

2.4 Facilitators of the Emergence of Zoonotic Viral Diseases

The factors that drive the emergence of zoonotic viral diseases are not quite different from the conventional ones. However, a few factors may be considered, including the pathogen, host or animal reservoir, environment, and cross-species transmission.

2.4.1 Wildlife Reservoirs as Drivers of Viral Haemorrhagic Diseases

Most zoonotic diseases of viral origin emanate from wildlife, resulting in viral spillover to humans and other animals in the environment. For example, bats are known and have been implicated in the transmission of Ebola and COVID-19 (to raccoon dogs as intermediate hosts); rodents such as Mastomys natalensis are involved in the transmission of Lassa fever; wild birds are involved in avian flu and a host of others. The population of wildlife in the world is numerous, and they are the principal reservoirs of pathogens, especially those of viral origin, including West

Nile virus, Nipah and Hantaviruses. A few domestic animal pathogens include rabies virus in dogs and cats (Bengis et al. 2004).

2.4.2 *Environmental Drivers, Including Climate Change*

Numerous environmental factors, most elicited by human activity, are responsible for the occasional outbreak of some endemic diseases in Africa. Human-animal interactions emanating from activities such as deforestation, urbanisation, wildlife poaching and trade have led to more frequent outbreaks recently (Shenge and Opayele 2020). In addition, the world is witnessing a series of climatic events which alter the life cycle of most arthropods by causing alterations in their natural habitat, leading to frequent outbreaks of vector-borne diseases, even in areas where outbreaks were uncommon in the past (Davies et al. 1985).

2.4.3 *Globalisation*

Socioeconomic engagements, including interactions through global travel, commercial enterprise, and unconventional farming, often provide opportunities for infectious agents to jump from animals to humans. For instance, exchanging goods and services involving infected animal skin and fur, livestock, and the pet trade, especially through import and export services, may introduce an infectious zoonotic agent into a new area (Gumusova et al. 2015).

2.5 One Health Approach to Prevention of Zoonoses

Important public health interventions are required for the prevention and control of zoonotic diseases to avert a possible pandemic, in addition to vaccination. Continuous surveillance at human, animal and environmental levels is always needed. At the human interface, adopting participatory surveillance that involves a bidirectional approach to disease reporting in communities and early warning signs and disease reporting in animals may be timely.

For contagious infectious diseases such as mpox, quarantine or isolation of infected individuals, followed by adequate treatment of cases, is recommended. Infected persons should be placed on antiviral therapy and other supportive care; they should be released when all symptoms have resolved. Globalisation through travel and trade of goods and services may serve as a possible port of entry for the virus into new areas. Prevention strategies targeting these should be stepped up, especially at the borders.

Animal reservoirs of the virus, especially those in the wild, must be appropriately secured to limit human interactions with them. Such an environment should be marked and made inaccessible to the public or secured against the escape of wildlife into cities. Control of zoonoses requires efficient barriers targeted at animal-to-human transmission levels and human-to-human transmission during an outbreak to reduce contact and improve environmental conditions.

2.6 Recommendations and Key Lessons for the Future

Most zoonotic viruses that cause haemorrhagic fever and arboviral infections (vector-borne) are RNA viruses, known for undergoing rapid mutation in their genomes, resulting in frequent variation that enhances their ability to adapt in their natural hosts, increase their pathogenicity, evade the immune system of their hosts, and unleash havoc on the infected body. As such, these viral infections, when not controlled, have the potential to cause a pandemic: Hence,

(i) Countries should enact laws protecting wildlife habitats and minimising interaction with people.
(ii) Identify well-equipped healthcare facilities where samples and infected persons can be isolated.
(iii) There is a need for continuous investment in research and development.
(iv) There should be increased resource mobilisation and scaling up of operational readiness for any outbreak.
(v) Promote sustainable agriculture by promoting global best practices.
(vi) Strengthen global surveillance systems, especially using genomics and related technology.
(vii) Encourage collaboration across sectors, involving all stakeholders using one health approach.
(viii) Each country should evaluate its readiness for a possible outbreak.

2.7 Recommendation

Globally, there is a need for global health agencies, nations and relevant stakeholders to optimise the preparedness for possible future pandemics by adopting a comprehensive One Health approach and integrated strategies built around human, animal and environmental health for effective prevention and control of viral haemorrhagic fever.

2.8 Conclusion

It has become apparent that humans are in constant war with emerging viral diseases, including haemorrhagic fever, which are caused by different viral pathogens. This, therefore, requires urgent strategies such as continuous surveillance, the design of potent vaccines, constant education, and other important scientific advancements to combat these health threats to the environment. Pathogens undergo genetic changes or mutations to adapt to new environments and cause diseases; humans, in the same vein, should adopt new technologies to either eradicate the pathogens or reduce outbreaks in animal and human populations in a very sustainable way, including embracing a One Health approach to disease prevention and control in its entirety. These gaps, when filled, will translate to reduced haemorrhagic disease outbreaks.

References

Africa CDC (2025) Lassa Fever. https://africacdc.org. Accessed 28 Jan 2025

Agbonlahor DE, Erah A, Agba IM, Oviasogie FE, Ehiaghe AF, Wankasi M, Eremwanarue OA, Ehiaghe IJ, Ogbu EC, Iyen RI, Abbey S, Tatfeng MY, Uhunmwangho J (2017) Prevalence of Lassa virus among rodents trapped in three South-South States of Nigeria. J Vector Borne Dis 54(2):146–150

Agbonlahor DE, Akpede GO, Happi CT, Tomori O (2021) 52 years of Lassa fever outbreaks in Nigeria, 1969-2020: an epidemiologic analysis of the temporal and spatial trends. Am J Trop Med Hygiene 105(4):974–985. https://doi.org/10.4269/ajtmh.20-1160

Akpede GO, Asogun DA, Okogbenin SA, Dawodu SO, Momoh MO, Dongo AE, Ike C, Tobin E, Akpede N, Ogbaini-Emovon E, Adewale AE, Ochei O, Onyeke F, Okonofua MO, Atafo RO, Odia I, Adomeh DI, Odigie G, Ogbeifun C, Muebonam E, Ihekweazu C, Ramharter M, Colubri A, Sarbeti PC, Happi CT, Günther S, Agbonlahor DE (2019) Caseload and case fatality of Lassa fever in Nigeria, 2001–2018: a specialist center's experience and its implications. Front Public Health 7:170. https://doi.org/10.3389/fpubh.2019.00170. Erratum in: Front Public Health 13;7:251. doi: 10.3389/fpubh.2019.00251

Bengis RG, Leighton FA, Fischer JR, Artois M, Mörner T, Tate CM (2004) The role of wildlife in emerging and re-emerging zoonoses. Rev Sci Tech 23(2):497–511

Bettini A, Lapa D, Garbuglia AR (2023) Diagnostics of Ebola virus. Front Public Health 11: 1123024. https://doi.org/10.3389/fpubh.2023.1123024

Butera Y, Mutesa L, Parker E, Muvunyi R, Umumararungu E, Ayitewala A et al (2024) Genomic and transmission dynamics of the 2024 Marburg virus outbreak in Rwanda. Nat Med 31(2): 422–426. https://doi.org/10.1038/s41591-024-03459-9

Center for Disease Prevention and Control (2025) Mpox in the United States and around the world: current situation. Accessed 3 Mar 2025

Davies FG, Linthicum KJ, James AD (1985) Rainfall and epizootic Rift Valley fever. Bull World Health Organ 63(5):941–943

Di Bari C, Venkateswaran N, Fastl C, Gabriël S, Grace D, Havelaar AH, Huntington B, Patterson GT, Rushton J, Speybroeck N, Torgerson P, Pigott DM, Devleesschauwer B (2023) The global burden of neglected zoonotic diseases: current state of evidence. One Health 17:100595. https://doi.org/10.1016/j.onehlt.2023.100595

Fisher-Hoch SP, Tomori O, Nasidi A, Perez-Oronoz GI, Fakile Y, Hutwagner L, McCormick JB (1995) Review of cases of nosocomial Lassa fever in Nigeria: the high price of poor medical practice. BMJ 311(7009):857–859. https://doi.org/10.1136/bmj.311.7009.857

Freuling CM, Breithaupt A, Müller T, Sehl J, Balkema-Buschmann A, Rissmann M, Klein A, Wylezich C, Höper D, Wernike K, Aebischer A, Hoffmann D, Friedrichs V, Dorhoi A, Groschup MH, Beer M, Mettenleiter TC (2020) Susceptibility of raccoon dogs for experimental SARS-CoV-2 infection. Emerg Infect Dis 26(12):2982–2985. https://doi.org/10.3201/eid2612.203733

Garry RF (2023) Lassa fever - the road ahead. Nat Rev Microbiol 21(2):87–96. https://doi.org/10.1038/s41579-022-00789-8

Ghebreyesus TA (2025) Evolving epidemiology of Mpox in Africa in 2024. N Engl J Med 392(7): 714–716. https://doi.org/10.1056/NEJMe2416384

Gumusova S, Sunbul M, Leblebicioglu H (2015) Ebola virus disease and the veterinary perspective. Ann Clin Microbiol Antimicrob 14(30). https://doi.org/10.1186/s12941-015-0089-x

Hawman DW, Feldmann H (2023) Crimean-Congo haemorrhagic fever virus. Nat Rev Microbiol 21(7):463–477. https://doi.org/10.1038/s41579-023-00871-9

Husseini S, Latham J (2022) Did West Africa's Ebola outbreak of 2014 have a lab origin? A review of the scientific evidence. Originally published online by Independent Science News, October 25, 2022

Ihekweazu C, Michael CA, Nguku PM, Waziri NE, Habib AG, Muturi M, Olufemi A, Dzikwi-Emennaa AA, Balogun MS, Visa TI, Dalhat MM, Atama NC, Umeokonkwo CD, Mshelbwala GM, Vakuru CT, Kabir J, Okolocha EC, Umoh JU, Olugasa B, Babalobi O, Lombin L, Cadmus S (2021) Nigeria Zoonotic Diseases Prioritization Group. Prioritisation of zoonotic diseases of public health significance in Nigeria using the one-health approach. One Health 13:100257. https://doi.org/10.1016/j.onehlt.2021.100257

Jacob ST, Crozier I, Fischer WA, Hewlett A, Kraft CS et al (2020) Ebola virus disease. Nat Rev Dis Primers 6(1):13. https://doi.org/10.1038/s41572-020-0147-3

Kuhn JH (2008) Filoviruses. A compendium of 40 years of epidemiological, clinical, and laboratory studies. Arch Virol Suppl 20:13–360

Lee AW, Liu K, Lhomme E, Blie J, McCullough J et al (2024) PREVAC study team. Immunogenicity and vaccine shedding after 1 or 2 doses of rVSVΔG-ZEBOV-GP Ebola vaccine (ERVEBO®): results from a phase 2, randomised, placebo-controlled trial in children and adults. Clin Infect Dis 78(4):870–879. https://doi.org/10.1093/cid/ciad693

Leroy EM, Kumulungui B, Pourrut X, Rouquet P, Hassanin A et al (2005) Fruit bats as reservoirs of Ebola virus. Nature 438(7068):575–576

Leroy EM, Epelboin A, Mondonge V, Pourut X, Gonzalex JP et al (2009) Human Ebola outbreak resulting from direct exposure to fruit bats in Luebo, Democratic Republic of Congo, 2007. Vector-Borne Zoonotic Dis 9(6):723–728

Ndembi N, Folayan MO, Komakech A, Mercy K, Tessema et al (2025) Evolving epidemiology of mpox in Africa in 202 4. N Engl J Med 392(7):666–676. https://doi.org/10.1056/NEJMoa2411368

Ozdarendeli A (2023) Crimean-Congo hemorrhagic fever virus: progress in vaccine development. Diagnostics 13(16):2708. https://doi.org/10.3390/diagnostics13162708

Pigott DM, Golding N, Mylne A, Huang Z, Henry AJ et al (2014) Mapping the zoonotic niche of Ebola virus disease in Africa. elife 3:e04395

Rasca LD, Kraft CS, Olinger GG, Hensley LE (2016) Viral hemorrhagic fever diagnostics. Clin Infect Dis 62(2):214–219. https://doi.org/10.1093/cid/civ792

Ristanović ES, Kokoškov NS, Crozier I, Kuhn JH, Gligić AS (2020) A forgotten episode of Marburg virus disease: Belgrade, Yugoslavia, 1967. Microbiol Mol Biol Rev 84(2):e00095–e00019. https://doi.org/10.1128/MMBR.00095-19

Shenge JA (2023) Genetics of viral resistance: clinical relevance and role in viral disease outbreak. In: Abia ALK, Essack SY (eds) Antimicrobial research and one health in Africa. Springer, Cham. https://doi.org/10.1007/978-3-031-23796-6_4

Shenge JA, Opayele AV (2020) The impact and control of emerging and re-emerging viral diseases in the environment: an African perspective. Curr Microbiol Res Afr 5:185–202. https://doi.org/10.1007/978-3-030-35296-7_7

Srivastava S, Sharma D, Kumar S, Sharma A, Rijal R et al (2023) Emergence of Marburg virus: a global perspective on fatal outbreaks and clinical challenges. Front Microbiol 14:1239079. https://doi.org/10.3389/fmicb.2023.1239079

Temur AI, Kuhn JH, Pecor DB, Apanaskevich DA, Keshtkar-Jahromi M (2021) Epidemiology of Crimean-Congo Hemorrhagic Fever (CCHF) in Africa-underestimated for decades. Am J Trop Med Hygiene 104(6):1978–1990. https://doi.org/10.4269/ajtmh.20-1413

Tomori O (2024) Neglected mpox resurges with virulence in Africa: will this be another neglected warning? J Public Health Afr 15(1):a730. https://doi.org/10.4102/jphia.v15i1.730

Wei H, Audet J, Wong G, He S, Huang X, Cutts T, Theriault S, Xu B, Kobinger G, Qiu X (2017) Deep-sequencing of Marburg virus genome during sequential mouse passaging and cell-culture adaptation reveals extensive changes over time. Sci Rep 7(1):3390. https://doi.org/10.1038/s41598-017-03318-3

World Health Organization. Mpox. Accessed 15 Jan 2024

World Health Organization, Zoonoses (2020). https://www.who.int/news-room/fact-sheets/detail/zoonoses. Accessed 26 Nov 2024

Worobey M, Levy JI, Malpica Serrano L, Crits-Christoph A, Pekar JE, Goldstein SA, Rasmussen AL, Kraemer MUG, Newman C, Koopmans MPG, Suchard MA, Wertheim JO, Lemey P, Robertson DL, Garry RF, Holmes EC, Rambaut A, Andersen KG (2022). The Huanan Seafood Wholesale Market in Wuhan was the early epicenter of the COVID-19 pandemic. Science 377(6609):951–959. https://doi.org/10.1126/science.abp8715. Erratum in: science. 383(6688): eadp1133. doi: 10.1126/science.adp1133

Worobey M et al (2024) Erratum for the Research Article "The Huanan Seafood Wholesale Market in Wuhan was the early epicenter of the COVID-19 pandemic". Science 383(6688):eadp1133. https://doi.org/10.1126/science.adp1133. Erratum for: Science. 377(6609):951–959. doi: 10.1126/science.abp8715

Chapter 3
African Swine Fever and Food Security

Terdsak Yano

3.1 The Agent of ASF and Its Global Distribution

The African Swine Fever, or ASF, is a high-impact disease in the pig industry globally. ASF is caused by the African Swine Fever Virus (ASFV). It is a linear, double-stranded DNA virus, a member of the family *Asfarviridae*, genus *Asfiviru.* ASFV is a large and complex virus. Its length is 170–193 kbp, and it contains around 50 structural proteins (Jia et al. 2017). The major component proteins include p72, p54, p30 and p17. These structural proteins help the virus attach, enter and replicate within the host cell. The complexity of ASFV affects vaccine development. The ASFV can survive in blood, faecal materials, and carcasses for extended periods. It can survive in Parma ham for 291 days (McKercher et al. 1987). It also survives longer at low-temperature conditions.

The ASF can be transmitted through direct contact with infected pigs, consumption of infected pork products, or contact with contaminated equipment, clothing, vehicles, and humans. ASFV can also be transmitted through a vector, the soft ticks *Ornithodoros* spp. Contaminated soil and water can be a source of ASF infection (Bergmann et al. 2021). Humans can carry ASFV from pork, pigs, faeces and urine. Environmental transmission can also occur when humans visit pig areas, interact with the animals and equipment directly, and fail to observe proper hygiene after the visit. Even though the viral load in these areas may be small, it can spread throughout the pig house.

ASF affects domestic or wild pigs, which are ASF reservoirs in Europe and Africa (Rademacher et al. 2022). The ASFV can spread from wild pigs to domestic pigs, especially when domestic and wild pigs share their habitat (Thanapongtharm et al. 2025). It was first reported in Kenya in 1921 and then spread to Europe in 1957

T. Yano (✉)
Faculty of Veterinary Medicine, Chiang Mai University, Chiang Mai, Thailand
e-mail: Terdsak.yano@cmu.ac.th

J. A. Shenge, A. L. K. Abia (eds.), *Viral Diseases and One Health in Africa*,
https://doi.org/10.1007/978-3-032-09613-5_3

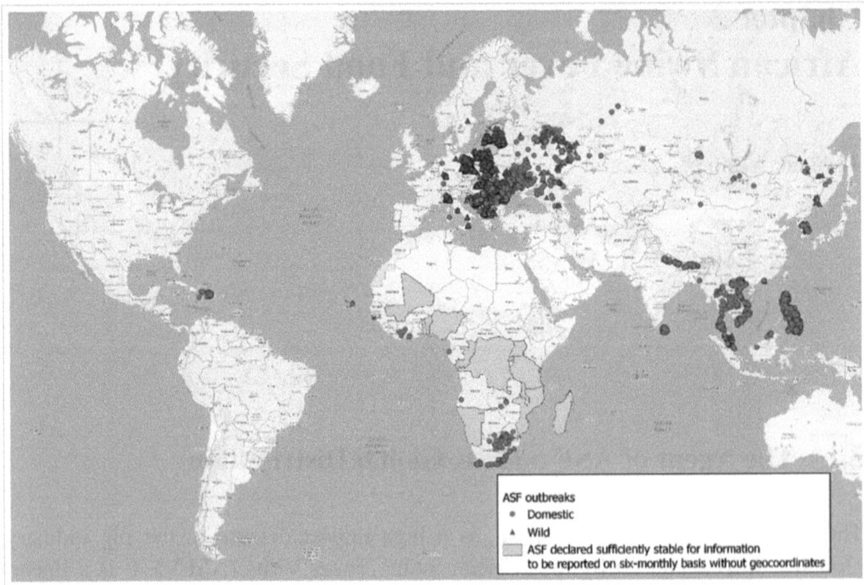

Fig. 3.1 The world map showing African swine fever (ASF) outbreaks reported in domestic and wild pigs worldwide from January 2022 until February 2025. (From https://www.woah.org/app/uploads/2025/04/asf-report-63-1-1.pdf). Brown circles indicate domestic outbreaks, while green triangles represent wild outbreaks. Regions shaded in light orange are declared stable for ASF information, reported biannually without geocoordinates. Outbreaks are concentrated in Europe, Asia, and parts of Africa

(Sánchez-Vizcaíno et al. 2019). The global outbreak started in 2007 in Eastern Europe, particularly in Georgia, Armenia, Azerbaijan, and Russia (Ito et al. 2023). In 2018, ASF was reported in China. It was the first ASF outbreak report in Asia. In 2020, the virus spread to Papua New Guinea in Oceania. ASF is a global threat (Fig. 3.1) because it has been reported in 64 countries across five continents and has killed more than 2,000,000 animals (WOAH 2025).

3.2 Clinical Signs and Lesions

ASF is a highly severe disease affecting pigs, with a case fatality rate reaching 100%. The incubation phase typically lasts between four and nineteen days, and the disease manifests in four clinical forms: peracute, acute, subacute, and chronic (Sánchez-Vizcaíno et al. 2019). The peracute form is most commonly observed in naïve populations, characterised by a sudden onset of high fever (>41 °C), lethargy, cutaneous erythema, and death within 4 days of infection. In contrast, the acute form presents with persistent high fever, depression, anorexia, vomiting,

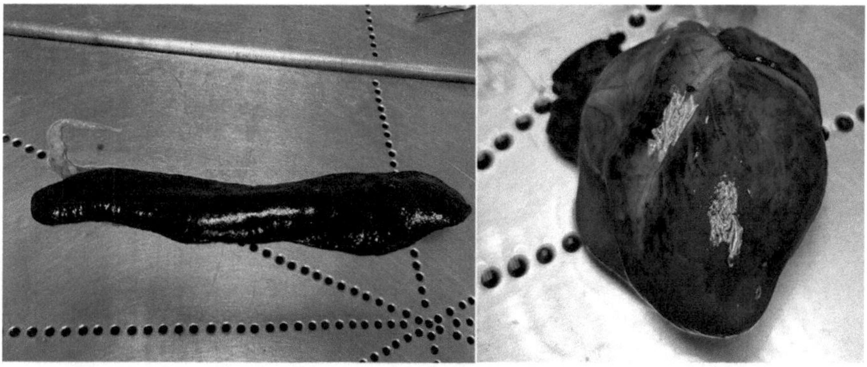

(a) (b)

Fig. 3.2 These two pictures the lesions of ASF in pigs. Hemorrhagic splenomegaly S (**a**) and petechial haemorrhages in the heart (**b**)

hemorrhagic diarrhoea (or occasionally constipation), and cutaneous haemorrhages on the extremities, ears, chest, abdomen, and perineum. Additional symptoms include dyspnea and coughing due to pulmonary oedema. Pregnant sows may experience abortions, stillbirths, or weak piglets. Mortality typically occurs within 7 days of symptom onset. While the acute form is predominant in outbreak areas, the subacute form is more common in endemic regions, exhibiting similar but milder clinical signs and a lower mortality rate. Key features include moderate to high fever, ascites, haemorrhages in multiple organs, and reproductive failures. The chronic form of ASF is marked by progressive emaciation, intermittent fever, respiratory distress, cutaneous necrosis, chronic ulcers, arthritis, and joint swelling (Murcia et al. 2009; Sánchez-Vizcaíno et al. 2014).

The lesion of ASF depends on the virulence of ASFV, most prominently in the acute form, characterised by severe hemorrhagic and inflammatory changes. The splenomegaly is often observed due to infarction and congestion (Fig. 3.2). Lymph nodes, particularly the mesenteric and hepatic lymph nodes, are hemorrhagic, swollen, and dark red or black (Fig. 3.3). Widespread petechial and ecchymotic haemorrhages appear on serosal surfaces of the heart (Fig. 3.2), kidneys, bladder, and lungs. The kidneys may show cortical petechiae, while the gallbladder often has oedema and haemorrhage, giving it a gelatinous, thickened wall. The gastrointestinal tract exhibits hemorrhagic gastritis and ileocecal valve haemorrhage, sometimes with bloody intestinal contents. Pulmonary oedema and hydropericardium (excess fluid around the heart) are also common. In chronic cases, lesions may include arthritis, pneumonia, and skin ulcers, though these are less distinctive (Geering et al. 2001; Sehl-Ewert et al. 2022; Cho et al. 2023).

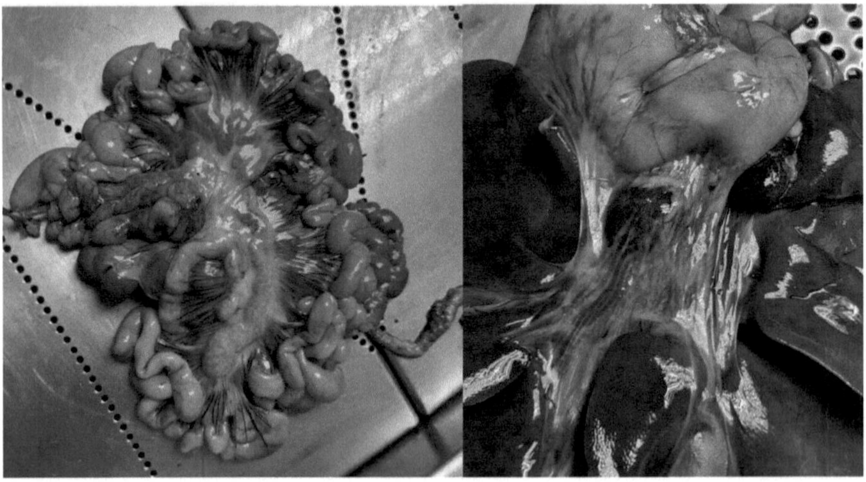

(a) (b)

Fig. 3.3 These two pictures showing the lesion of ASF in pigs. Swollen. Mesenteric (**a**) and hepatic lymph nodes (**b**), which are hemorrhagic and swollen. The pictures indicate the active lymph nodes which stimulated bi ASFV

3.3 ASF Effect on Food Security

From 2007 until 2025, the ASF has been spreading throughout the globe, with 64 countries reporting the ASF outbreak (WOAH 2025). The disease affects not only animals but also the socioeconomic environment. The ongoing ASF pandemic has precipitated a multidimensional global crisis with far-reaching economic, social, and food security consequences. Since its explosive spread from 2018 onward, this highly contagious viral disease has decimated pork industries across continents, with particularly devastating impacts in China, where between 25% and 35% of the national swine herd was culled, resulting in economic losses exceeding $141 billion and fundamentally altering global meat trade dynamics (Berthe 2020). The reduction of pigs affects the import of raw materials for animal feed, particularly soybeans, in China (Schmidhuber 2019). The repercussions extended throughout Asian markets, where smallholder farmers representing approximately 80% of pork producers in countries like Vietnam and the Philippines faced catastrophic losses, creating lucrative black markets for smuggled pork. Per capita pork consumption in Vietnam dropped by 25% (Nguyen-Thi et al. 2021). In Thailand, despite a reduction in the number of pigs, the pork price remained lower than the previous year. While official imports represent less than 1% of domestic production, authorities note that undocumented pork smuggling continues to exert downward pressure on prices, creating market distortions despite improved domestic supply conditions. This price adjustment reflects Thailand's gradual recovery from ASF disruptions, though the swine sector has not fully regained its pre-crisis production capacity or farmer participation levels (Kasikorn Research Center 2023).

The socioeconomic fallout has been severe and multifaceted (Mohan et al. 2021). Pork processing industries across affected regions experienced workforce reductions. At the same time, small-scale farmers encountered prohibitive barriers to restocking due to the combined effects of financial constraints, persistent environmental contamination (Dixon et al. 2020), and limited access to disease-free breeding stock. Smallholder farmers are a vulnerable group that ASF negatively impacts. In Timor-Leste, 70% of households keep pigs for unexpected expenses, particularly health and education. During the ASF outbreak in 2019, they risked losing their pig, which adversely affected their livelihood (Smith et al. 2019). The environmental consequences have been equally concerning. The ASFV can spread through contaminated soil, where infected carcasses are buried (Duc et al. 2022), raising significant concerns about groundwater contamination and methane emissions.

This crisis has exposed critical vulnerabilities in global food systems, demonstrating how a single animal disease can trigger cascading effects across economic markets, labour systems, and nutritional security. The ASF pandemic underscores the urgent need for coordinated international responses that address animal health and the interconnected socioeconomic and environmental dimensions of such outbreaks. Future strategies must incorporate lessons from this ongoing crisis to build more resilient food production systems capable of withstanding similar shocks.

3.4 How to Prevent ASF at the Farm and National Level

ASF has no effective drug to cure it, unlike bacteria. Immunisation is a major tool against the virus; however, the vaccine has low effectiveness in producing immunity. Other control measures have been introduced at the farm level to prevent the ASFV from being introduced into the farm, especially sanitation and disinfection. Conventional biosecurity measures are insufficient to stop the virus. Personal hygiene, including bathing and changing clothes and boots before entering the pig area or houses, is crucial for reducing the spread of the virus from contaminated personnel to pigs. Pork and pig products cannot be brought into the farm since the virus can survive in pork and pig products for an extended period. Cleaning the pig pen thoroughly, i.e. scraping and sweeping, then washing with low-pressure water, can reduce the spread of the virus inside the pen. Insects and pests must be eliminated to reduce ASFV spread from one house to another.

Monitoring stamping out of infected pigs needs to be done as early as possible. Infrared cameras can be applied to screen the potentially infected pigs, then confirmed with a PCR test. The partial depopulation of individual pigs can reduce the number of subclinical pigs on the farm. The restocking gilt must be separated from the sows. A separate house is ideal. These gills are the uninfected pigs that will replace the sows, possibly exposed to the virus. When the uninfected pigs increase in number, the farm will be free soon.

ASF outbreak farms have virus contamination in the walls, floors, water, soil, equipment, feed, and pig skin (Li et al. 2022). Drug or vaccine injection can carry the virus into the pig's body. Avoiding injection with a needle should be considered. If it cannot be avoided, the aseptic technique of injection by applying povidone iodine, instead of 70% alcohol, on the injection site must be done. The injector must wear gloves when injecting a pig that must stay still and on the correct injection site. Finally, mucosal immunity stimulation can be performed in a pig herd to increase nonspecific immunity that prevents viral invasion.

At the national level, ASF prevention measures require a comprehensive, multi-sectoral approach centred on strict biosecurity, surveillance, movement control, and rapid response systems. Since no effective vaccine is commercially available, the cornerstone of prevention lies in implementing rigorous biosecurity measures across all production systems, including commercial farms and backyard operations, emphasising disinfection protocols, controlled access, and prohibition of swill feeding. A robust surveillance system combining active monitoring of high-risk populations and passive reporting by veterinarians and farmers is essential for early detection, supported by rapid diagnostic capabilities through PCR and ELISA testing. Movement restrictions and zoning strategies, including quarantine measures for infected premises and establishment of ASF-free zones, are critical to contain outbreaks, complemented by prompt stamping-out policies with proper carcass disposal and fair compensation to ensure farmer compliance. Wild boar populations must be managed through population control, habitat fencing, and carcass removal to break the transmission cycle between wildlife and domestic pigs. Concurrently, nationwide public awareness campaigns should educate stakeholders on ASF recognition, biosecurity practices, and the dangers of the illegal pork trade. International collaboration through border controls, import restrictions, and data sharing with global organisations enhances cross-border protection. Finally, preparedness through contingency planning and regular simulation exercises ensures swift, coordinated responses to potential outbreaks. This integrated strategy forms the foundation for national ASF control when combining prevention, surveillance, and response mechanisms (FAO 2023; Dixon et al. 2020).

References

Bergmann H, Schulz K, Conraths FJ, Sauter-Louis CA (2021) Review of environmental risk factors for African swine fever in European wild boar. Animals. https://doi.org/10.3390/ani11092692

Berthe F (2020) The global economic impact of ASF. Panorama, 1. Available at: https://bulletin.woah.org/?panorama=02-2-2-2020-1-economic

Cho KH, Hong SK, Kim DY, Jang MK, Kim JH, Lee H, Kim EM, Park JH, Suh TY, Choi JG, Yoo DS, Kang HE, Kim YH (2023) Pathogenicity and pathological characteristics of African swine fever virus strains from pig farms in South Korea from 2022 to January 2023. Pathogens 12(9): 1158. https://doi.org/10.3390/pathogens12091158

Dixon LK, Stahl K, Jori F, Vial L, Pfeiffer DU (2020) African swine fever epidemiology and control. Annu Rev Anim Biosci 8:221–246. https://doi.org/10.1146/annurev-animal-021419-083741

Duc HM, Ngan PH, Son HM, Lan NT, Van Hung L, Ha CT, Hoa NT, Lam TQ, Van Thang N, Flory GA, Hutchinson M (2022) The use of composting for the disposal of African swine fever virus-infected swine carcasses. Transbound Emerg Dis 69(5):e3036–e3044

FAO (2023) African swine fever prevention, detection and control in resource-limited settings. FAO Animal Production and Health Guidelines No. 35. Rome. https://doi.org/10.4060/cc7491en

Geering WA, Penrith ML, Nyakahuma D (2001) Manual on the preparation of African swine fever contingency plan. the Food and Agriculture Organization. Available at: https://www.fao.org/4/Y0510E/Y0510E02.htm#ch2.5

Ito S, Kawaguchi N, Bosch J, Aguilar-Vega C, Sánchez-Vizcaíno JM (2023) What can we learn from the five-year African swine fever epidemic in Asia? Front Vet Sci 10:1273417. https://doi.org/10.3389/fvets.2023.1273417

Jia N, Ou Y, Pejsak Z, Zhang Y, Zhang J (2017) Roles of African swine fever virus structural proteins in viral infection. J Vet Res 61(2):135–143. https://doi.org/10.1515/jvetres-2017-0017

Kasikorn Research Center (2023) The trend of pork prices in Thailand in 2023. Available at: https://www.kasikornresearch.com/en/analysis/k-social-media/Pages/Pig-Price-FB-18-08-2023.aspx

Li Z, Chen W, Qiu Z, Li Y, Fan J, Wu K, Li X, Zhao M, Ding H, Fan S et al (2022) African swine fever virus: a review. Life 12:1255. https://doi.org/10.3390/life12081255

McKercher PD, Yedloutschnig RJ, Callis JJ, Murphy R, Panina GF, Civardi A et al (1987) Survival of viruses in "Prosciutto di Parma" (Parma Ham). Can Inst Food Sci Technol J 20(4):267–272. https://doi.org/10.1016/s0315-5463(87)71198-5

Mohan NH, Misha MM, Gupta VK (2021) Consequences of African swine fever in India: beyond economic implications. Transbound Emerg Dis 68:3009–3011

Murcia P, Donachie W, Palmarini M (2009) Viral pathogens of domestic animals and their impact on biology, medicine and agriculture. In: Schaechter M (ed) Encyclopedia of microbiology, 3rd edn. Academic, pp 805–819. https://doi.org/10.1016/B978-012373944-5.00368-0

Nguyen-Thi T, Pham-Thi-Ngoc L, Nguyen-Ngoc Q, Dang-Xuan S, Lee HS, Nguyen-Viet H, Padungtod P, Nguyen-Thu T, Nguyen-Thi T, Tran-Cong T, Rich KM (2021) An assessment of the economic impacts of the 2019 African swine fever outbreaks in Vietnam. Front Vet Sci 8: 686–691

Rademacher C, Brown J, Karriker L (2022) Impact of human behavior on the spread of African swine fever virus: what every veterinarian should know. J Am Vet Med Assoc 260:1413–1417. https://doi.org/10.2460/javma.22.06.0250

Sánchez-Vizcaíno JM, Mur L, Gomez-Villamandos JC, Carrasco L (2014) An update on the epidemiology and pathology of African swine fever. J Comp Pathol. https://doi.org/10.1016/j.jcpa.2014.09.003

Sánchez-Vizcaíno JM, Laddomada A, Arias ML (2019) African swine fever virus. In: Zimmerman JJ, Karriker LA, Ramirez A, Schwartz KJ, Stevenson GW, Zhang J (eds) Diseases of swine, 11th edn. Wiley, pp 443–452

Schmidhuber J (2019) African swine fever challenges for some, opportunities for others? Food Outlook – Biannual report on global food markets. Rome, pp 65–72

Sehl-Ewert J, Deutschmann P, Breithaupt A, Blome S (2022) Pathology of African swine fever in Wild Boar Carcasses naturally infected with German virus variants. Pathogens 11(11):1386. https://doi.org/10.3390/pathogens11111386

Smith D, Cooper T, Pereira A, Jong JBDC (2019) Counting the cost: the potential impact of African swine fever on smallholders in Timor-Leste. One Health 8:100109. https://doi.org/10.1016/j.onehlt.2019.100109

Thanapongtharm W, Wiratsudakul A, Gilbert M et al (2025) Spatial prediction of wild boar distribution in Thailand applications for African swine fever prevention and control. Sci Rep 15:9987. https://doi.org/10.1038/s41598-025-94922-1

WOAH (World Organisation for Animal Health) (2025) African Swine (ASF) Situation Report 63. Available at: https://www.woah.org/app/uploads/2025/04/asf-report-63-1-1.pdf

Chapter 4
Rift Valley Fever: An Emerging and Reemerging Zoonotic Viral Disease of Public Health Concern in Africa

Arthur O. Oragwa, Emmanuel T. Obishakin, Faith C. Oragwa, and Daniel O. Oluwayelu

4.1 Introduction

Rift Valley fever (RVF) is a zoonotic arthropod-borne viral (ARBO-viral) disease that presents various severe clinical manifestations in humans and different species of domestic and wild animals. The disease was first officially described around the Rift Valley area of Kenya during an outbreak involving a high rate of abortion and sudden mortality among sheep in 1930 (Daubney et al. 1931; Daubney and Hudson 1932). However, records show that clinical diseases similar to, and most likely, RVF were experienced intermittently by humans and livestock as early as 1912, but not investigated. Such outbreaks were erroneously attributed to other infections, including malaria (for humans) and diverse bacterial infections (for animals). They were, therefore, not studied adequately until the large outbreak of 1930 (Daubney and Hudson 1932). Subsequently and gradually, the disease spread to most African

A. O. Oragwa (✉)
Department of Veterinary Microbiology, Faculty of Veterinary Medicine, University of Jos, Jos, Plateau State, Nigeria
e-mail: oragwaa@unijos.edu.ng

E. T. Obishakin
Biotechnology Division, National Veterinary Research Institute, Vom, Plateau State, Nigeria

F. C. Oragwa
Department of Health Science Education, Faculty of Education, University of Nigeria, Nsukka, Enugu State, Nigeria

D. O. Oluwayelu
Department of Veterinary Microbiology, Faculty of Veterinary Medicine, University of Ibadan, Ibadan, Oyo State, Nigeria

Centre for Control and Prevention of Zoonoses, University of Ibadan, Ibadan, Nigeria
e-mail: do.oluwayelu@ui.edu.ng

J. A. Shenge, A. L. K. Abia (eds.), *Viral Diseases and One Health in Africa*,
https://doi.org/10.1007/978-3-032-09613-5_4

countries (Tomori 1980; Shope et al. 1982; Shope 1985; Gerdes 2004). At the dawn of the new millennium, RVF spread to Yemen and Saudi Arabia within the Arabian Peninsula (Ahmad 2000; Abdo-Salem et al. 2006) and later to other parts of the Asian continent (Azhar et al. 2010). Tezcan-Ulger et al. (2019) recently reported serologic evidence of the disease in Europe. At the moment, the disease is gradually assuming a global dimension, with substantial public health implications.

4.2 Aetiology of Rift Valley Fever

RVF is caused by RVF virus (RVFV), recently renamed *Phlebovirus riftense* by the International Committee on the Taxonomy of Viruses (ICTV). The most recent virus classification update by the ICTV categorised RVFV as a species under the Genus *Phlebovirus*, Family *Phenuiviridae*, Order *Hareavirales*, Class *Bunyaviricetes*, Subphylum *Polyploviricotina*, Phylum *Negarnaviricota*, Kingdom *Orthornavirae* and Realm *Riboviria* (ICTV 2025). Beyond the taxon species, RVFV is further classified into genotypes or lineages. Presently, 15 recognised RVFV genotypes/lineages are indicated as Lineages A to O (van Schalkwyk and Romito 2019; van Vuren et al. 2019). Additionally, RVFV is classified into Group V of Baltimore's classification scheme because it possesses a negative-sense single-stranded RNA genome.

4.2.1 Morphology of Rift Valley Fever Virus

The RVFV virion is composed basically of a tripartite genome (nucleic acid material), a protein coat, and a surrounding membrane called the envelope (Nichol et al. 2005; Harrison 2013), but without the matrix protein (Huiskonen et al. 2009). Other virion components include the enzymes, the glycoproteins, and sometimes, antigenomes, i.e. replicative intermediates (Ikegami et al. 2005). The virion measures about 100 nm (±10 nm) in diameter (Ellis et al. 1979; Freiberg et al. 2008), which is within average compared to other viruses. The envelope contains the glycoproteins of the virus, the Gn and Gc, which are necessary for attachment to initiate virus infection. These glycoproteins are incorporated into the envelope of the virion in a regular fashion, just like some other phleboviruses (Fig. 4.1) (von Bonsdorff and Pettersson 1975). It was initially thought that the particle is either spherical or pleomorphic in shape, but some subsequent and more detailed studies revealed that the virion has a symmetrical pattern that is consistent with an icosahedron (Huiskonen et al. 2009; Sherman et al. 2009).

The genome of RVFV measures approximately 11.9 kilobases. Like the genomes of other members of the *Phenuiviridae* family, it is segmented, consisting of three segments designated as Large (L), Medium (M) and Small (S) segments (Bishop et al. 1980; Rice et al. 1980; Schmaljohn and Nichol 2007) based on their relative sizes (Fig. 4.2). These segments are packaged into the virion bound by several

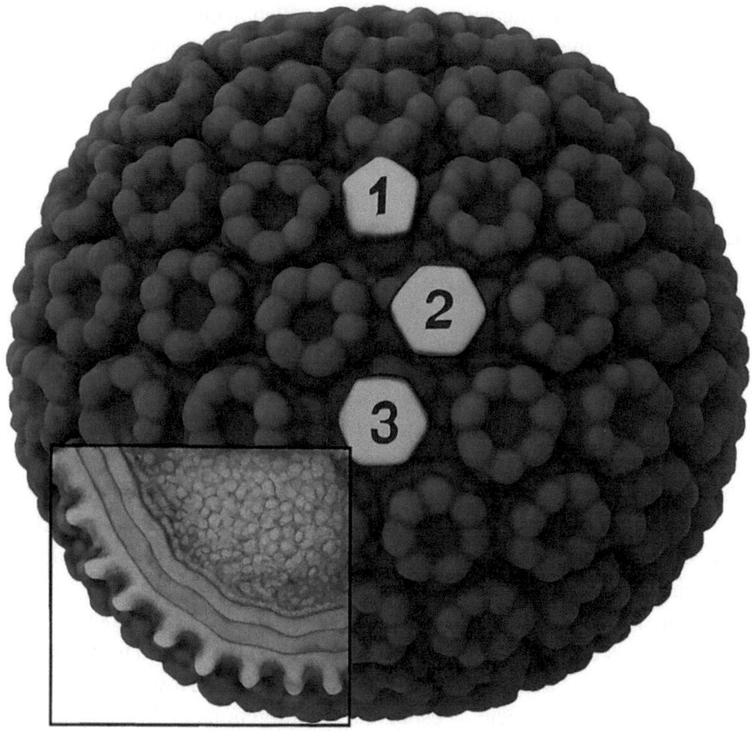

Fig. 4.1 3-dimensional image of Rift Valley fever virus virion

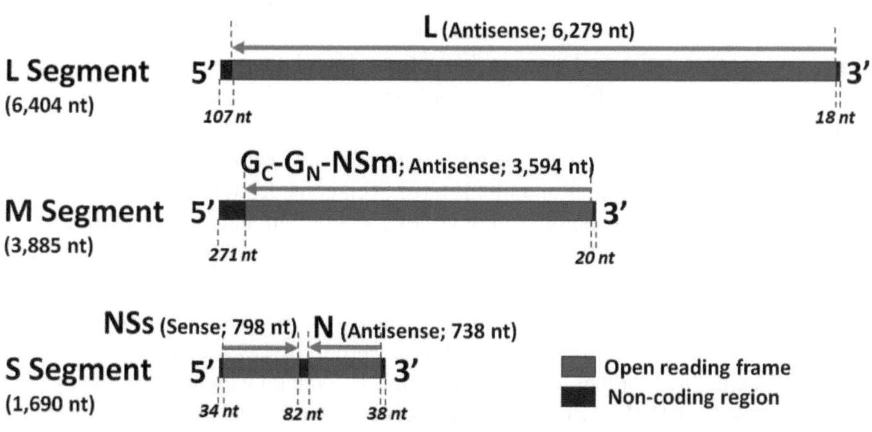

Fig. 4.2 Genome organisation of Rift Valley fever virus MP12 strain. The lengths of the overall segments and those of the coding and flanking non-coding regions are indicated. L = Viral RNA-dependent RNA polymerase, G_C = Glycoprotein located at the C-terminus of the precursor molecule, G_N = Glycoprotein located at the N-terminus of the precursor molecule, NSm = M segment-derived non-structural protein, NSs = S segment-derived non-structural protein. N = Nucleoprotein

amounts of viral proteins [nucleoprotein (N) together with the virus-encoded polymerase (L)] and can therefore be referred to as ribonucleoproteins (RNPs). Both the large and medium segments are minus sense, but the small segment is ambisense. Each RVFV genome segment comprises section(s) that code for functional protein (s) and those that do not. The coding region(s) contain the open reading frame (s) (ORFs) and are flanked at both ends (5′ and 3′ ends) by the non-coding regions, also called the untranslated regions (UTRs) (Schmaljohn and Nichol 2007) (Fig. 4.2).

4.3 Hosts and Transmission of Rift Valley Fever Virus

Being a zoonosis, RVF affects both humans and animals and presents with a variety of clinical signs depending on factors like the species and age of the affected. Studies show that a wide variety of animal species can be infected, including but not limited to cattle, sheep, goats, dromedaries, buffaloes, elephants, antelopes, and rodents. However, some animals do not develop severe diseases; the Old World monkeys, dogs, and cats only have a short viraemic phase.

Apart from these vertebrate hosts, mosquitoes of different genera can also be infected, serving as the vectors. The transmission of the virus was initially thought to involve only the *Aedes* and *Culex* species of mosquitoes. However, further studies revealed that many other species, besides those indigenous to the African continent, are involved in the virus transmission cycle (Moutailler et al. 2008; Turell et al. 2010). Consequently, the chances of its emergence and eventual endemicity in virgin geographic regions are increasing (Turell et al. 1988), with the possibility that it might eventually become a global health threat. Additionally, apart from mosquitoes, some other arthropod vectors have been found to possess the potential to replicate the virus, notable among which are *Culicoides* midges, phlebotomine sand flies, and *Amblyomma* ticks (Sang et al. 2010; Oragwa et al. 2024). However, the contribution of these vectors to RVF outbreaks has yet to be fully determined. Furthermore, a large number of animals have been considered as possible reservoirs of RVFV in the environment, including several wild animal species (Olive et al. 2012; Gaudreault et al. 2015) and several reptile and amphibian species (Rissmann et al. 2020, 2021).

Transmission of RVFV, both in humans and animals, is possible during blood meals by infected mosquitoes or through exposure to diseased animals' tissues and fluids. Placental membranes and other materials associated with aborted foetuses are laden with lots of RVFV virions and can serve as sources of infection for humans and other animals or even for long-term environmental contamination (Theiler 1957; Craig et al. 1967). Both modes of transmission play essential roles in spreading RVFV. Specifically, contact with tissues, blood and other bodily fluids of infected animals can serve as a means of RVFV transmission to occupationally exposed individuals, especially butchers and abattoir workers (Oragwa et al. 2022). Also, bites of infected mosquitoes are significant for the spread of the virus between animal herds within short and even long distances (Chevalier et al. 2004). Vertical transmission of the virus in humans and animals (Arishi et al. 2006; Antonis et al. 2013) and accidental laboratory transmissions (Kitchen 1934) have also been documented. In addition, transmission through needle inoculation, blood transfusion or organ transplant is possible. The emergence and/or re-emergence of RVFV in a geographical location can be aided by the translocation of diseased livestock and/or infected vectors (Pfeffer and Dobler 2010). Additionally, RVFV reservoirs, along with the vectors, play important roles in the maintenance of the virus in the environment and contribute to its re-emergence in enzootic circulations at regional levels (Favier et al. 2006).

4.4 Pathogenesis of Rift Valley Fever

The pathogenesis of RVF varies considerably depending on the portal of entry of the virus and the species of the exposed animal. For instance, mice that received intraperitoneal inoculation of the virus suffer more serious disease than those that received intradermal inoculation due to better virus replication in the liver cells (Gommet et al. 2011). Conversely, reasonable viraemia may not always be produced by intraperitoneal inoculation of the virus in sheep (Ikegami and Makino 2011). Overall, natural exposure to RVFV following mosquito bites and virus deposition results in its transportation from the mosquito bite site to the lymph nodes via the lymphatics. The initial virus replication occurs in the lymph nodes, from where the virus is distributed to different target body organs via the blood (primary viraemia). The target organs for virus replication include the liver, spleen, and brain (Flick and Bouloy 2005); the clinical signs and symptoms seen in the affected animal largely depend on the organs and systems of the body affected.

It has been reported that RVF pathogenesis is driven mainly by two non-structural proteins of the virus, namely the NSs and NSm proteins, which are encoded by its small and medium genomic segments, respectively (Billecocq et al. 2004; Won et al. 2007). The NSs protein causes neurologic and hepatic disorders, leading to the death of the affected animal, and is therefore considered the major virulence factor of the virus (Bird et al. 2007a). It is also responsible for the evasion of the host immune system through its interference with host mRNA transcription, thereby inhibiting the production of critical antiviral cytokines like interferon-γ (Billecocq et al. 2004; Ikegami et al. 2009). On the other hand, the NSm suppresses apoptosis, usually induced by a competent immune system to destroy RVFV-infected cells to terminate the replication of the virus (Won et al. 2007).

4.5 Clinical Signs and Symptoms of Rift Valley Fever

The type and severity of the clinical manifestations of RVF vary reasonably owing to some inherent factors of the affected host, including age, species and immune status, and concurrent infections. Following exposure to the virus, the incubation period may last 4–7 days in humans and 1–6 days in other animals, typically shorter in neonatal, young and immunocompromised animals (Smith et al. 1972; Abdulkadir 1989). These neonatal and young animals may experience a brief episode of fever followed by depression resulting from abdominal pain and anorexia. The affected animal may die within one day (Smith et al. 1972; Ikegami and Makino 2011). Adult animals may develop fever suddenly, which climaxes typically between the second and fourth days. The animal may also have other signs like nasal discharges that may be mucopurulent or bloody, lacrimation, salivation, anorexia, and diarrhoea, which may be fetid or bloody. Pregnant animals may abort or have malformed foetuses, while dairy cattle may have dysgalactia (Tomori 1979; Zeller et al. 1997; Morrill 2001). Mortality rates may be almost 100% in neonatal lambs and about 5–10% in mature cattle populations.

Humans usually experience a milder form of the disease, which generally presents with malaria-like and/or influenza-like symptoms, including fever, malaise, myalgia, headache, etc. The affected humans typically recover fully with no residual complications, usually within one week of clinical disease. However, occasionally, RVF in humans may degenerate into haemorrhagic fever, causing renal failure, jaundice resulting from severe liver damage, encephalitis, ocular lesions, etc. Such haemorrhagic fever can result in high case fatality rates, which, in some instances, can be as high as 50% (Madani et al. 2003; Kahlon et al. 2010).

4.6 Epidemiology of Rift Valley Fever

4.6.1 Geographical Spread of Rift Valley Fever in Africa

Rift Valley fever was first reported in Kenya in 1930, from where it spread to most countries of Africa. It was reported outside Africa for the first time in 2000 following an outbreak in Saudi Arabia and Yemen (Ahmad 2000). In Africa, RVF outbreaks and evidence of the disease have been reported at different times in most countries, especially sub-Saharan African countries. Table 4.1 shows some of the major RVF outbreaks recorded so far at various times and in different geographic locations within Africa.

Table 4.1 Records of RVF outbreaks in Africa

SN	Country	Dates of outbreaks	References
1.	Central African Republic	2019–2020	WHO (2019a)
2.	Egypt	1977–1978, 1993–1994, 1997–1998, 2003	Abdel-Wahab et al. (1978), Davies (2010)
3.	Gambia	1999, 2002	WHO (2018a)
4.	Kenya	1930–1931, 1950–1951, 1997–1998, 2006–2007, 2018–2019, 2020–2021	Daubney et al. (1931), Murithi et al. 2011; WHO (2018b, 2021)
5.	Libya	2019–2020	Mahmoud et al. (2021)
6.	Madagascar	1979, 1990–1991, 2008–2009	Morvan et al. (1991), Andriamandimby et al. (2010)
7.	Mauritania	1987, 1998–1999, 2002, 2010, 2012, 2020	Diallo et al. (2005), Soumare et al. (2012), Caminade et al. (2014)
8.	Mayotte	2018–2019	WHO (2019b)
9.	Mozambique	1969	Valadão (1969)
10.	Namibia	1955, 1974–1975, 2010	Monaco et al. (2013)
11.	Niger Republic	2016	Lagare et al. (2019)
12.	Somalia	1997–1998, 2007	Ahrens (1998), Anonymous (2007)
13.	South Africa	1950–1953, 1974–1976, 1999, 2008–2011, 2018	van Velden et al. (1977), Archer et al. (2013), van Vuren et al. (2019)
14.	Sudan	1973, 1976, 2007, 2019–2020	WHO (2018b, 2019c)
15.	Tanzania	1947, 1957, 1960, 1963, 1968, 1977–1978, 1989, 1997–1998, 2006–2007	WHO (2018b)
16.	Uganda	2016, 2018–2019	Luke et al. (2019)
17.	Zambia	1973–1974,1976, 1985	Hussein et al. (1987), Dautu et al. (2012)
18.	Zimbabwe	1955, 1957, 1969–1970, 1976	Swanepoel (1981)

4.6.2 *Seasonality of Rift Valley Fever Transmission and Outbreaks*

Since mosquitoes and other arthropod vectors transmit RVF, the peak of virus transmission is expected to coincide with the season of the year marked with the highest vector activities. In most parts of Africa, vector activities are at their peaks during the rainy season, usually late rainy season (Okorie et al. 2014). This may coincide with different months of the year in various countries. Overall, RVF outbreaks usually commence around or shortly after peak rainfall. Sindato et al. (2014) reported that most outbreaks in Tanzania between 1977 and 2007 were preceded by or coincided with maximum total monthly rainfall records. Alhaji et al. (2018) reported a statistically significant association of RVF with late rainy season (July–

September) in Nigeria. Conversely, Oragwa et al. (2023) reported a higher detection rate of the virus during the dry season compared to the rainy season and suggested that RVFV transmission could be an all-year-round event in Nigeria. Seasonality is only essential when considering transmission through infected arthropod vectors. Other modes of transmission, including contact with aborted materials, tissue, blood and other bodily fluids of infected animals and consumption of unpasteurised contaminated milk, do not necessarily have any seasonal connections.

4.6.3 Emergence and Re-emergence of Rift Valley Fever

RVF has the capacity to emerge and reemerge in a geographical location. Sometimes, the disease can cross considerable geographical barriers and emerge in distant places. This capacity of the virus to "jump" to such a virgin environment is made possible through the movement of infected vectors and/or viraemic animals (Pfeffer and Dobler 2010). This is made possible by the increasing transportation speed and connectivity between different geographical locations (i.e. the globalisation of travel). Indeed, international livestock trade has been a significant means of movement of viraemic animals and, thus, RVF to new territories. For instance, the first RVF outbreak in Egypt that occurred between 1977 and 1978 was suspected to have been introduced via viraemic sheep brought into the country from Sudan, travelling along Lake Nasser (Gad et al. 1986); the first report of the disease in Nigeria was from Merino sheep imported from South Africa (Ferguson 1959).

The re-emergence of the disease in an environment after an initial outbreak has continued to be recorded. Many African countries have recorded multiple episodes of RVF outbreaks, including Kenya, Tanzania, South Africa, Mauritania, Egypt, Madagascar, Sudan, Zambia, and Zimbabwe, among others (Table 4.1). There are two modes of RVF re-emergence in an environment: renewed replication and transmission of RVFV already existing in the environment or through fresh reintroduction of the virus into the environment. The earlier mode is usually driven by the preservation of the virus in the reservoir hosts or through vertically infected eggs of *Aedes* mosquitoes. So far, particular species of wild animals, including buffaloes and deer (Beechler et al. 2015; Gaudreault et al. 2015), as well as amphibians and reptiles like lizards, turtles, etc. (Rissmann et al. 2020, 2021), are suspected to serve as reservoirs of the virus in an environment. Vertically infected *Aedes* mosquito eggs can remain dormant for several years to decades in dry mud (O'Malley 1990) and hatch at the return of unusually heavy rainfalls and attendant floods. Vertically infected progeny *Aedes* mosquitoes initiate the virus transmission to susceptible hosts and the contributions of other mosquito species and other means of virus transmission lead to full-blown RVF outbreaks.

The latter mode of RVF re-emergence, i.e. fresh RVFV reintroduction to an environment, resembles the initial emergence and is driven by the introduction of viraemic animals or infected vectors. In some instances, the newly introduced strains may differ from the already established strain in the environment. This is evidenced

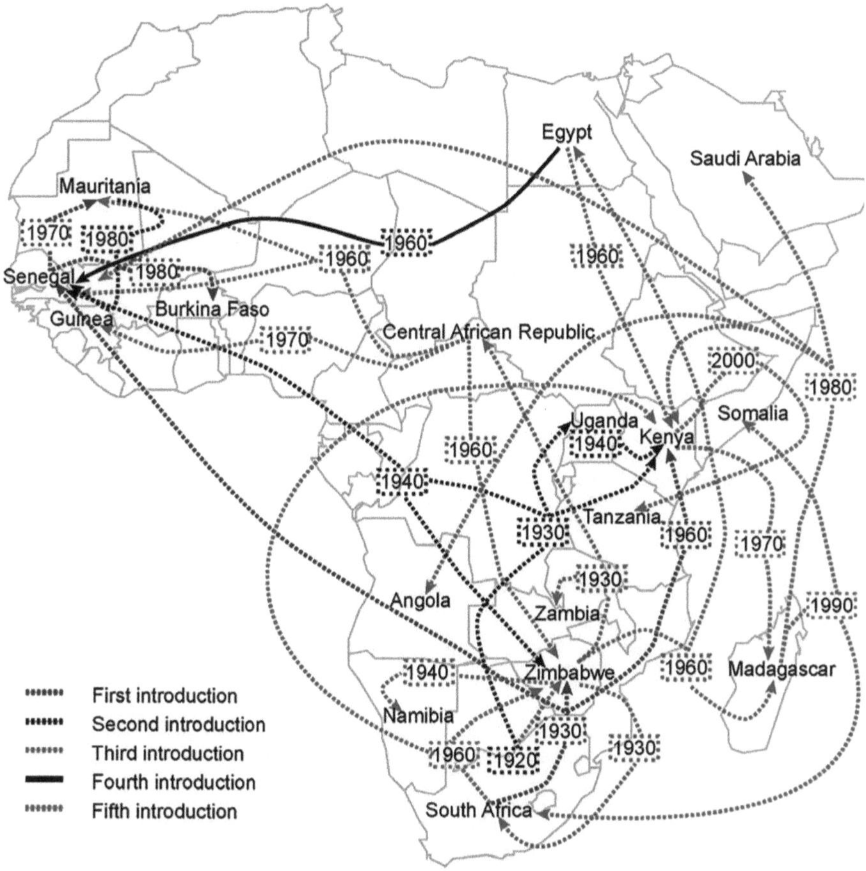

Fig. 4.3 Multiple introductions of RVFV into different countries of Africa. (Source: Soumare et al. (2012))

by the co-circulation of RVFV strains belonging to multiple lineages in a particular geographic location. The re-emergence of RVFV following multiple introductions into many African countries is summarised in Fig. 4.3.

4.6.4 Molecular Epidemiology of Rift Valley Fever Virus

Most countries in Africa, particularly those in sub-Saharan Africa, have experienced varying numbers of RVF outbreaks and evidence of the disease to date. A comparison of the genomes of the RVFV strains reported at different times from different geographical locations and different hosts reveals high genomic fidelity. The RVFV genomic sequences are highly conserved. Accordingly, the virus exhibits minimal antigenic diversity, resulting in its existence as a single serotype (Bird et al. 2007b;

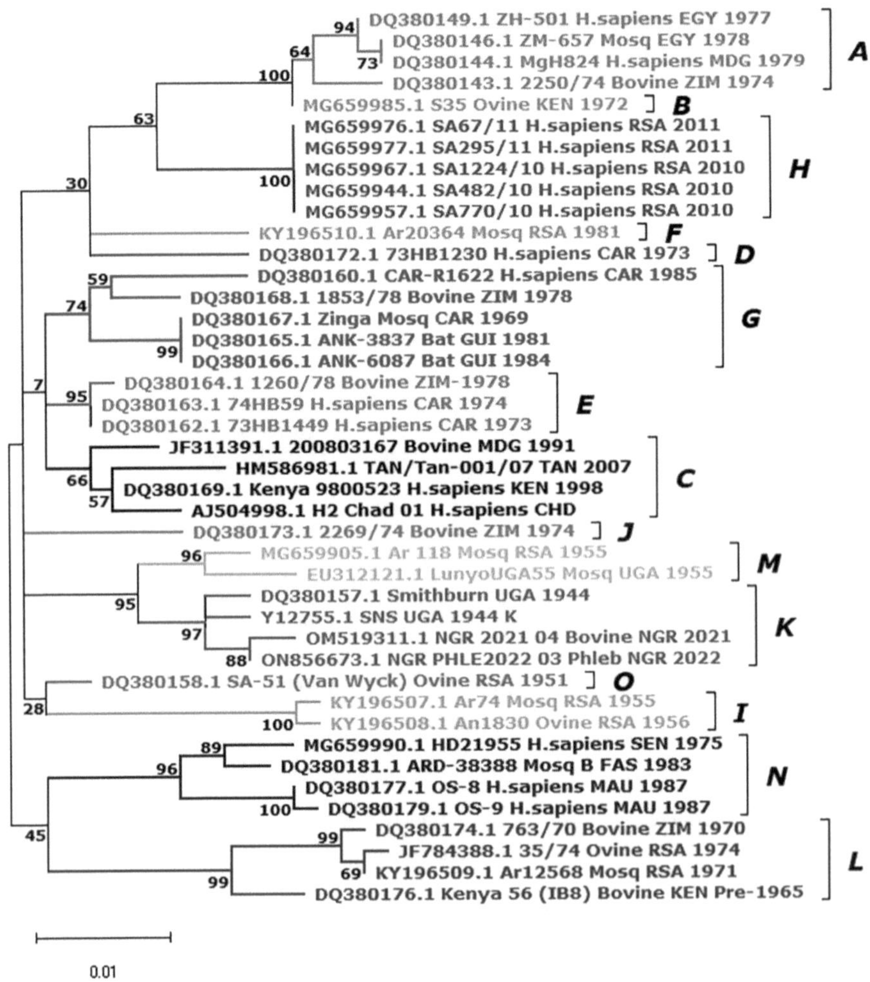

Fig. 4.4 Phylogenetic presentation of the clustering pattern of the 15 RVFV Lineages (A-O) representatives based on their S-segment. B FAS Burkina Faso; CAR Central African Republic; CHD Chad; EGY Egypt; GUI Guinea; KEN Kenya; MAU Mauritania; MDG Madagascar; NGR Nigeria; RSA South African Republic; SEN Senegal; TAN Tanzania; UGA Uganda; ZIM Zimbabwe

Maluleke et al. 2019). According to Bird et al. (2007b), this finding is attributable to a possibly reduced ability of the RVFV genome to cope with mutations, a concept described as an inherently slow clock. This notwithstanding, RVFV strains have been segregated into 15 genotypes (lineages) based on their discrete clustering on the phylogenetic tree. These lineages are alphabetically named Lineages A to O (Fig. 4.4) (Grobbelaar et al. 2011; van Vuren et al. 2019; van Schalkwyk and Romito 2019). It has been observed that the phylogenetic trees constructed based on the nucleotide sequences of the whole genomes and each of the L, M and S segments of

Table 4.2 Established RVFV lineages and African countries in which they have been reported

SN	Lineage	Countries
1.	A	Egypt, Madagascar, Zimbabwe
2.	B	Kenya, Zimbabwe
3.	C	Angola, Chad, Kenya, Madagascar, Mauritania, Saudi Arabia, Somalia, South Africa, Sudan, Tanzania, Uganda, Zimbabwe
4.	D	CAR
5.	E	CAR, Zimbabwe, Zambia
6.	F	South Africa
7.	G	CAR, Guinea, Senegal, Zimbabwe
8.	H	Namibia, South Africa
9.	I	South Africa
10.	J	Zimbabwe
11.	K	China, Kenya, Nigeria, South Africa, Uganda, Zimbabwe
12.	L	Egypt, Kenya, South Africa, Zimbabwe
13.	M	South Africa, Uganda
14.	N	Burkina Faso, Mauritania, Senegal
15.	O	South Africa

RVFV strains representing the established lineages share similar topologies. Occasionally, this may not hold, as some strains may have their different segments clustering with representatives of different lineages. This can be considered evidence of reassortment, with the parent strains belonging to different lineages (Bird et al. 2007b). To further simplify the process of RVFV genotyping, Juma et al. (2022) developed a user-friendly RVFV genotyping tool, which has a web-based interface and a command line (https://www.genomedetective.com/app/typingtool/rvfv/).

The clustering pattern of the representative strains of the RVFV lineages is shown in Fig. 4.4, while Table 4.2 shows some of the countries where the respective lineages have been reported so far. Apart from Lineages D (Central African Republic), J (Zimbabwe), F, I, and O (South Africa), which have been reported in only one country each, other lineages are circulating in multiple countries, with some located far apart within the continent. The geographic circulation of the individual lineages is not restricted, and Lineage C has the widest spread, reaching the different regions of the African continent and beyond (Table 4.2).

4.6.5 Consequences of Rift Valley Fever Outbreaks

Various undesirable outcomes in human and livestock populations have always accompanied Rift Valley fever outbreaks. Although some exposed humans may not exhibit any clinical disease, others may manifest some severe clinical signs, necessitating hospitalisation. In some occasions, the disease may degenerate into haemorrhagic fever syndrome, with high chances of culminating in the death of the affected individual. Some infected persons may also suffer ocular and neurological complications (Alrajhi et al. 2004; Al-Hazmi et al. 2005). In such situations, the case fatality rates estimated at 0.5–2% (Meegan et al. 1981) may rise to as high as 50% (Madani et al. 2003; Kahlon et al. 2010). Among the animals, outbreaks can lead to varying degrees of abortions, foetal malformation in the affected herds, and death, especially in younger animals. Fatality rates may differ significantly depending on the species and age of affected animals, ranging from 5–10% among mature cattle to nearly 100% among neonatal lambs (Ikegami and Makino 2011).

The first RVF epizootic of 1930 in Kenya reportedly resulted in the death of more than 1200 ewes and 3500 lambs, with large numbers of abortions among the pregnant animals (Daubney et al. 1931). Altogether, several million livestock and more than 2000 human lives have been reportedly lost, along with several hundred thousand human infections in Kenya alone between 1912 and 2007 (Murithi et al. 2011). These numbers must have further increased as more outbreaks have continued to be recorded in the country. In Egypt, the major outbreak recorded in 1977 resulted in the loss of about 600 human lives, with about 20,000 to 200,000 clinical diseases (Abdel-Wahab et al. 1978; Davies 2010). In addition, many other African countries have different records of losses associated with RVF outbreaks among humans and animals. Apart from the loss of livestock, RVF endemicity in any geographic location results in trade restrictions, thereby negatively affecting the income of poor farmers and the economy of the affected countries. A good example is the adverse effects of such an export ban on Somalia and other countries of the Horn of Africa (Ahrens 1998). Additionally, the loss of livestock to RVF can adversely affect crop farming, especially in rural farming localities where these animals are used for ploughing and transporting farm produce. Meat and milk production can also be adversely affected, considering RVF infection can cause dysgalactia in lactating animals (Nielsen et al. 2020).

4.7 Prevention, Control and Management of Rift Valley Fever

Effective prevention and control strategies against RVF are based on appropriately controlling the arthropod vectors capable of transmitting the virus and restricting indiscriminate movement and importation of susceptible animals, especially from RVF-endemic localities. There is also a need to educate occupationally exposed individuals (such as veterinarians, butchers, livestock keepers, and abattoir workers) who are at higher risk of contracting the disease through contact with tissues, blood, and other bodily fluids of infected animals. Additionally, the general public needs to be informed about the risks associated with consuming unpasteurized milk. Newly acquired animals should also be quarantined before introduction into livestock farms. Moreover, adopting mass RVF vaccination campaigns at local, national, and regional levels would greatly help control the disease. Currently, both live-attenuated and killed vaccines exist for use in animals only. The live-attenuated vaccine reportedly induces long-lasting protection but should be used with caution, especially in pregnant animals, as it can cause congenital malformations and abortions in pregnant sheep (Morrill 2001; Hunter et al. 2002). Conversely, human RVF vaccines are yet to be commercially available. The management of the disease, especially in humans, is achieved through symptomatic treatment.

References

Abdel-Wahab KS, El Baz LM, El-Tayeb EM, Omar H, Ossman MA, Yasin W (1978) Rift Valley fever virus infections in Egypt: Pathological and virological findings in man. Trans R Soc Trop Med Hyg 72:392–396. https://doi.org/10.1016/0035-9203(78)90134-7

Abdo-Salem S, Gerbier G, Bonnet P, Al-Qadasi M, Tran A, Thiry E et al (2006) Descriptive and spatial epidemiology of Rift Valley fever in Yemen, 2000-2001. Ann N Y Acad Sci 1081:240–242

Abdulkadir IA (1989) Rift Valley fever. In: Infectious diseases of livestock in Nigeria. Ahmadu Bello University Press Limited, Zaria, pp 195–197

Ahmad K (2000) More deaths from Rift Valley fever in Saudi Arabia and Yemen. Lancet 356:1422. https://doi.org/10.1016/S0140-6736(05)74068-X

Ahrens JD (1998) Cessation of livestock exports severely affects the pastorals economy of Somali Region. UNDP Emergencies Unit for Ethiopia Mission: 31 March to April 1998

Alhaji NB, Babalobi OO, Wungak Y, Ularamu HG (2018) Participatory survey of Rift Valley fever in nomadic pastoral communities of north-central Nigeria: The associated risk pathways and factors. PLoS Negl Trop Dis 12:e0006858

Al-Hazmi A, Al-Rajhi AA, Abboud EB, Ayoola EA, Al-Hazmi M, Saadi R et al (2005) Ocular complications of Rift Valley fever outbreak in Saudi Arabia. Fortschr Ophthalmol 112:313–318

Alrajhi AA, Al-Semari A, Al-Watban J (2004) Rift Valley fever encephalitis. Emerg Infect Dis 10: 554–555

Andriamandimby SF, Randrianarivo-Solofoniaina AE, Jeanmaire EM, Ravololomanana L, Razafimanantsoa LT, Rakotojoelinandrasana T et al (2010) Rift Valley fever during rainy seasons, Madagascar, 2008 and 2009. Emerg Infect Dis 16(6):963–970. https://doi.org/10.3201/eid1606.091266

Anonymous (2007) 14 die after Rift Valley Fever breaks out in southern Somalia. https://web.archive.org/web/20070930154712/http://www.shabelle.net/news/ne2114.htm. Accessed 29 Aug 2024

Antonis AFG, Kortekaas J, Kant J, Vloet RPM, Vogel-Brink A, Stockhofe N et al (2013) Vertical transmission of Rift Valley fever virus without detectable maternal viremia. Vector Borne Zoonotic Dis 13(8):601–606. https://doi.org/10.1089/vbz.2012.1160

Archer BN, Thomas J, Weyer J, Cengimbo A, Landoh DE, Jacobs C et al (2013) Epidemiological investigations into outbreaks of Rift Valley fever in humans, South Africa, 2008-2011. Emerg Infect Dis 19(12):1918–1925. https://doi.org/10.3201/eid1912.121527

Arishi HM, Aqeel AY, Al Hazmi MM (2006) Vertical transmission of fatal Rift Valley fever in a newborn. Ann Trop Paediatr 26:251–253

Azhar EI, Madani TA, Kao M, Jamjoom GA (2010) A seroepidemiological study of Rift Valley fever virus among slaughterhouses' workers in Saudi Arabia. Int J Med Med Sci 2:111–115

Beechler BR, Bengis R, Swanepoel R, Paweska JT, Kemp A, Jansen van Vuren P et al (2015) Rift Valley fever in Kruger national park: do buffalo play a role in the inter-epidemic circulation of virus? Transbound Emerg Dis 62:24–32. https://doi.org/10.1111/tbed.12197

Billecocq A, Spiegel M, Vialat P, Kohl A, Weber F, Bouloy M et al (2004) NSs protein of Rift Valley fever virus blocks interferon production by inhibiting host gene transcription. J Virol 78: 9798–9806

Bird BH, Albarino CG, Nichol ST (2007a) Rift valley fever virus lacking Nsm proteins retains high virulence in vivo and may provide a model of human delayed onset neurologic disease. Virology 362:10–15

Bird BH, Khristova ML, Rollin PE, Ksiazek TG, Nichol ST (2007b) Complete genome analysis of 33 ecologically and biologically diverse Rift Valley fever virus strains reveals widespread virus movement and low genetic diversity due to recent common ancestry. J Virol 18(6):2805–2816. https://doi.org/10.1128/JVI.02095-06

Bishop DHL, Calisher C, Casals J, Chumadov MP, Gaidamovich SYA, Hannoun C et al (1980) Bunyaviridae. lntervirology 14:125–143

Caminade C, Ndione JA, Diallo M, MacLeod DA, Faye O, Ba Y et al (2014) Rift Valley fever outbreaks in Mauritania and related environmental conditions. Int J Environ Res Public Health 11:903–918. https://doi.org/10.3390/ijerph110100903

Chevalier V, Mondet B, Diaite A, Lancelot R, Fall AG, Poncon N (2004) Exposure of sheep to mosquito bites: Possible consequences for the transmission risk of Rift Valley fever in Senegal. Med Vet Entomol 18:247–255

Craig DE, Thomas WJ, DeSanctis AN (1967) Stability of Rift Valley fever virus at 4°C. Appl Microbiol 15:446–447

Daubney R, Hudson JR (1932) Rift Valley fever. Lancet 1:611–612

Daubney R, Hudson JR, Gamham PC (1931) Enzootic hepatitis or Rift Valley fever: An undescribed virus disease of sheep, cattle and man from East Africa. J Path Bacteriol 34:545–579

Dautu G, Sindato C, Mweene AS, Samui KL, Roy P, Noad R, at. (2012) Rift Valley fever: Real or perceived threat for Zambia? Onderstepoort J Vet Res 79(2):94–99. http://www.scielo.org.za/scielo.php?script=sci_arttext&pid=S0030-24652012000200022&lng=en&tlng=en

Davies FG (2010) The historical and recent impact of Rift Valley fever in Africa. Am J Trop Med Hygiene 83:73–74. https://doi.org/10.4269/ajtmh.2010.83s2a02

Diallo M, Nabeth P, Ba K, Sall AA, Ba Y, Mondo M et al (2005) Mosquito vectors of the 1998–1999 outbreak of Rift Valley Fever and other arboviruses (Bagaza, Sanar, Wesselsbron and West Nile) in Mauritania and Senegal. Med Vet Entomol 19:119–126. https://doi.org/10.1111/j.0269-283X.2005.00564.x

Ellis DS, Simpson DIH, Stamford S, Wahab KSEA (1979) Rift Valley fever virus: Some ultra-structural observations on material from the outbreak in Egypt 1977. J Gen Virol 42:329–337

Favier C, Chalvet-Monfray K, Sabatier P, Lancelot R, Fontenille D, Dubois MA (2006) Rift Valley fever in West Africa: the role of space in endemicity. Trop Med Int Health 11:1878–1888. https://doi.org/10.1111/j.1365-3156.2006.01746.x

Ferguson W (1959) Identification of Rift Valley fever in Nigeria. Bull Epizoot Dis Afr 7:317–318

Flick R, Bouloy M (2005) Rift Valley fever virus. Curr Mol Med 5(8):827–834

Freiberg AN, Sherman MB, Morais MC, Holbrook MR, Watowich SJ (2008) Three-dimensional organisation of Rift Valley fever virus revealed by cryoelectron tomography. J Virol 82:10341–10348

Gad AM, Feinsod FM, Allam IH, Eisa M, Hassan AN, Soliman BA et al (1986) A possible route for the introduction of Rift Valley fever virus into Egypt during 1977. J Trop Med Hyg 89:233–236

Gaudreault NN, Indran SV, Bryant PK, Richt JA, Wilson WC (2015) Comparison of Rift Valley fever virus replication in North American livestock and wildlife cell lines. Front Microbiol 6: 664

Gerdes GH (2004) Rift Valley fever. Rev Sci Tech 23:613–623

Gommet C, Billecocq A, Jouvion G, Hasan M, Zaverucha do Valle T, Guillemot L et al (2011) Tissue tropism and target cells of NSs-deleted Rift Valley fever virus in live immunodeficient mice. PLoS Negl Trop Dis 5:e1421

Grobbelaar AA, Weyer J, Leman PA, Kemp A, Paweska JT, Swanepoel R (2011) Molecular epidemiology of Rift Valley fever virus. Emerg Infect Dis 17:2270–2266. https://doi.org/10.3201/eid1712.111035
Harrison SC (2013) In: Fields Virology BN, Fields DMK, Howley PM (eds) Principles of virus structure, 6th edn. Wolters Kluwer, Lippincott William and Wilkins Health, Philadelphia, pp 52–86
Huiskonen JT, Overby AK, Weber F, Grunewald K (2009) Electron cryo–microscopy and single–particle averaging of Rift Valley fever virus: evidence for GN–GC glycoprotein heterodimers. J Virol 83:3762–3769
Hunter P, Erasmus BJ, Vorster JH (2002) Teratogenicity of mutagenised Rift Valley fever virus (MVP 12) in sheep. Onderst J Vet Res 69:95–98
Hussein NA, Chizyuka RZ, Kasiazek TG, Scott R, Boulos BAM (1987) Epizootic of Rift Valley fever in Zambia, 1985. Vet Rec 121:111. https://doi.org/10.1136/vr.121.5.111
Ikegami T, Makino S (2011) The Pathogenesis of Rift Valley fever. Viruses 3:493–519. https://doi.org/10.3390/v3050493
Ikegami T, Won S, Peters CJ, Makino S (2005) Rift Valley fever virus NSs mRNA is transcribed from an incoming anti-viral-sense S RNA segment. J Virol 79:12106–12111
Ikegami T, Narayanan K, Won S, Kamitani W, Peters CJ, Makino S (2009) Rift Valley fever virus NSs protein promotes post-transcriptional downregulation of protein kinase pkr and inhibits eif2alpha phosphorylation. PLoS Pathog 5:e1000287
International Committee on Taxonomy of Viruses (ICTV) (2025) ICTV 2024 Master Species List (MSL#40). https://ictv.global/. Accessed 12 April 2025
Juma J, Fonseca V, Konongoi SL, van Heusden P, Roesel K, Sang R et al (2022) Genomic surveillance of Rift Valley fever virus: from sequencing to lineage assignment. BMC Genomics 23:520. https://doi.org/10.1186/s12864-022-08764-6
Kahlon SS, Peters CJ, LeDuc J, Muchiri EM, Muiruri S, Njenga MK et al (2010) Severe Rift Valley fever may present with a characteristic clinical syndrome. Am J Trop Med Hygiene 82:371–375. https://doi.org/10.4269/ajtmh.2010.09-0669
Kitchen SF (1934) Laboratory infections with the virus of Rift Valley fever. Am J Trop Med 14: 547–564
Lagare A, Fall G, Ibrahim A, Ousmane S, Sadio B, Abdoulaye M et al (2019) First occurrence of Rift Valley fever outbreak in Niger, 2016. Vet Med Sci 5:70–78. https://doi.org/10.1002/vms3.135
Luke N, Balinandi S, Mulei S, Kyondo J, Tumusiime A, Klena J et al (2019) Ten outbreaks of Rift Valley fever in Uganda 2016-2018: epidemiological and laboratory findings. Int J Infect Dis 79: 4
Madani TA, Al-Mazrou YY, Al-Jeffri MH, Mishkhas AA, Al-Rabeah AM, Turkistani AM et al (2003) Rift Valley fever epidemic in Saudi Arabia: Epidemiological, clinical, and laboratory characteristics. Clin Infect Dis 37:1084–1092
Mahmoud AS, Sawesi OK, El-Waer OR, Bennour EM (2021) Rift valley fever in Africa with the emerging interest in Libya. Int J One Health 7(2):237–245. www.onehealthjournal.org/Vol.7/No.2/13.pdf
Maluleke MR, Phosiwa M, van Schalkwyk A, Michuki G, Lubisi BA, Kegakilwe PS et al (2019) A comparative genome analysis of Rift Valley fever virus isolates from foci of the disease outbreak in South Africa in 2008-2010. PLoS Negl Trop Dis 13:e0006576
Meegan JM, Watten RH, Laughlin LW (1981) Clinical experience with Rift Valley fever in humans during the 1977 Egyptian epizootic. Contrib Epidemiol Biostat 3:114–123
Monaco F, Pinoni C, Cosseddu GM, Khaiseb S, Calistri P, Molini U et al (2013) Rift Valley fever in Namibia, 2010. Emerg Infect Dis 9:12. https://doi.org/10.3201/eid1912.130593
Morrill JC (2001) Rift valley fever in animals and humans. In: Goodman DE (ed) Zoonoses, animal diseases that affect man. Christian Veterinary Missions, Seattle, pp 49–56
Morvan J, Saluzzo JF, Fontenille D, Rollin PE, Coulanges P (1991) Rift Valley fever on the east coast of Madagascar. Res Virol 142(6):475–482

Moutailler S, Krida G, Schaffner F, Vazeille M, Failloux AB (2008) Potential vectors of Rift Valley fever virus in the Mediterranean region. Vector Borne Zoonotic Dis 8(6):749–753. https://doi.org/10.1089/vbz.2008.0009

Murithi RM, Munyua P, Ithondeka PM, Macharia JM, Hightower A, Luman ET et al (2011) Rift Valley fever in Kenya: history of epizootics and identification of vulnerable districts. Epidemiol Infect 139(3):372–380. https://doi.org/10.1017/S0950268810001020

Nichol ST, Beaty BJ, Elliott RM, Goldbach RW, Plyusnin A, Tesh RB (2005) The Bunyaviridae. In: Fauquet C, Mayo MA, Maniloff LSM, Desselberger U, Ball LA (eds) Virus taxonomy. Classification and nomenclature of viruses. VIIIth report of the International Committee on Taxonomy of Viruses. Elsevier Academic Press, London, pp 695–716

Nielsen SS, Alvarez J, Bicout DJ, Calistri P, Depner K, Drewe JA et al (2020) Rift Valley fever: risk of persistence, spread and impact in Mayotte (France). EFSA J 18(4):6093. https://doi.org/10.2903/j.efsa.2020.6093

O'Malley CM (1990) Aedesvexans (Meigen): An old foe. Proc N J Mosquito Control Assoc:90–95

Okorie PN, Popoola K, Awobifa OM, Ibrahim KT, Ademowo GO (2014) Species composition and temporal distribution of mosquito populations in Ibadan, Southwest Nigeria. J Entomol Zool Stud 2(4):164–169

Olive MM, Goodman SM, Reynes JM (2012) The role of wild mammals in the maintenance of Rift Valley fever virus. J Wildl Dis 48:241–266

Oragwa AO, Oragwa FC, Oluwayelu DO (2022) Serologic evidence of silent circulation of Rift Valley fever virus among occupationally exposed persons in northern Nigeria. J Infect Dev Ctries 16(5):881–888. https://doi.org/10.3855/jidc.15367

Oragwa AO, Obishakin ET, Oluwayelu DO (2023) Molecular detection and characterisation of Rift Valley fever virus in humans and domestic ruminants in Nigeria. Microbe 1:100016. https://doi.org/10.1016/j.microb.2023.100016

Oragwa AO, Obishakin ET, Oluwayelu DO (2024) Molecular detection and characterisation of Rift Valley fever virus in arthropod vectors in Nigeria. Microbe 5,100198. https://doi.org/10.1016/j.microb.2024.100198

Pfeffer M, Dobler G (2010) Emergence of zoonotic arboviruses by animal trade and migration. Parasit Vectors 3:35. https://doi.org/10.1186/1756-3305-3-35

Rice RJ, Erlick BJ, Rosato RR, Eddy GE, Mohanty SB (1980) Biochemical characterisation of Rift Valley fever virus. Virology 157:31–39

Rissmann M, Kley N, Ulrich R, Stoek F, Balkema-Buschmann A, Eiden M et al (2020) Competency of amphibians and reptiles and their potential role as reservoir hosts for Rift Valley fever virus. Viruses 12:1206. https://doi.org/10.3390/v12111206

Rissmann M, Lenk M, Stoek F, Szentiks CA, Eiden M, Groschup MH (2021) Replication of Rift Valley fever virus in amphibian and reptile-derived cell lines. Pathogens 10:681. https://doi.org/10.3390/pathogens10060681

Sang R, Kioko E, Lutomiah J, Warigia M, Ochieng C, O'Guinn M et al (2010) Rift Valley fever virus epidemic in Kenya, 2006/2007: the entomologic investigations. Am J Trop Med Hygiene 83:28–37. https://doi.org/10.4269/ajtmh.2010.09-0319

Schmaljohn C, Nichol ST (2007) Bunyaviridae. In: Knipe DM et al (eds) Fields virology, 5th edn. Lippincott Williams & Wilkins, Philadelphia, pp 1741–1789

Sherman MB, Freiberg AN, Holbrook MR, Watowich SJ (2009) Single-particle cryo-electron microscopy of Rift Valley fever virus. Virology 387:11–15

Shope RE (1985) Rift Valley fever. In: Fields BN (ed) Fields virology, vol 1, 1st edn. Haven Press, New York, pp 1055–1088

Shope RE, Peters CJ, Davies EG (1982) The spread of Rift Valley fever and approaches to its control. Bull World Health Organ 60(3):299–304

Sindato C, Karimuribo ED, Pfeiffer DU, Mboera LE, Kivaria F, Dautu G et al (2014) Spatial and temporal pattern of Rift Valley fever outbreaks in Tanzania; 1930 to 2007. PLoS One 9(2): e88897. https://doi.org/10.1371/journal.pone.0088897

Smith HA, Jones TC, Hunt RD (1972) Diseases caused by viruses- Rift Valley fever. In: Veterinary pathology, 4th edn. Lea and Febiger, Philadelphia, pp 471–474

Soumare POL, Freire CCM, Faye O, Diallo M, de Oliveira JVC, Zanotto PMA et al (2012) Phylogeography of Rift Valley fever virus in Africa reveals multiple introductions in Senegal and Mauritania. PLoS One 7(4):e35216. https://doi.org/10.1371/journal.pone.0035216

Swanepoel R (1981) Observations on Rift Valley fever in Zimbabwe. Contrib Epidemiol Biostat 3: 383–391

Tezcan-Ulger S, Kurnaz N, Ulger M, Aslan G, Emekdas G (2019) Serological evidence of Rift Valley fever virus among humans in Mersin province of Turkey. J Vector Borne Dis 56:373–379

Theiler M (1957) Action of sodium desoxycholate on arthropod-borne viruses. Proc Soc Exp Biol Med 96:380–382

Tomori O (1979) Clinical, virological and serological response of the West African dwarf sheep to experimental infection with different strains of Rift Valley fever virus. Res J Vet Sci 26:152–159

Tomori O (1980) Rift Valley fever virus infection in man in Nigeria. J Med Virol 5:343–350

Turell MJ, Faran ME, Cornet M, Bailey CL (1988) Vector competence of Senegalese Aedes fowleri (Diptera: Culicidae) for Rift Valley fever virus. J Med Entomol 25:262–266

Turell MJ, Wilson WC, Bennett KE (2010) Potential for North American mosquitoes (Diptera: Culicidae) to transmit Rift Valley fever virus. J Med Entomol 47:884–889

Valadão FG (1969) Nota prévia sobre a ocorrência de uma nova doença em Moçambique—a doença do vale do Rift. Veterin Moçamb 2:13–20

van Schalkwyk A, Romito M (2019) Genomic characterisation of Rift Valley fever virus, South Africa, 2018. Emerg Infect Dis 25(10):1979–1981. www.cdc.gov/eid. https://doi.org/10.3201/eid2510.181748

van Velden DJ, Meyer JD, Olivier J, Gear JH, McIntosh B (1977) Rift Valley fever affecting humans in South Africa: a clinicopathological study. S A Med J 51(24):867–871. ISSN 0256-9574

van Vuren PJ, Kgaladi J, Msimang V, Paweska JT (2019) Rift Valley fever re-emergence after 7 years of quiescence, South Africa, May 2018. Emerg Infect Dis 25(2):338–341. www.cdc.gov/eid. https://doi.org/10.3201/eid2502.181289

Von Bonsdorff CH, Pettersson R (1975) Surface structure of Uukuniemi virus. J Virol 16:1296–1307

Won S, Ikegami T, Peters CJ, Makino S (2007) NSm protein of Rift Valley fever virus suppresses virus-induced apoptosis. J Virol 81:13335–13345

World Health Organisation (WHO) (2018a) Rift Valley fever-Gambia. https://www.who.int/emergencies/disease-outbreak-news/item/26-february-2018-rift-valley-fever-gambia-en. Accessed 29 Aug 2024

World Health Organisation (WHO) (2018b) Rift Valley fever. https://www.who.int/news-room/fact-sheets/detail/rift-valley-fever. Accessed 29 Aug 2024

World Health Organisation (WHO) (2019a) Weekly bulletin on outbreaks and other emergencies, week 35 (26 August—1 September, 2019). https://iris.who.int/bitstream/handle/10665/326846/OEW35-260801092019. Accessed 29 Aug 2024

World Health Organisation (WHO) (2019b) Rift Valley fever-Mayotte (France). https://web.archive.org/web/20190701132213/https://www.who.int/csr/don/13-may-2019-rift-valley-fever-mayotte-france/en/. Accessed 29 Aug 2024

World Health Organisation (WHO) (2019c) Rift Valley fever-Sudan. https://www.who.int/emergencies/disease-outbreak-news/item/2019-DON205. (Accessed; August 29, 2024)

World Health Organisation (WHO) (2021) Rift Valley fever-Kenya; Disease outbreak news, 12 February 2021. https://www.who.int/csr/don/12-february-2021-rift-valley-fever-kenya/en/. Accessed 29 Aug 2024

Zeller HG, Fontenille D, Traore-Lamizana M, Thiongane Y, Digoutte JP (1997) Enzootic activity of Rift Valley fever virus in Senegal. Am J Trop Med Hygiene 56(3):265–272

Chapter 5
Challenges and Constraints Regarding Control and Prevention of Dog-Mediated Human Rabies Using the One Health Approach in Africa

Hafiz Muhammad Usman, Abdul Subhan, Muhammad Mubashar Beig, Muhammad Hassnain, Waqas Ahmad, Amber Arshad, and Muhammad Younus

5.1 Introduction

Dog-mediated rabies is an acute encephalitis or meningoencephalitis viral disease caused by single-stranded RNA viruses of the genus *Lyssavirus* (from the Greek word "lyssa", meaning "rage"), having family Rhabdoviridae (from the Greek word rhabdo", meaning "rod") (Müller and Freuling 2020). It is bullet-shaped and has helical symmetry, with a length of about 180 nm and a diameter of about 75 nm. One end is rounded, and the other end is planar (Shite et al. 2015). More than 17 Lyssaviruses have been known to cause rabies, but the rabies virus is the most important member of the genus (Leon et al. 2021). The rabies virus has a similar

H. M. Usman · A. Subhan
Department of Pathobiology, Section of Microbiology, University of Veterinary and Animal Sciences, Lahore, Jhang, Pakistan

M. M. Beig
Faculty of Veterianry Science, University of Veterinary and Animal Sciences, Lahore, Pakistan

M. Hassnain
University of Veterinary and Animal Sciences, Lahore, Narowal, Pakistan

W. Ahmad (✉)
Department of Clinical Sciences, University of Veterinary and Animal Sciences, Lahore, Narowal, Pakistan
e-mail: waqas.hussain@uvas.edu.pk

A. Arshad
Department of Community Medicine, Shalamar Medical and Dental College, Lahore, Pakistan

M. Younus
Department of Pathobiology, University of Veterinary and Animal Sciences, Lahore, Narowal, Pakistan

J. A. Shenge, A. L. K. Abia (eds.), *Viral Diseases and One Health in Africa*,
https://doi.org/10.1007/978-3-032-09613-5_5

morphology, cell biology, and life cycle to the vesicular stomatitis virus (VSV) in the genus *Vesiculovirus*. Both share the same family, and the vesicular stomatitis virus can infect mammalian hosts (humans and animals) and cause foetal encephalomyelitis (Murphy et al. 1995). Rabies is a disease that can affect multiple hosts, but dogs, cats, and wild animals like foxes, jackals, wolves, bats, raccoons, and skunks are the natural hosts of the rabies virus (Ruan 2017). In 1885, Pasteur, Roux, and their colleagues developed the human rabies vaccine and did the first anti-rabies treatment (Shite et al. 2015).

According to the WHO, every year, at least 59,000 people die due to rabies worldwide, with almost 98% being dog-mediated and mostly occurring in developing countries in Africa and Asia (Nadal and Radhakrishnan 2023). The case fatality rate of rabies is also higher than that of any infectious disease (Rupprecht et al. 2017). Almost 99% of deaths due to rabies occur from the bite of rabid dogs in developing countries (Caffrey et al. 2019; Hampson et al. 2015). The incubation period of rabies varies, but in domestic animals, it ranges from 3 to 12 weeks, but can be from several days to months and may exceed up to 6 months (Shite et al. 2015).

Despite the availability of effective vaccines for humans and animals, rabies results in annual economic losses of over $8.6 billion because of several factors. These include poor vaccination coverage in high-risk areas, a lack of knowledge and restricted availability of human and animal vaccinations. To effectively control rabies, these obstacles must be removed by utilising a "One Health" strategy that emphasises widespread dog vaccination and easily accessible post-exposure prophylaxis for people (Hampson et al. 2015; Adesina et al. 2020). Some countries have made substantial strides in establishing robust national rabies control programs characterised by systematic vaccination campaigns, surveillance mechanisms, and public awareness initiatives (Moore 2019; Hanlon et al. 1999; Haselbeck et al. 2021). Conversely, others face challenges in resource allocation and infrastructure development. However, integrating effective strategies leads to varied progress spectra (Haselbeck et al. 2021). For example, Nyasulu and colleagues (2021) evaluated 2775 records, comprising 43 investigations (Nyasulu et al. 2021). His computerised research included studies that censored 543,714 bite sufferers. Victims under the age of fifteen made up the majority of the casualties. Based on preventive and control strategies, the investigations revealed significant variations existed in rabies morbidity (21) and fatality (15) throughout Africa (16). The others were management and control (7), surveillance (09), surveillance and prevention (5), and surveillance, prevention, and control (6) (Nyasulu et al. 2021).

With the support of the World Health Organization (WHO), the World Organization for Animal Health (WOAH), the Food and Agriculture Organization of the United Nations (FAO), and GARC, many countries are working to eliminate rabies under "One Health" concept which is a very collaborative and broad approach with researchers in environmental, animal and human health (Lavan et al. 2017). However, developing countries do not successfully apply different approaches adopted by developed countries to eliminate rabies due to the high cost of vaccines, cultural and religious objections to various preventive measures, and insufficient facilities to manage canine rabies (Haupt 1999). For example, Ethiopia is one of the developing countries that has very prevalent canine rabies and faces different challenges each year; more than 2700 people die from rabies, resulting in significant financial losses caused by a lack of resources, a national rabies management strategy, and low canine vaccination rates. Research shows that almost 98% of human cases of rabies are caused by dogs, with prevalence rates as high as 78% in cities like Addis Ababa (Belete et al. 2021).

Although rabies is fatal, it can be controlled and prevented through different effective and scientific measures (Shwiff et al. 2013; Franka et al. 2013). To eliminate rabies, there must be a restriction on the transmission of the rabies virus among animals, mainly dogs. The incidence of dog-dog and dog-to-human rabies virus transmission can be effectively reduced by improving the immunity level of dogs, good management practices of dogs, and increasing awareness among humans (Lv et al. 2023). The WHO stated that the immunisation coverage of dogs must be above 70%, which can effectively inhibit rabies virus transmission (Coleman and Dye 1996). The incidence of human rabies can also be reduced by decreasing the number of stray dogs. Countries adopt different approaches to the awareness of rabies and their unique surveillance and prevention (Franka et al. 2013). Thirty-nine (39/54, 70.4%) African countries have officially started vaccination programs for animal vaccination against rabies. Fifteen (15) out of fifty-four (54) countries mainly focused on the vaccination of dogs, while 10 other countries vaccinated both dogs and cats (Scott et al. 2015).

However, to control rabies, there are preventive measures to be adopted and post-exposure prophylaxis in humans; still, the costliest measure of prevention is the continuous vaccination of dogs (Belotto et al. 2005; Schneider et al. 2007). The global quadripartite mission led by the WHO, the World Organization for Animal Health (OIE), the FAO, and the Global Alliance for Rabies Control (GARC) has the goal of eliminating the dog-mediated human rabies by 2030 (Khelef and Nel 2016). Many control measures successfully eliminate dog-mediated human rabies, such as vaccination programs for dogs, control of the dog population, access to human vaccines, and public awareness. Dog vaccination should be the priority because dogs are the main source of virus transmission (Wallace et al. 2020).

5.2 Challenges and Constraints

In 2010, Lembo et al. stated four common reasons for Africa's unsuccessful control of canine rabies. These include limited resources for monitoring and controlling rabies, epidemiological restrictions, such as uncertainties about the necessary immunisation coverage levels, easy access to the dogs for vaccination, and poor focus on disease control (Lembo et al. 2010). For control and elimination, collaboration and coordination are deficient throughout Africa, within and between nations (Haselbeck et al. 2021). There are many challenges to the stray dog population, including a lack of education and awareness among dog owners, high vaccine prices, insufficient veterinary services, easy access to vaccines, and limited resources. Yoak et al. also concluded that the main barrier to controlling rabies is the unawareness that dogs require rabies vaccines. They also reported that many owners are unwilling to travel more than 1 km to vaccinate their dogs (Yoak et al. 2021).

5.2.1 *Widespread Host Range*

The wide host range of rabies is one of the main challenges to its control in Africa (Shite et al. 2015). Several vulnerable species make control strategies more difficult, particularly in Africa, where wildlife is essential in rabies transmission(Shite et al. 2015). Several studies reported the involvement of wildlife in the rabies outbreak. It is more challenging to control rabies in wildlife populations due to habitat fragmentation and animal-human conflict. Habitat fragmentation due to human activity can increase the overlap between wildlife and domestic populations, promoting rabies transmission among many species (Schell et al. 2021; Long et al. 2020). Moreover, conflicts between humans and wildlife, including attacks on humans or livestock theft, may lead to the senseless killing of wild animals, worsening the rabies epidemic(Constable et al. 2016).

Recent studies also show that the rabies virus can be replicated in vitro in many cold-blooded animals, but no data have been reported yet showing its replication in vivo (Barecha et al. 2017). Generally, dogs and cats are the primary source of rabies, but wild animals also transmit the disease. This disease (Constable et al. 2016) also affects warm-blooded animals like cattle, sheep, pigs, and horses. The broad host range of rabies in Africa significantly impedes control efforts, making the application of comprehensive and multidisciplinary strategies necessary for effectively stopping the disease's spread (Constable et al. 2016).

5.2.2 *Socioeconomic Challenges and Poor Rabies Prophylaxis*

Rabies causes an estimated loss of $ 8.6 billion per year globally (Hampson et al. 2015). Livestock losses in Africa and Asia are estimated to be $12.3 million annually, with five deaths per 100,000 cattle (Lembo et al. 2010). The economic costs of rabies in a country can be determined by immunisation of pets, inspection of animal bites, quarantine facilities of the animals that bite or are suspected of being infected, vaccine costs, staff training, treatment plans, and diagnosis expenses (Habib et al. 2020).

Sub-Saharan Africa is a very diversified region made up of 13 small nations with a small population, little human capital, and a small land area, as well as low-, lower-middle-, upper-middle-, and a few high-income countries, 22 of which are fragile or afflicted by violence (Moore 2021). Three critical facets of health are directly impacted by the socioeconomic position of residents in a given setting: health care, exposure to the environment, and health behaviour. One aspect of socioeconomic status is poverty. Appropriate post-exposure prophylaxis can prevent rabies in humans, but it is not always accessible or economical in nations with limited resources (Hampson et al. 2019). Anti-rabies clinics (ARCs) that are easily accessible, reasonably priced, and equipped are crucial for successfully preventing rabies in victims of animal bites. However, maintaining a steady supply and storage of rabies vaccines and immunoglobulins poses enormous issues in a continent the size and geographic diversity of Africa (Rupprecht and Salahuddin 2019). Due to financial limitations, rabies prevention in low- and middle-income countries like Tanzania, Nigeria and Gabon is significantly hampered by variations in Post-Exposure Prophylaxis (PEP) availability outside of urban areas (Sreenivasan et al. 2019; Smith et al. 2019). Certain rabies-endemic nations have noted that their low financial resources prevent them from offering free PEP. One major issue impeding the efficient control of rabies in people is the non-availability of PEP at rural health centres, primarily due to a lack of government funding support for rabies prevention and control (Wentworth et al. 2019). Gabon's veterinary services lack the resources to conduct community-based surveillance or provide rabies diagnoses (Mbilo et al. 2021).

Post-Exposure Prophylaxis (PEP) helps prevent human rabies deaths; according to a recent Ethiopian study, the method is expensive and can only shield people who can get to medical facilities quickly and access PEP provisions (Ali 2022). Referencing financial constraints and a lack of knowledge regarding rabies, 25.3% (418/1655) of potentially exposed individuals in Tanzania's Serengeti and Ngorongoro districts did not seek treatment. 15.3% (189/1237) of those who sought care afterwards did not start PEP because of expense.

In Nigeria, dog vaccinations and PEP are not readily available in rural areas, mainly due to the government's lack of funding for rabies prevention and control (Abubakar et al. 2024). Without PEP, there is a higher risk of developing rabies following viral exposure, which might lead to higher medical costs and even death.

Strict estimates have the overall cost of care around $40 in Africa and $49 in Asia, which, respectively, equal 5.8% and 3.9% of the gross national product per capita annually (Hampson et al. 2008). Most of Africa suffers from PEP shortages, which further increase costs by forcing bite victims to travel to multiple places for treatment, causing unnecessary delays (Shim et al. 2009). In Northern Tanzania, where PEP patients pay for themselves, the median delay for those who commenced PEP was two days; in Southern Tanzania, where PEP was free of charge, the median delay for those who initiated PEP was zero days. This illustrates how cost affects rabies management (Changalucha et al. 2019).

5.2.3 *Diagnosis Challenges and Insufficient Diagnostic Surveillance*

Rapid and reliable diagnosis of rabies cases is hindered by the lack of diagnostic facilities, trained personnel, and other veterinary infrastructure in many African countries, i.e. East African countries like Ethiopia and Tanzania and West African countries like Nigeria and Ghana. Access to diagnostic techniques for rabies, including the polymerase chain reaction (PCR), rapid immunochromatographic testing (RICT), and direct fluorescent antibody test (DFA), is restricted in some regions of Africa. As a result, diagnosing and controlling might take more time. The other challenging factor in the diagnosis of rabies is the long incubation period of rabies, which varies in every case (on average 20–60 days, rarely 5–6 days, and can be up to 7 years), and the lack of clinical symptoms(Jackson et al. 2003). Ineffective surveillance systems can be caused by delays in data transmission, bureaucratic obstacles, and a lack of incentives for reporting (Asaaga et al. 2023). It is more challenging to perhaps increase rabies surveillance in Africa due to the absence of digital diagnostic tools (Coetzer et al. 2019).

Most African countries' national surveillance systems do not effectively detect rabies. An additional detrimental effect on rabies surveillance and attempts to assess the incidence of rabies is a general lack of competence for rabies diagnosis (Mbilo et al. 2021). The foundation of effective surveillance in cases of zoonotic rabies is confirmatory laboratory diagnosis (Franka and Wallace 2018). Comprehensive surveillance systems for rabies in humans and animals are lacking in Nigeria, Uganda, and Kenya. A recent worldwide study on surveillance systems in rabies-endemic nations, of which 49 of the 54 African nations are classified as having a moderate-to-high risk of human rabies, found that at least 16 of the 23 countries that participated in the study found their surveillance systems to be inefficient (Taylor and Knopf 2015). Even though most African countries now require reporting of animal-bite injuries and cases of both animal and human rabies. Inadequate or nonexistent surveillance makes national epidemiological data untrustworthy (Taylor et al. 2017).

Due to inadequate resources and expertise, restricted access to approved diagnostic tests, and challenges in collecting brain samples, laboratory analysis results in a low count of confirmatory human rabies cases (Banyard et al. 2013). Thus, since rabies can manifest in several ways, and incorrect diagnoses are frequent (Broban et al. 2018), there is a lack of reporting accuracy on rabies morbidity and fatality statistics among African nations. Accurate estimation of disease prevalence is hampered by small-scale research combined with data fluctuations throughout time and geographical areas (Nyasulu et al. 2021). Although the NTD Master Plan in Nigeria has more complex methods, the lack of prevalence and incidence data on rabies presents serious concerns in controlling and preventing DMR (Nigeria 2015).

In Gabon, a country in the Central African region, there is no specialised framework for rabies, and efforts to combat the disease are disorganised.

Additionally, the few epidemiological data that are currently accessible are only gathered in Libreville, the country's capital (Mbilo et al. 2021).

According to data on diagnostic activities, there is no established diagnostic capacity in Guinea-Bissau (Nyasulu et al. 2021).

Observed clinical symptoms were the only basis for rabies diagnosis in both animals and people in Benin until 2018. The Central Veterinary Laboratory (CVL) of Parakou possessed the necessary equipment (De Benedictis et al. 2011) to conduct two tests that were recommended; nevertheless, they were unable to establish a rabies diagnostic service due to a shortage of specialised reagents and personnel (Nel 2013). There was no internationally renowned laboratory involved in proficiency testing programs, no RABV variants were molecularly characterised in circulation in Benin, there was an inability to test suspected rabid samples in the lab (though that was supposed to change after the workshop), and no secondary diagnostic tests were available to confirm the diagnosis of suspected rabid samples (Djegui et al. 2022).

In sub-Saharan Africa, the frequency of dog bite injuries and rabies cases that go unreported is often significant. To reduce unreported dog bite injuries and rabies cases in Sub-Saharan Africa, increased public awareness, improved monitoring, greater access to healthcare, and community involvement (Savadogo et al. 2022; Smith et al. 2019).

5.2.4 *Constraints of Vaccine Accessibility and Immunisation Campaign Effectiveness*

In Nigeria and other African countries, the main restriction in the development of vaccines is the high prices of supplies, chemicals, biologicals, consumables, and additional materials (Oladipo et al. 2023). The concentrations of betapropiolactone and acytylethyleneimine used for inactivating the virus are usually high. Furthermore, an inconsistent power supply is a serious problem for producing, maintaining, and transporting vaccines on an industrial scale (Shittu et al. 2016). The cost associated with vaccine production is another issue, as developing new vaccines requires almost \$300 – \$800 million (Gouglas et al. 2018).

The primary obstacles to dog rabies vaccination campaigns are vaccine accessibility and dogs' high degree of mobility, which is mainly caused by human-mediated dog transport and virtually certainly results in the pathogen's reintroduction of rabies at the local and national levels (Freuling et al. 2013). An annual mass vaccination program against rabies must immunise at least 70% of dogs in an endemic area to eradicate the disease (Coleman and Dye 1996).

In Africa, the proportion of dogs immunised through free vaccination programs is significantly higher than that of owner-paid vaccination coverage (Wera et al. 2013). A high vaccination rate may not always ensure effective rabies control. According to studies, African dogs receiving a rabies vaccination have fewer zero-conversions. For example, the study found that only 71.9% of Nigerian dogs who received the rabies vaccination acquired neutralising antibodies against the virus. The duration since vaccination, the technical effectiveness of the administered vaccine, and the dogs' age, sex, and nutritional state all affect the antibody titer (Kennedy et al. 2007).

The immunisation effort in Africa encountered several difficulties, such as resource shortages or logistical issues with transportation, which resulted in some vaccine sites being missed or unreachable. Employee morale was badly impacted by poor compensation for newly hired immunisation workers, extra work, and late payment of daily allowances. Moreover, during the rollout phase, teams were occasionally unavailable to run awareness initiatives (Athingo et al. 2020). The following groups were indirect stakeholders: international institutions (FAO, WHO, OIE, World Animal Health Organization, Pan African Rabies Control Network, Rabies-free World Africa, and Regional Animal Health Centre (RAHC); media; education actors; local authorities; hygiene officers; human health workers; and NGOs (Savadogo et al. 2022). This demonstrates the complexity of dog vaccination by emphasising the variety of stakeholders engaged and the necessity of considering stakeholders from other relevant sectors, including politics, education, environment management and sanitation, security, and community. The interaction between various stakeholder levels, which makes it imperative to include all stakeholders in the board process, is one of the main causes of the inadequate coverage of vaccines in African states (Savadogo et al. 2020).

5.2.5 Increasing Population of Free-Roaming Dogs

Numerous studies indicate that most African dogs are owned yet wander freely (Lembo et al. 2010). Free-roaming dogs often travel freely in search of food and shelter, posing a higher risk of inflicting bite injuries to pedestrians and animals. Lack of preventive measures for rabies and non-vaccinated free-roaming dogs are the two main factors for higher mortality in Africa (Warembourg et al. 2021). Furthermore, in countries like Ethiopia, Nigeria, Tanzania, and Kenya, religious and cultural beliefs hamper efforts to regulate free-roaming dog populations. For example, religious beliefs may prevent dog culling or stringent management, whereas cultural traditions may promote unfettered dog ownership (Conan et al. 2015; Smith et al. 2019). This results in a high prevalence of rabies in those countries where the non-vaccinated dog population is uncontrolled (Morters et al. 2014). Reliably covering 70% of the dog population in such areas thus presents a significant challenge (Nyasulu et al. 2021; Hammami et al. 2018). When the vaccination rates for dogs were reviewed throughout African nations, the results showed that only six countries—South Africa, Tanzania, Algeria, Morocco, and Egypt—achieved vaccination rates of 63%, 37.24%, 23.7%, 25%, and 23.7%, respectively. The percentage of dogs vaccinated in all other African countries was less than 18%, and in many situations, it was less than 5% (Conan et al. 2017). The overall low coverage has been attributed to the cost of vaccination, which dog owners feel reluctant to cover, arguing that the government must cover this cost; owners often do not think they will directly benefit financially or health-wise from vaccinating their dogs against rabies (Cleaveland et al. 2003; Lapiz et al. 2012; Minhaj et al. 2023).

5.2.6 *Lack of Awareness in Community and Health Professionals*

Most African countries, particularly those in Western and Central Africa, do not enforce case reporting, so epidemiological statistics on rabies are inadequate (Dodet 2009). This is due to several factors, including a lack of understanding of rabies and the high cost of PEP therapy. Inadequate community-level educational outreach has left people unaware of how to protect themselves from animal attacks and how to manage bites and other potential rabies exposures (Nyasulu et al. 2021).

Market dynamics, involved stakeholders, public health awareness, and the basic disease trajectory are also the four major root causes of dog-mediated rabies (Rupprecht and Salahuddin 2019; Shite et al. 2015). There is still a misconception about the disease, particularly in rural communities and socioeconomically underprivileged areas. When asked why dogs bite people, 84% of the respondents in a recent study gave an answer related to Hadkai Mata (a local deity); the remaining respondents gave biological or ethological explanations (e.g. a feature of dog behaviour, pups' protection, reaction to danger, and aggression triggered by rabies)(Nadal et al. 2022). A study conducted in the Upper Eastern region of Ghana revealed that some communities may associate rabies with supernatural forces rather than viral infection (Awuni et al. 2019). In the Ethiopian Bale Mountains, the largely Muslim community's resistance to handling dogs contributed to the comparatively low coverage levels of parenteral dog vaccination. A similar phenomenon was recorded in Maasai villages in northwest Tanzania, where people are not accustomed to caring for and controlling dogs (Müller et al. 2023).

Significant knowledge gaps in nearly every facet of the disease, including prevention, transmission, and treatment, were found in medical and veterinary health experts in a study conducted in Chad (Mbaipago et al. 2020). Dog bite victims also exhibited low compliance due to the paramedical staff's improper communication of the significance of finishing the entire anti-rabies PEP regimen (Changalucha et al. 2019).

According to a study, the residence of dog owners influenced their understanding of rabies. For example, dog owners in Bolgatanga Municipality were 7.89 times more likely to understand the disease better than those in Bawku Municipality. Residents of Bawku Municipality were 29% less likely to vaccinate their pets against rabies (Awuni et al. 2019). According to a survey in the Tanzanian city of Dodoma, 75.5% of dog owners knew that canine rabies vaccinations were available, while 24.5% did not. According to the responses from dog owners in the area, only 44.7% of them tended to vaccinate their dogs against rabies. This suggests that most dog owners in the area were not vaccinating their pets against the rabies virus, despite the awareness of the disease (Mussa 2022).

A study conducted in KwaZulu-Natal, South Africa, showed that 86% of people had heard about the disease but were unaware of the aftermath of rabies. Few said that they did not know the source of the disease or what the preventive measures were. However, some people knew vaccination was essential for safety (Hergert and Nel 2013). One study in Addis Ababa, Ethiopia, showed that only a few people had the basics of rabies and knew it was a fatal disease. Thirty-four percent of people in the study knew the clinical signs of rabies in humans and animals (Abraham Ali et al. 2013). People mainly from rural areas only seek PEP once they are exhausted from traditional medical treatment, usually after the death of a family member (Asefa Deressa et al. 2010).

Tadele Kabeta conducted a study at The Jimma Town Anti-rabies Health Center (JTAHC) located in Jimma Town, the Jimma Zone seat in the Ethiopian Oromia National Region. The target sample for this cross-sectional survey was guardians or victims of animal bites who visited JTAHC for the first time between July 20, 2012, and March 12, 2013. The study evaluated participants' knowledge about rabies, attitudes toward the disease's risk to the public's health, and strategies for preventing and treating the sickness. Only 384 people were part of the study, and the results show that participants did not know the basics of the disease (Gelgie et al. 2022).

5.2.7 *Limited Finance, Skilled Personnel, and Material Resources*

One major flaw in disease monitoring systems is the occurrence of underreporting, especially in areas where rabies is widespread (Sofeu et al. 2018). Examining this phenomenon requires thoroughly investigating the causes of missing data (Research, 2019). The underrepresentation of cases in surveillance systems makes accurate epidemiological estimates difficult to achieve (Broban et al. 2018). This is partly due to gaps in reporting processes, low awareness of the reporting requirements for rabies, and inadequate reporting infrastructure (Okell et al. 2013). The assessment of current techniques for identifying rabies cases is critical to the efficacy of disease surveillance (Mbilo et al. 2021; Franka and Wallace 2018). A detailed examination of laboratory results, clinical diagnoses, and community reporting is all included in this. Evaluating these methods' sensitivity and specificity is crucial to guaranteeing accurate and dependable data collection and enabling prompt reactions to possible outbreaks (Léchenne et al. 2016; Rupprecht et al. 2018). Technological barriers, such as inadequate data storage, outdated software, and restricted connectivity in isolated regions, hinder the timely gathering and evaluation of rabies information (Mbilo 2021).

Rabies is considered a neglected disease since most governments do not think it is a serious health issue. People who are aware that widespread dog vaccinations can successfully eradicate human rabies frequently ask questions regarding the planning and execution of control programs because they are unsure of how to carry this out in Africa's complex social and political environments (Fahrion et al. 2017). Hardly 1.5% of funds allocated to rabies-related projects benefit veterinary field services, which are occasionally overloaded due to many other pressing concerns (Mbilo et al. 2021). Organisations do not know where to start or how to accomplish this, so they wait for foreign aid and facilitation.

Still, there are inspiring stories of Africans fighting rabies despite having few resources. For example, in Kenya, a district was motivated by the mother of a child who died from rabies, and 300,000 dogs were vaccinated because of her passionate campaigning (Le Roux et al. 2018). Africa, along with the rest of the world, must realise that all the resources required to eradicate the disease already exist and have been applied successfully across the continent, such as eliminating rinderpest and smallpox (Roeder et al. 2013).

5.2.8 Community Pressure/Social Non-governmental Organizations' Response

Rabies Free Burkina Faso, a non-profit organisation established on September 28, 2020, targets rabies elimination using a One Health approach. Rabies Free Burkina Faso's interventions include raising awareness, training and One Health capacity building, dog rabies vaccination, seeking vaccines and supporting communities, including financial resources to ensure bite victims receive PEP, research, community engagement, and joint outbreak investigation with competent authorities (Savadogo et al. 2023). Success stories highlight Rabies Free Burkina Faso's capacity to assist animal and human health authorities with rabies control and One Health development. Unfortunately, Rabies Free Burkina Faso and other rabies control organisations are chronically underfunded despite the illness becoming a national concern (Savadogo et al. 2023). This leads to insufficient dog vaccination coverage and post-exposure prophylaxis shortages. Therefore, the national integrated strategic plan must encourage collaboration and coordination among stakeholders, including civil society groups such as Rabies Free Burkina Faso.

5.2.9 Extending the One Health Project from Small Scale to Large Scale

Operationalising a "One Health" model requires more surveillance to improve early case finding and inform rabies control and prevention. Integrated Bite Case Management (IBCM) was tested in Tanzania to enhance intersectional interaction between veterinary and medical specialists. Government employees have been taught to use IBCM, including medical experts' bite victim risk assessments, livestock field officers' rabid animal investigations, and a mobile app for integration (Townsend et al. 2013). After a year, IBCM was implemented in 20 areas in four Tanzanian regions (Wallace et al. 2015). Bites patients who presented to medical institutions varied by location, but when IBCM was established, the number of people at high risk of developing rabies more than doubled nationwide. Based on clinical signs, animal fate, and fast diagnostic tests, 49% of over 800 high-risk studies were likely canine rabies cases. Rabies was possible, although 20% of biting animals were unknown. The data strengthen the case for using IBCM to monitor large canine vaccination campaigns and establish the absence of rabies in endemic countries(Sommerville 2011). The main impediments to implementation are the lack of resources for livestock field officers to investigate, the perceived difficulties of real-time recording, and the poor rabies training of health experts. IBCM greatly improved case identification and sector communication (Lushasi et al. 2020).

5.2.10 Navigating Administrative Hurdles

Initiatives to prevent rabies must successfully negotiate administrative roadblocks, which are frequently found at both the organisational and governmental levels (Haselbeck et al. 2021; Mbilo et al. 2021). For government organisations tasked with controlling rabies, a lack of funds is a major obstacle (Ogun et al. 2010). Comprehensive execution of rabies management techniques is hampered by the frequent underfunding of vaccination programs, public awareness campaigns, and surveillance initiatives (Lembo et al. 2010). Administrative bottlenecks that impede the timely execution of well-designed plans further worsen the problem by creating administrative bottlenecks in the enforcement and implementation of policies. Government departments and agencies must coordinate and collaborate to effectively control rabies. However, obstacles to successful interagency cooperation might obstruct the smooth implementation of integrated policies (Nel et al. 2012; Okello et al. 2015).

5.2.11 Enhancing Policy and One Health Approaches

A key component of changing policy is advocating for increased legislative support for One Health initiatives (Fasina et al. 2021). Given the interdependence of animal, human, and environmental health, One Health initiatives require governmental support to compel cooperation among many sectors (Alimi and Wabacha 2023). Clear legislative frameworks that require cross-sectoral collaboration, resource sharing, and information exchange should be emphasised in recommendations for policy changes (Acharya et al. 2020). Increasing governmental backing for the One Health strategy gives it legitimacy and lays the groundwork for ongoing, well-coordinated efforts to eradicate dog-mediated human rabies (Acharya et al. 2021). Achieving sustainable impact also requires resolving policy gaps and inconsistencies related to dog-mediated human rabies in Africa (Research, 2019). Policies should be carefully examined to find any discrepancies, coverage gaps, or implementation issues that might impede the effective control of rabies (Tiwari et al. 2021). Suggestions for modifications must include specific ways to address these problems, guaranteeing that policies are sound in theory, workable and efficient in practice (Scott et al. 2020). The framework for rabies control can be strengthened by adjusting policies in response to reality on the ground, which will help to produce long-lasting and significant results (Mbilo et al. 2021).

Organisational barriers complicate rabies control efforts (Van de Burgwal et al. 2017; Octaria et al. 2018). Health and veterinary organisations often face limitations in capacity and resources, impacting their ability to actively contribute to control initiatives (Mbilo et al. 2021). Challenges in inter-organisational communication and cooperation further impede collaborative efforts. However, innovative solutions and best practices offer avenues for overcoming these organisational barriers (Haselbeck et al. 2021; Léchenne et al. 2021).

5.3 Conclusions

Reaching regional, national, and international goals requires identifying the major obstacles to implementing the One Health approach for rabies prevention and control measures. Dog-mediated human rabies often requires serious commitment, legislative involvement, budgets, and cooperation of various stakeholders under the platform of One Health at the regional and national levels in endemic countries. Research has shown multiple levels where improvements and necessary efforts are needed to enhance and make this approach more effective. Similar problems and challenges arose in Asian countries due to cultural, economic, and technological connections between administrative and scientific institutions. Many Asian and African countries have also demonstrated their ability to overcome these challenges and streamline the pathway to eradicate dog-mediated human rabies by the end of 2030. The quadripartite vision, mission, and ongoing large-scale mass-dog vaccination initiatives are believed to provide day-to-day proof that this zoonotic disease can be decreased and eliminated by 2030, which is both feasible and optimistic.

References

Abubakar AT, Al-Mustapha AI, Oyewo M, Ibrahim A, Abdulrahim I, Yakub JM, Elelu N, Nguku P, Balogun MS, Awosanya EJ, Kia GSN (2024) Prospects for dog rabies elimination in Nigeria by 2030. Zoonoses Public Health 71:1–17

Acharya KP, Acharya N, Phuyal S, Upadhyaya M, Lasee SJ (2020) One-health approach: a best possible way to control rabies. One Health 10:100161
Acharya KP, Subedi D, Wilson RT (2021) Rabies control in South Asia requires a One Health approach. One Health 12:100215
Adesina M, Olufadewa I, Ogah Y, Nwachukwu N (2020) Incidence and mortality from a neglected tropical disease (rabies) in 28 African countries. Folia Vet 64:46–51
Ali JA (2022) Prevention and control of rabies in animals and humans in Ethiopia. Health Sci J 16: 1–10
Ali A, Ahmed EY, Sifer D (2013) A study on knowledge, attitude and practice of rabies among residents in Addis Ababa, Ethiopia. Ethiopian Vet J 17:19–35
Alimi Y, Wabacha J (2023) Strengthening coordination and collaboration of One Health approach for zoonotic diseases in Africa. J One Health Outlook 5:10
Asaaga FA, Sriram A, Chanda MM, Hoti SL, Young JC, Purse BV (2023) 'It doesn't happen how you think, it is very complex!' Reconciling stakeholder priorities, evidence, and processes for zoonoses prioritisation in India. Front Public Health 11:123456
Asefa Deressa AD, Abraham Ali AA, Mekoro Beyene MB, Selassie B, Yimer E, Kedir Hussen KH (2010) The status of rabies in Ethiopia: a retrospective record review. Ethiop J Health Dev 24: 143–150
Athingo R, Tenzin T, Shilongo A, Hikufe E, Shoombe KK, Khaiseb S, van der Westhuizen J, Letshwenyo M, Torres G, Mettenleiter TC (2020) Fighting dog-mediated rabies in Namibia—implementation of a rabies elimination program in the northern communal areas. Trop Med Infect Dis 5:12
Awuni B, Tarkang E, Manu E, Amu H, Ayanore MA, Aku FY, Ziema SA, Bosoka SA, Adjuik M, Kweku M (2019) Dog owners' knowledge about rabies and other factors that influence canine anti-rabies vaccination in the Upper East Region of Ghana. Trop Med Infect Dis 4:115
Banyard AC, Hayman DT, Freuling CM, Müller T, Fooks AR, Johnson N (2013) Bat rabies. Rabies:215–267
Barecha CB, Girzaw F, Kandi RV, Pal M (2017) Epidemiology and public health significance of rabies. Public Health Rev 5:55–67
Belete S, Meseret M, Dejene H, Assefa A (2021) Prevalence of dog-mediated rabies in Ethiopia: a systematic review and meta-analysis from 2010 to 2020. One Health Outlook 3:1–8
Belotto A, Leanes L, Schneider M, Tamayo H, Correa E (2005) Overview of rabies in the Americas. Vaccine Res 111:5–12
Broban A, Tejiokem MC, Tiembre I, Druelles S, L'Azou M (2018) Bolstering human rabies surveillance in Africa is crucial to eliminating canine-mediated rabies. PLoS Negl Trop Dis 12:e0006367
Caffrey N, Rock M, Schmidtz O, Anderson D, Parkinson M, Checkley SL (2019) Insights about the epidemiology of dog bites in a Canadian city using a dog aggression scale and administrative data. Animals 9:324
Changalucha J, Steenson R, Grieve E, Cleaveland S, Lembo T, Lushasi K, Mchau G, Mtema Z, Sambo M, Nanai A, Govella NJ, Dilip A, Sikana L, Ventura F, Hampson K (2019) The need to improve access to rabies post-exposure vaccines: lessons from Tanzania. Vaccine 37:A45–A53
Cleaveland S, Kaare M, Tiringa P, Mlengeya T, Barrat J (2003) A dog rabies vaccination campaign in rural Africa: impact on the incidence of dog rabies and human dog-bite injuries. Vaccine 21: 1965–1973
Coetzer A, Scott TP, Noor K, Gwenhure LF, Nel LH (2019) A novel integrated and labile eHealth system for monitoring dog rabies vaccination campaigns. Vaccine 7:108
Coleman PG, Dye C (1996) Immunisation coverage required to prevent outbreaks of dog rabies. Vaccine 14:185–186
Conan A, Akerele O, Simpson G, Reininghaus B, van Rooyen J, Knobel D (2015) Population dynamics of owned, free-roaming dogs: implications for rabies control. PLoS Negl Trop Dis 9: e0004177

Conan A, Geerdes JA, Akerele OA, Reininghaus B, Simpson GJ, Knobel D (2017) Census and vaccination coverage of owned dog populations in four resource-limited rural communities, Mpumalanga province, South Africa. J S Afr Vet Assoc 88:1–7

Constable PD, Hinchcliff KW, Done SH, Grünberg W (2016) Veterinary medicine: a textbook of the diseases of cattle, horses, sheep, pigs and goats. Elsevier Health Sciences, Amsterdam

De Benedictis P, De Battisti C, Dacheux L, Marciano S, Ormelli S, Salomoni A, Caenazzo ST, Lepelletier A, Bourhy H, Capua I, Cattoli G (2011) Lyssavirus detection and typing using pyrosequencing. J Clin Microbiol 49:1932–1938

Djegui F, Gourlaouen M, Coetzer A, Adjin R, Tohozin R, Leopardi S, Mauti S, Akpo Y, Gnanvi C, Nel LH, De Benedictis P (2022) Capacity building efforts for rabies diagnosis in resource-limited countries in sub-Saharan Africa: a case report of the Central Veterinary Laboratory in Benin (Parakou). Front Vet Sci 8:987654

Dodet B (2009) The fight against rabies in Africa: from recognition to action. Vaccine 27:5027–5032

Fahrion AS, Taylor LH, Torres G, Müller T, Dürr S, Knopf L, De Balogh K, Nel LH, Gordon-Cillo MJ, Abela-Ridder B (2017) The road to dog rabies control and elimination—what keeps us from moving faster? Front Public Health 5:103

Fasina FO, Fasanmi OG, Makonnen YJ, Bebay C, Bett B, Roesel K (2021) The One Health landscape in sub-Saharan African countries. One Health 13:100325

Federal Ministry of Health Nigeria (2015) Neglected tropical diseases Nigeria multi-year master plan 2015–2020. Federal Ministry of Health, Abuja

Franka R, Wallace R (2018) Rabies diagnosis and surveillance in animals in the era of rabies elimination. Rev Sci Tech 37:359–370

Franka R, Smith TG, Dyer JL, Wu X, Niezgoda M, Rupprecht CE (2013) Current and future tools for global canine rabies elimination. Antivir Res 100:220–225

Freuling CM, Hampson K, Selhorst T, Schröder R, Meslin FX, Mettenleiter TC, Müller T (2013) The elimination of fox rabies from Europe: determinants of success and lessons for the future. Philos Trans R Soc B 368:20120142

Gelgie AE, Cavalerie L, Kaba M, Asrat D, Mor SM (2022) Rabies research in Ethiopia: a systematic review. One Health 15:100450

Gouglas D, Le TT, Henderson K, Kaloudis A, Danielsen T, Hammersland NC, Robinson JM, Heaton PM, Røttingen J-A (2018) Estimating the cost of vaccine development against epidemic infectious diseases: a cost minimisation study. Lancet Glob Health 6:e1386–e1396

Habib A, Principe U, Ashraf Z, Imran M (2020) Epidemiology of rabies and the control challenges. Biomed Res Ther 2:1201–1204

Hammami P, Lancelot R, Domenech J, Lesnoff M (2018) Ex-ante assessment of different vaccination-based control schedules against the peste des petits ruminants virus in sub-Saharan Africa. PLoS One 13:e0190296

Hampson K, Dobson A, Kaare M, Dushoff J, Magoto M, Sindoya E, Cleaveland S (2008) Rabies exposures, post-exposure prophylaxis and deaths in a region of endemic canine rabies. PLoS Negl Trop Dis 2:e339

Hampson K, Coudeville L, Lembo T, Sambo M, Kieffer A, Attlan M, Barrat J, Blanton JD, Briggs DJ, Cleaveland S (2015) Estimating the global burden of endemic canine rabies. PLoS Negl Trop Dis 9:e0003709

Hampson K, Ventura F, Steenson R, Mancy R, Trotter C, Cooper L, Abela-Ridder B, Knopf L, Ringenier M, Tenzin T (2019) The potential effect of improved provision of rabies post-exposure prophylaxis in Gavi-eligible countries: a modelling study. Lancet Infect Dis 19:102–111

Hanlon CA, Olson JG, Clark CJ (1999) Prevention and education regarding rabies in human beings. J Am Vet Med Assoc 215:1276–1280

Haselbeck AH, Rietmann S, Tadesse BT, Kling K, Kaschubat-Dieudonné ME, Marks F, Wetzker W, Thöne-Reineke C (2021) Challenges to the fight against rabies—the landscape of policy and prevention strategies in Africa. Int J Environ Res Public Health 18:1736

Haupt W (1999) Rabies–risk of exposure and current trends in prevention of human cases. Vaccine 17:1742–1749

Hergert M, Nel LH (2013) Dog bite histories and response to incidents in canine rabies-enzootic KwaZulu-Natal, South Africa. PLoS Negl Trop Dis 7:e2059

Jackson AC, Warrell MJ, Rupprecht CE, Ertl HC, Dietzschold B, O'Reilly M, Leach RP, Fu ZF, Wunner WH, Bleck TP (2003) Management of rabies in humans. Clin Infect Dis 36:60–63

Kennedy LJ, Lunt M, Barnes A, McElhinney L, Fooks AR, Baxter DN, Ollier WE (2007) Factors influencing the antibody response of dogs vaccinated against rabies. Vaccine 25:8500–8507

Khelef N, Nel L (2016) Aiming for elimination of dog-mediated human rabies cases by 2030. Vet Rec

Lapiz SMD, Miranda MEG, Garcia RG, Daguro LI, Paman MD, Madrinan FP, Rances PA, Briggs DJ (2012) Implementation of an intersectoral program to eliminate human and canine rabies: the Bohol Rabies Prevention and Elimination Project. PLoS Negl Trop Dis 6:e1891

Lavan RP, King AIM, Sutton DJ, Tunceli K (2017) Rationale and support for a one health program for canine vaccination as the most cost-effective means of controlling zoonotic rabies in endemic settings. Vaccine 35:1668–1674

Le Roux K, Kotze J, Perrett K (2018) Elimination of dog-mediated human rabies: the burden of human rabies in Africa. Revue Scientifique et Technique (International Office of Epizootics) 37: 607–615

Léchenne M, Naïssengar K, Lepelletier A, Alfaroukh IO, Bourhy H, Zinsstag J, Dacheux L (2016) Validation of a rapid rabies diagnostic tool for field surveillance in developing countries. PLoS Negl Trop Dis 10:e0005010

Léchenne M, Traore A, Hattendorf J, Kallo V, Oussiguere A, Tetchi M, Moyengar R, Traore AK, Moto DD, Ngandolo R (2021) Increasing rabies data availability: the example of a One Health research project in Chad, Côte d'Ivoire and Mali. *Acta Trop* 215:105808

Lembo T, Hampson K, Kaare MT, Ernest E, Knobel D, Kazwala RR, Haydon DT, Cleaveland S (2010) The feasibility of canine rabies elimination in Africa: dispelling doubts with data. PLoS Negl Trop Dis 4:e626

Leon B, González SF, Solís LM, Ramirez-Cardoce M, Moreira-Soto A, Cordero-Solorzano JM, Hutter SE, Gonzalez-Barrientos R, Rupprecht CE (2021) Rabies in Costa Rica: next steps towards controlling bat-borne rabies after its elimination in dogs. Yale J Biol Med 94:311

Long RB, Krumlauf K, Young AM (2020) Characterising trends in human–wildlife conflicts in the American Midwest using wildlife rehabilitation records. PLoS One 15:e0238805

Lushasi K, Steenson R, Bernard J, Changalucha JJ, Govella NJ, Haydon DT, Hoffu H, Lankester F, Magoti F, Mpolya EA, Mtema Z, Nonga H, Hampson K (2020) One Health in practice: using integrated bite case management to increase detection of rabid animals in Tanzania. Front Public Health 8:13

Lv M-M, Sun X-D, Jin Z, Wu H-R, Li M-T, Sun G-Q, Pei X, Wu Y-T, Liu P, Li L (2023) Dynamic analysis of rabies transmission and elimination in mainland China. One Health 17:100615

Mbaipago N, Mindekem R, Oussiguere A, Moyengar R, Naïssengar K, Madjadinan A, Zinsstag J, Léchenne M (2020) Rabies knowledge and practices among human and veterinary health workers in Chad. Acta Trop 202:105180

Mbilo C (2021) Rabies in sub-Saharan Africa: one health-based surveillance strategy in the Kongo central province (Democratic Republic of the Congo) and disease transmission in N'Djamena (Chad). University of Basel, PhD Thesis

Mbilo C, Coetzer A, Bonfoh B, Angot A, Bebay C, Cassamá B, De Benedictis P, Ebou MH, Gnanvi C, Kallo V, Lokossou RH, Manjuba C, Mokondjimobe E, Mouillé B, Mounkaila M, Ndour APN, Nel L, Olugasa BO, Pato P, Pyana PP, Rerambyath GA, Roamba RC, Sadeuh-Mba SA, Suluku R, Suu-Ire RD, Tejiokem MC, Tetchi M, Tiembre I, Traoré A, Voupawoe G, Zinsstag J (2021) Dog rabies control in West and Central Africa: a review. Acta Trop 224: 105459

Minhaj FS, Bonaparte SC, Boutelle C, Wallace RM (2023) Analysis of available animal testing data to propose peer-derived quantitative thresholds for determining adequate surveillance capacity for rabies. Sci Rep 13:3986

Moore SM (2019) Rabies: current preventive strategies. Vet Clin N Am Small Anim Pract 49:629–641

Moore M (2021) Glimpses of fiscal states in sub-Saharan Africa. WIDER Working Paper

Morters MK, McKinley TJ, Restif O, Conlan AJ, Cleaveland S, Hampson K, Whay HR, Damriyasa IM, Wood JLN (2014) The demography of free-roaming dog populations and applications to disease and population control. J Appl Ecol 51:1096–1106

Müller T, Freuling CM (2020) Rabies in terrestrial animals. In: Sing A (ed) Rabies. Elsevier, pp 67–98

Müller T, Rupprecht CC, Fooks AR, Both L, Smith SP, Gibson AP, Lohr F, Fahrion A, Freuling CM (2023) Elimination of rabies: a missed opportunity. In: Sing A (ed) Zoonoses: infections affecting humans and animals. Springer International Publishing, Cham, pp 123–140

Murphy F, Fauquet C, Bishop D, Ghabrial S, Jarvis A, Martelli G, Mayo M, Summers M (1995) Virus taxonomy: Sixth report of the International Committee on Taxonomy of Viruses. Arch Virol 10:350–354

Mussa ML (2022) Determinants on preventing transmission of canine rabies disease for local dogs in Tanzania: a case study of Dodoma City. The Open University of Tanzania

Nadal D, Radhakrishnan S (2023) Global dog and human rabies control efforts from ancient times to 2030 and beyond. In: One health for dog-mediated rabies elimination in Asia: a collection of local experiences. CABI, Wallingford

Nadal D, Hampson K, Lembo T, Rodrigues R, Vanak AT, Cleaveland S (2022) Where rabies is not a disease: bridging healthworlds to improve mutual understanding and prevention of rabies. Front Vet Sci 9:867266

Nel LH (2013) Discrepancies in data reporting for rabies, Africa. Emerg Infect Dis 19:529–533

Nel L, Scott T, Wright N, Mollentze N, Markotter W, Sabeta C, Le Roux K (2012) Rabies and rabies control in African regions. In: Compendium of the OIE Global Conference on Rabies Control, 7–9 September 2011, Incheon-Seoul (Republic of Korea). World Organisation for Animal Health, Paris, p 51

Nyasulu PS, Weyer J, Tschopp R, Mihret A, Aseffa A, Nuvor SV, Tamuzi JL, Nyakarahuka L, Helegbe GK, Ntinginya NE (2021) Rabies mortality and morbidity associated with animal bites in Africa: a case for integrated rabies disease surveillance, prevention and control—a scoping review. BMJ Open 11:e048551

Octaria R, Salyer SJ, Blanton J, Pieracci EG, Munyua P, Millien M, Nel L, Wallace RM (2018) From recognition to action: a strategic approach to foster sustainable collaborations for rabies elimination. PLoS Negl Trop Dis 12:e0006756

Ogun A, Okonko I, Udeze A, Shittu I, Garba K, Fowotade A, Adewale O, Fajobi E, Onoja B, Babalola E (2010) Feasibility and factors affecting global elimination and possible eradication of rabies in the world. J Gen Mol Virol 2:1–27

Okell C, Pinchbeck G, Stringer A, Tefera G, Christley R (2013) A community-based participatory study investigating the epidemiology and effects of rabies to livestock owners in rural Ethiopia. Prev Vet Med 108:1–9

Okello A, Welburn S, Smith J (2015) Crossing institutional boundaries: mapping the policy process for improved control of endemic and neglected zoonoses in sub-Saharan Africa. Health Policy Plan 30:804–812

Oladipo EK, Olufemi SE, Ojo TO, Adediran DA, Idowu AF, Idowu UA, Onyeaka H (2023) Africa (COVID-19) vaccine technology transfer: where are we? Life 13:1886

Roeder P, Mariner J, Kock R (2013) Rinderpest: the veterinary perspective on eradication. Philos Trans R Soc B 368:20120139

Ruan S (2017) Spatiotemporal epidemic models for rabies among animals. Infect Dis Model 2:277–287

Rupprecht CE, Salahuddin N (2019) Current status of human rabies prevention: remaining barriers to global biologics accessibility and disease elimination. Expert Rev Vaccines 18:629–640
Rupprecht C, Kuzmin I, Meslin F (2017) Lyssaviruses and rabies: current conundrums, concerns, contradictions and controversies. F1000Res 6:184
Rupprecht CE, Fooks AR, Abela-Ridder B, World Health Organization (2018) Laboratory techniques in rabies, vol 1. WHO, Geneva
Savadogo M., Koné P, Dahourou LD, Manishimwe R, Sow A, Nébié L, Antoine-Moussiaux N, Doulkom B, Bada-Alambedji R (2020) Rabies epidemiology and community knowledge, attitudes and practices in Burkina Faso. (Manuscript/Report — source details incomplete; please verify publisher or journal)
Savadogo M, Renmans D, Alambedji RB, Tarnagda Z, Antoine-Moussiaux N (2022) Using causal loop analysis to explore pathways for zoonosis control in low-income setting: the case of dog rabies vaccination in Burkina Faso. Prev Vet Med 203:105623
Savadogo M, Dahourou LD, Ilboudo AK, Ilboudo SG, Zangré H, Tarnagda G, Souli Z, Combari AHB, Diarra R, Bidima M, Traoré MGB, Mandé CD, Sondo KA, de Balogh K (2023) The Rabies Free Burkina Faso initiative: an example of how one health-oriented civil society organisations can contribute towards the achievement of the rabies zero by 30 goal. One Health Outlook 5:9
Schell CJ, Stanton LA, Young JK, Angeloni LM, Lambert JE, Breck SW, Murray MH (2021) The evolutionary consequences of human–wildlife conflict in cities. Evol Appl 14:178–197
Schneider MC, Belotto A, Adé MP, Hendrickx S, Leanes LF, Rodrigues MJF, Medina G, Correa EJ (2007) Current status of human rabies transmitted by dogs in Latin America. Cad Saude Publica 23:2049–2063
Scott TP, Coetzer A, de Balogh K, Wright N, Nel LH (2015) The Pan-African Rabies Control Network (PARACON): a unified approach to eliminating canine rabies in Africa. Antivir Res 124:93–100
Scott TP, Coetzer A, Nel LH (2020) Strategies for the elimination of dog-mediated human rabies by 2030. In: Rabies. Elsevier, Amsterdam
Shim E, Hampson K, Cleaveland S, Galvani AP (2009) Evaluating the cost-effectiveness of rabies post-exposure prophylaxis: a case study in Tanzania. Vaccine 27:7167–7172
Shite A, Guadu T, Admassu B (2015) Challenges of rabies. Int J Basic Appl Virol 4:41–52
Shittu E, Harnly M, Whitaker S, Miller R (2016) Reorganising Nigeria's vaccine supply chain reduces need for additional storage facilities, but more storage is required. Health Aff 35:293–300
Shwiff S, Hampson K, Anderson A (2013) Potential economic benefits of eliminating canine rabies. Antivir Res 98:352–356
Smith LM, Hartmann S, Munteanu AM, Dalla Villa P, Quinnell RJ, Collins LM (2019) The effectiveness of dog population management: a systematic review. Animals 9:1020
Sofeu CL, Broban A, Njifou Njimah A, Blaise Momo J, Sadeuh-Mba SA, Druelles S, L'Azou M, Tejiokem MC (2018) Improving systematic rabies surveillance in Cameroon: a pilot initiative and results for 2014–2016. PLoS Negl Trop Dis 12:e0006597
Sommerville I (2011) Software engineering, 9th edn. Pearson Education India, New Delhi
Sreenivasan N, Li A, Shiferaw M, Tran C, Wallace R, Blanton J, Knopf L, Abela-Ridder B, Hyde T, Siddiqi U (2019) Overview of rabies post-exposure prophylaxis access, procurement and distribution in selected countries in Asia and Africa, 2017–2018. Vaccine 37:A6–A13
Taylor L, Knopf L (2015) Surveillance of human rabies by national authorities—a global survey. Zoonoses Public Health 62:543–552
Taylor LH, Hampson K, Fahrion A, Abela-Ridder B, Nel LH (2017) Difficulties in estimating the human burden of canine rabies. Acta Trop 165:133–140
Tiwari HK, Gogoi-Tiwari J, Robertson ID (2021) Eliminating dog-mediated rabies: challenges and strategies. Anim Dis 1:1–13

Townsend SE, Lembo T, Cleaveland S, Meslin FX, Miranda ME, Putra AAG, Haydon DT, Hampson K (2013) Surveillance guidelines for disease elimination: a case study of canine rabies. Comp Immunol Microbiol Infect Dis 36:249–261

Van de Burgwal L, Neevel A, Pittens C, Osterhaus A, Rupprecht C, Claassen E (2017) Barriers to innovation in human rabies prophylaxis and treatment: a causal analysis of insights from key opinion leaders and literature. Zoonoses Public Health 64:599–611

Wallace RM, Reses H, Franka R, Dilius P, Fenelon N, Orciari L, Etheart M, Destine A, Crowdis K, Blanton JD (2015) Establishment of a canine rabies burden in Haiti through the implementation of a novel surveillance program. PLoS Negl Trop Dis 9:e0004245

Wallace RM, Cliquet F, Fehlner-Gardiner C, Fooks AR, Sabeta CT, Setién AA, Tu C, Vuta V, Yakobson B, Yang D-K (2020) Role of oral rabies vaccines in the elimination of dog-mediated human rabies deaths. Emerg Infect Dis 26:1

Warembourg C, Fournié G, Abakar MF, Alvarez D, Berger-González M, Odoch T, Wera E, Alobo G, Carvallo ETL, Bal VD (2021) Predictors of free-roaming domestic dogs' contact network centrality and their relevance for rabies control. Sci Rep 11:12898

Wentworth D, Hampson K, Thumbi SM, Mwatondo A, Wambura G, Chng NR (2019) A social justice perspective on access to human rabies vaccines. Vaccine 37:A3–A5

Wera E, Velthuis AG, Geong M, Hogeveen H (2013) Costs of rabies control: an economic calculation method applied to Flores Island. PLoS One 8:e83654

Yoak AJ, Haile A, O'Quin J, Belu M, Birhane M, Bekele M, Murphy S, Medley A, Vincent E, Stewart D (2021) Barriers and opportunities for canine rabies vaccination campaigns in Addis Ababa, Ethiopia. Prev Vet Med 187:105256

Chapter 6
Vaccine Utilisation in the Prevention of Viral Diseases in Africa

Muhammad Hassnain, Abdul Subhan, Muhammad Mubashar Beig, Waleed Akram, Faseeh Ahmad, Sana Mushtaq, and Waqas Ahmad

6.1 Introduction

Vaccine-preventable diseases (VPDs) continue to pose a serious threat to public health, especially in sub-Saharan Africa. The VPDs are caused by infectious bacteria and viruses that cause mild to severe pathological diseases, which vaccinations can prevent (Sibanda et al. 2023). VPDs affect more than 30 million children in Africa under the age of five, demonstrating the significant impact these diseases have on the continent. Over 500,000 people lost their lives as a result of restricted access to

M. Hassnain
University of Veterinary and Animal Sciences, Lahore, Narowal Campus, Pakistan

A. Subhan
Faculty of Veterinary Science, University of Veterinary and Animal Sciences, Lahore, Lahore, Pakistan

M. M. Beig
Institute of Microbiology, University of Veterinary and Animal Sciences, Lahore, Pakistan

W. Akram
Department of Pathobiology, Section of Parasitology, University of Veterinary and Animal Sciences, Lahore, Jhang, Pakistan

F. Ahmad
Genome Breeding Technologies Private Limited, Genome Breeding Technologies Pvt Ltd, Okara, Okara, Pakistan

S. Mushtaq
Department of Pharmacology, Institute of Pharmacy, Faculty of Pharmaceutical and Allied Health Sciences, Lahore College for Women University, Lahore, Pakistan

W. Ahmad (✉)
Department of Clinical Sciences, University of Veterinary and Animal Sciences, Lahore, Narowal Campus, Narowal, Pakistan
e-mail: waqas.hussain@uvas.edu.pk

J. A. Shenge, A. L. K. Abia (eds.), *Viral Diseases and One Health in Africa*,
https://doi.org/10.1007/978-3-032-09613-5_6

vaccination services, accounting for 58% of all VPD-related deaths worldwide (Butera et al. 2018). One in five African children still does not have access to all of the life-saving recommended vaccines that the World Health Organization (WHO) globally advocates, endangering not just the health of families but also the stability of African economies and social justice (Bon et al. 2023). There are still frequent outbreaks of VPDs in many African nations. Epidemics linked to VPDs typically occur in regions with low vaccination rates (Niyongabo et al. 2024). Principal VPDs impacting the African region include the following but are not limited to cholera, yellow fever, influenza, Malaria, polio, rotavirus, typhoid fever, rabies, and COVID-19 (Wariri et al. 2021).

Reduced vaccination coverage has been associated with increased VPD outbreaks in Africa (Shapira et al. 2021). Africa saw a 400% increase in measles infections between January and March 2022 compared to the same timeline in 2021, indicating a surge in vaccine-preventable disease outbreaks. In addition, there has been a rise in the number of impacted countries in recent years, contributing to the frequency of polio and yellow fever epidemics (Africa 2022). The new coronavirus SARS-CoV-2—a zoonotic virus—is the cause of COVID-19, which primarily affects the respiratory system and causes symptoms that range from minor respiratory problems to acute respiratory distress syndrome and severe pneumonia (ARDS) (Cascella et al. 2023). Increased human-animal contact brought on by rapid urbanisation, the degradation of natural habitats, wildlife hunting, livestock husbandry, climate change, and shifting ecosystems are some of the factors that speed up the introduction of these disorders (Ahmad et al. 2024).

The frequency of VPDs is higher in African nations for several reasons, such as poor sanitation, restricted access to healthcare, low vaccination coverage, and climate change (Le Polain de Waroux et al. 2013; Wiysonge et al. 2012). Research has revealed obstacles to reaching high immunisation rates, which are worsened by unstable political environments and logistical limitations (Oyo-Ita et al. 2023). Through contaminated food and water sources, diseases like hepatitis A and E can spread more easily when there is poor sanitation (Jacobsen and Wiersma 2010). Dengue and yellow fever are mosquito-borne illnesses that benefit from urbanisation and climate change (Anoopkumar and Aneesh 2022). To combat VPDs in Africa, comprehensive public health policies are needed due to the additional facilitation of disease spread provided by population movement and environmental changes (Rocklöv et al. 2020). Understanding the impact of VPDs on public health is vital to addressing the many challenges these diseases pose to healthcare systems and communities throughout Africa. This is evident as we delve into the detailed discussion of VPDs, which includes COVID-19, Japanese encephalitis virus, polio, hepatitis A and E, rabies, yellow fever, and dengue in African countries.

6.1.1 COVID-19

The new coronavirus SARS-CoV-2, the cause of COVID-19, has affected African nations to differing degrees. Despite an initial variation in the distribution of cases, a tendency of increasing incidence and intermittent peaks has been noted throughout the continent. On February 14, 2020, Egypt announced the first COVID-19 case in Africa (Medhat and El Kassas 2020). The virus spread throughout the continent in three months, and by May 2020, it had reached most African countries (Lone and Ahmad 2020). The 55 Member States of the African Union (AU) have reported 12,860,292 COVID-19 cases and 258,884 deaths (CFR: 2.01%), as per the current available data. This represents nearly 2% of all cases and 4% of all fatalities recorded worldwide (Mckay et al. 2024).

Significant COVID-19 variations have been identified during the history of the virus in African nations. The Beta variant was first found in South Africa in February 2020. The Beta variant presents difficulties for containment efforts and vaccination efficacy due to alterations linked to enhanced transmissibility and possible immune response evasion (Rotondo et al. 2021). The *Eta variant* (Pango lineage B.1.525) of SARS-CoV-2 was first identified in Nigeria in December 2020 (Ozer et al. 2022). The Delta form, which was discovered in India in December 2020 and later extended to several nations, including those in Africa, is another noteworthy variation (Dhawan et al. 2022). Finally, the Omicron form was discovered for the first time in South Africa in November 2021. Concerns have been raised due to Omicron's numerous mutations, particularly those in the spike protein, which could affect immunological evasion, transmissibility, and vaccination efficacy (Dhama et al. 2023). Due to inadequate genetic surveillance capacity, unequal resource availability, and logistical problems, African countries have encountered difficulties throughout the epidemic in identifying, monitoring, and responding to volatile organic compounds (VOCs) (Tegally et al. 2022).

The COVID-19 pandemic has therefore affected the socioeconomic aspects of countries, particularly in Africa. To fight the COVID-19 pandemic worldwide, several potent COVID-19 vaccines are given. The majority of African nations have relatively few immunisation programmes in place. In 2022, 448,942,809 COVID-19 vaccine doses were delivered in Africa, marking a 39.9% increase from the previous year. Cumulatively, as of December 31, 2022, 769,784,340 doses were delivered, with 66.5% from COVAX, 20.7% from bilateral donations, and 9.4% from AVAT, highlighting the diverse sources of vaccine procurement and distribution in Africa (Mboussou et al. 2023). To further evaluate the combined effect of immunisation and the decrease in SARS-CoV-2 transmission brought about by control measures, a numerical sensitivity analysis was conducted on the control reproduction number (Rn). The findings show that to contain the pandemic, each African country needed to vaccinate at least 60% of its population (Montcho et al. 2023b).

Furthermore, immunisation, in addition to preventive measures, has been highlighted as a critical tactic to battle COVID-19 successfully (Oghenebrume et al. 2023). Numerous COVID-19 vaccines, including AstraZeneca, Pfizer-BioNTech, and Johnson & Johnson, were rolled out across Africa, as planned by the WHO through COVAX (Md Khairi et al. 2022). Vaccination then advanced in late 2022, with Mauritius and Seychelles achieving more than 70% coverage of people vaccinated, underlining the significance of these immunisations in shielding public health from the virus (Vilches et al. 2021). Moreover, public health education programs improved community knowledge, encouraged preventive actions, and helped to contain the pandemic overall, highlighting the significance of coordinated strategies in the fight against COVID-19 (Tambo et al. 2021).

6.1.2 Poliomyelitis

The polio virus is a member of the *Enterovirus* family that causes poliomyelitis. It affects primarily children under five years of age and causes acute flaccid paralysis in affected persons. Vaccination is the only effective method to prevent this disease, as there is currently no known medical cure (Uwishema et al. 2022; Hull et al. 1994). It is recognised that the poliovirus primarily affects humans and does not have a substantial zoonotic component (Nichol and Magnus 2018). Following a 20-year years of vaccination, surveillance, and other preventive measures, public health experts gained valuable experience in 1980 when smallpox was officially eradicated. This experience helped in understanding how to interrupt the natural transmission of a viral pathogen and eventually eradicate it (WHO 2010). Over 220 million children have been successfully vaccinated against the poliovirus since its discovery, which is hugely commendable.

Up until 2012, the majority of cases of polio worldwide occurred in Africa (Patterson 2018). One of the three wild poliovirus (WPV) serotypes—types 1 (WPV1), type 2 (WPV2), or type 3 (WPV3)—causes paralytic polio. Each serotype has a different epidemiology, case-to-infection ratio, immune response, and vaccination features (Patel and Cochi 2017). Significant immunity to one serotype does not result in immunity to the other serotypes (Concepcion et al. 2021). The most widely used vaccine, the Oral Poliovirus Vaccine (OPV), uses an inactivated virus with minimal or no pathogenicity. In contrast, the Injected Poliovirus Vaccine (IPV) confers immunity through a killed specimen. On the other hand, when the inactivated virus of OPV replicates in the gut, it may experience mutations. Seldom can these mutations make the virus more transmissible and virulent (Rachlin et al. 2022).

When unvaccinated people are infected with these vaccine-derived variants, they become circulating vaccine-derived polioviruses (cVDPV) and can infect the same way as naturally occurring wild polioviruses (WPV). The aim of eliminating the poliovirus worldwide is in jeopardy due to the swift growth of cVDPV2 transmission. The type 2 live vaccine may need to be reintroduced into routine immunisation if the spread of cVDPV2 is not stopped, which would be a significant setback to the objective of eliminating polioviruses (Cooper et al. 2022). Outbreaks of circulating vaccine-derived type 2 poliovirus (cVDPV2) throughout Africa are due to reduced population immunity to type 2 poliovirus as a result of the trivalent oral poliovirus vaccination being discontinued worldwide (Pons-Salort et al. 2016).

In 2016, one of the major steps toward the improvement of the polio control programme globally was undertaken in terms of changing from the trivalent oral poliovirus vaccine (tOPV) to the bivalent oral poliovirus vaccine (bOPV), also known as "Switch". This transition sought to reduce the risks associated with the type 2 component of OPV, which has been found to cause vaccine-derived poliovirus outbreaks. When switching from tOPV to bOPV, which only eliminates types 1 and 3 polioviruses, the authorities wanted to prevent cVDPV of type 2, indirectly strengthening the approach to a polio-free global strategy (Mohanty et al. 2023). As per the reports of the Independent Monitoring Board of the Global Polio Eradication Initiative, this initiative to shift from tOPV to bOPV is still in place (Donaldson et al. 2024). To effectively combat the poliovirus in Africa, addressing these issues calls for a comprehensive strategy that includes raising immunisation rates as one of the other factors (Ezezika et al. 2022).

6.1.3 Dengue

Dengue is a mosquito-borne viral disease transmitted by mosquitoes of the genus *Aedes* and its species, *Aedes aegypti*. The virus belongs to the family *Flaviviridae*, genus *Flavivirus* and has four serotypes (DENV-1 to DENV-4). It affects people from both tropical and subtropical areas, causing about 100 to 400 million cases per year globally (Abdul Rahman et al. 2024). Symptoms may range from mild flu-like to the most critical conditions resulting in Dengue Shock Syndrome (DSS).

Vaccine development for dengue is challenging because of its serotypes (Miller 2010). The sole registered available vaccine is Dengavaxia (CYD-TDV) (Thomas and Yoon 2019). The live attenuated Recombinant Vaccine for dengue fever is a chimeric vaccine with features of both the dengue virus and the yellow fever 17D strain, containing the structural prM and envelope of all four DENV groups, from DENV 1 to DENV 4. This strategy seeks to initiate a responsive and powerful immunogenic reaction against the dengue virus as well as to capitalise on the safety aspects of the yellow fever vaccine to present a reliable strategy for total vaccine protection against dengue viral infections in affected areas (Deng et al. 2020).

Immunisation has affected dengue virus (DENV) transmission and the severity of diseases predominantly through live attenuated vaccines in Africa. The efficacy of these vaccines can be as high as 79.6%, and while there is some suggestion that primed individuals who have been exposed to dengue through prior infection seem to have better vaccine efficacy at 89.2% compared to those without previous exposure (75.3%) (Thomas 2023). The difference in vaccine effectiveness indicates that past dengue exposure enhances the resulting impact by offering the best efficiency (Akter et al. 2024).

6.1.4 *Rabies*

The global campaign to eradicate dog-mediated rabies is a continuous and challenging undertaking, with notable successes in certain areas and enduring difficulties in others. Although rabies is a significant disease burden in Africa, little is known about successfully eradicating the illness in individual nations (Broban et al. 2018; Haselbeck et al. 2021). These authors draw attention to the difficulties in preventing and controlling rabies in the area, which include a dearth of political will and faulty surveillance data. Specific initiatives in Tunisia and Nigeria aimed at controlling and eradicating rabies through comprehensive canine vaccination campaigns and enhanced surveillance measures (Ripani et al. 2017; Mshelbwala et al. 2021). However, the effectiveness of these initiatives in eradicating rabies is unclear from the available data. The human rabies death rate increased by 13.6% between 2012 and 2015, but then declined by 23.41% between 2015 and 2018, indicating that control measures were somewhat effective during this period. Post-exposure prophylaxis has been a concern, with 360 PEP treatments per 100,000 inhabitants per year and stressing supposed exposure (Kalthoum et al. 2021).

Current statistics indicate that some states in Nigeria have achieved vaccination rates of over 80%, aligning with their visions for Nigerian cities. However, in rural areas, access remains a significant challenge due to inadequate logistics and limited health education (Ajoke et al. 2014). Therefore, more investigation is required to determine which African nations have successfully eradicated rabies. Numerous factors affect the effectiveness of rabies elimination efforts in African countries. Research emphasises the necessity for thorough and ongoing dog vaccination, increased public awareness, and access to high-quality human rabies vaccines. Effective vaccination tactics and community engagement are also necessary. Researchers emphasise that top-down interventions are essential for engaging with project organisation and community participation (Bardosh et al. 2014). "One Health" approach, focused on achieving sustainable herd immunity in dogs through community-based immunisation and educational initiatives, should be implemented. (Franka et al. 2013). The importance of political will and sustained dog vaccination initiatives in North Africa, as well as the effectiveness of central-point vaccination in rural Tanzania, should be regarded as examples for other countries. These studies underscore the importance of tailored, community-oriented approaches for eliminating rabies in Africa (Ripani et al. 2017; Kaare et al. 2009).

6.1.5 *Yellow Fever*

Expanding vaccination use, stopping worldwide transmission, and controlling outbreaks are the main goals of the WHO's Eliminate Yellow Fever Epidemics (EYE) plan (Chen and Wilson 2020). Mass vaccination initiatives have successfully prevented yellow fever-associated mortality, with about 10,000 deaths being avoided in 2018 (Gaythorpe et al. 2020). However, initiatives to eradicate yellow fever in Africa face a difficult situation (Adogo and Ogoh 2019).

It took a combination of variables for yellow fever to be successfully eradicated in nations like Brazil and Cuba. These included determining that the *Aedes aegypti* mosquito is the disease's vector, implementing mosquito control measures, and creating potent immunisation plans (Camargo 1967; Chaves-Carballo 2005). Nevertheless, there is still a chance of re-emergence, especially in high-risk regions like West Africa and the Equatorial region of Latin America (Ndeffo-Mbah and Pandey 2020). Ongoing efforts are required to address this by customising vaccination plans to the unique risk profiles of endemic nations (Ndeffo-Mbah and Pandey 2020; Bifani et al. 2020).

Numerous studies have demonstrated that immunisation programs play an essential role in preventing yellow fever in Africa. The preventive mass vaccination efforts successfully lower the illness load; these campaigns have reduced fatalities by 47%. Widespread vaccination initiatives aimed at prevention have resulted in a 34% decrease in the likelihood of yellow fever outbreaks. The fact that routine yellow fever vaccination is more effective in preventing cases and deaths than emergency control further supports the cost-effectiveness of these measures (Monath and Nasidi 1993). The potential significance of upcoming large vaccination initiatives for prevention suggests that they might prevent millions of diseases (Gaythorpe et al. 2020).

Yellow fever keeps resurfacing in countries like Nigeria, despite a reliable vaccine, causing outbreaks and fatalities. Controlling these outbreaks requires quick action through emergency vaccination campaigns (Adogo and Ogoh 2019). To effectively reduce yellow fever, African governments must take the initiative and focus on routine immunisation and large-scale vaccine efforts, with assistance from international organisations (Tomori 2002). Africa has a high illness burden from yellow fever, which seriously threatens public health, especially for young people (Monath 2006; Tomori 2002). The disease has resurfaced in the past 20 years, resulting in significant morbidity and death. One of the main causes of the region's ongoing outbreaks of yellow fever is the lack of or sporadic use of the vaccine (Baba and Ikusemoran 2017). Still, there has been a lot of progress in integrating the yellow fever vaccine into regular pediatric vaccination schedules in Africa (Monath 2006). Research has demonstrated that widespread immunisation programs can reduce disease prevalence (Garske et al. 2014). These results show the significance of consistent endeavors in yellow fever vaccination campaigns and initiatives to prevent the spread of the disease throughout Africa.

6.1.6 Hepatitis

African countries exhibit notable differences in the prevalence and risk factors of hepatitis A, B, and E, exacerbated by variable health care and sanitation standards, risk factors, and immunisation efforts, especially in the northern regions (Kamal et al. 2010). This complicates the current state of hepatitis A, B, and E eradication initiatives on the continent (Sonderup and Spearman 2022). Despite the development of efficient antiviral medication and universal immunisation, the prevalence of hepatitis B remains high in sub-Saharan Africa (Spearman et al. 2017). It is imperative that the HBV birth-dose vaccine be used globally and that vaccination coverage be 100% to effectively prevent future infections (Spearman et al. 2017). The implications of hepatitis B virus infection for eliminating viral hepatitis in sub-Saharan Africa are significant, with a need to scale up coverage of hepatitis B birth dose and early childhood vaccination (Amponsah-Dacosta 2021).

Numerous studies have shown how affordable different hepatitis immunisation plans are in Africa. For example, routinely providing a newborn dose of the hepatitis B virus (HBV) vaccine in Ethiopia was very cost-effective (Das 1999; Margolis et al. 1995; Memirie et al. 2020). The most cost-effective option was universal vaccination against the hepatitis A virus (HAV). Despite improvements in hepatitis B control in Africa, with certain nations achieving high vaccination rates (Breakwell et al. 2017), issues persist, including inadequate understanding of immunisation protocols and unstable vaccine supply. The necessity of successfully integrating HBV immunisation into current programmes is emphasised by Kew (1996). Furthermore, there is a pressing need for operational and research programmes to eliminate these obstacles to control and possible solutions (Lemoine et al. 2015). Healthcare workers in Africa are at risk of infection due to inadequate uptake of the hepatitis B vaccination, even after it was made universal (Auta et al. 2018). Concentrating on preventive measures, such as the widespread use of the HBV birth-dose vaccine and complete vaccination coverage, is imperative to meet the WHO's 2030 hepatitis B elimination targets (Spearman et al. 2017).

6.2 Global Collaborative Initiatives Engaged in African Countries

Global collaborative initiatives have significantly impacted the control and prevention of VPDs in Africa, including diseases such as COVID-19, polio, hepatitis A, B, and E, Japanese encephalitis, dengue, yellow fever, and rabies. These initiatives helped to strengthen VPD surveillance activities, prioritise surveillance staff, and adapt to changes in health-seeking behaviours during the COVID-19 pandemic (Bigouette et al. 2022). The existing global health infrastructure, particularly the World Health Organization (WHO), has played a central role in guiding targeted and coordinated international disease responses, highlighting both strengths and vulnerabilities (Lee et al. 2022).

Lessons from the Global Polio Eradication Initiative (GPEI) addressed the need to map barriers systematically, strategies to overcome VPDs, and unintended consequences (Deressa et al. 2020). Factors associated with successful surveillance programmes include involving local communities and frontline implementers in the planning and implementation process (Osaghae et al. 2022). The introduction and implementation of hepatitis B vaccination programs require ongoing support and interventions to achieve control (Hollinger et al. 2007). The successful withdrawal of oral polio vaccines (OPV) required intense global coordination and planning, including forecasting vaccine needs, scaling production, and training health workers (Ramirez Gonzalez et al. 2017). Strengthening vaccine service delivery at national and sub-national levels is crucial for achieving universal health coverage (UHC), and strategies include reaching hard-to-reach populations, expanding disease-focused programs, building community trust, and promoting multi-sectoral collaboration (Olateju et al. 2022).

6.3 Impediments and Difficulties in Accessing Vaccines to Treat VPDs in Africa

Several barriers and challenges hinder the availability of vaccines for VPDs in Africa, notably reduced availability, which significantly impacts public health. These are complex, encompassing supply chain complications, restricted funding, health infrastructure deficiencies, vaccine reluctance, and germane policies. A current and critical issue is weak vaccine distribution logistics. Most African countries largely depend on organisations like the COVAX for vaccines, for instance, which have been exposed as being poorly equipped during health crises. For example, as the world reacted to the COVID-19 outbreak, many countries had a vaccine shortage. In contrast, the wealthiest countries took the doses, leaving African countries with limited vaccines to use for their citizens (Wei et al. 2023). Further, other factors that influence vaccine stock include chemical imbalances, such as delayed transportation of vaccines from depots to health facilities (Mkamba et al. 2023).

Another major challenge is inadequate financial resources to support the vaccination efforts. Unfortunately, most African administrations spend poorly on any immunisation programme, although the scarce available cash tends to be spent only on the early stages of immunisation drives (Mkamba et al. 2023). When the disease is on the rise or there is a high demand for vaccines, funding gaps surface as an impediment to targeting hard-to-reach populations and specific risk groups. Another report pointed out that about 60% of the total spending on mass immunisation programmes goes towards overheads rather than the actual cost of vaccination commodities (Saidu et al. 2024).

The weak health systems also hinder mass vaccination, as evidenced by the weaknesses in healthcare systems. Inefficient storage and distribution of vaccines remain major challenges in most areas, as they are vital in retaining the cold chain essential for vaccine effectiveness (Mirza et al. 2024). This is particularly evident in rural areas where health facilities are scarce. In addition, human resources constraints, including a lack of adequate staffing and poor training of the health care providers, lead to ineffective campaigns in otherwise effective vaccination (Ekezie et al. 2024).

The issue of vaccine hesitancy persists in many African countries to this day. False information on the safety and effectiveness of vaccines might cause the public to decline vaccination programmes (Alie et al. 2024). Some of the reasons why people did not come out to take the COVID-19 vaccine include a lack of trust in the government as well as the pharmaceutical companies which developed the vaccines, cultural beliefs, and fear of being used for experiments similar to the ones that were carried out by the Nazi's during the Second World War. This hesitancy can become a massive barrier to effective vaccination with available vaccines, hence counterproductive for public health (Unfried and Priebe 2024).

6.4 Future Perspective and Recommendations

Effective strategies for controlling and preventing the spread of Japanese encephalitis virus, dengue, yellow fever, and rabies in Africa include vaccination, good hygiene practices, respiratory etiquette, the use of personal protective equipment, social distancing, staying informed, maintaining environmental hygiene, and implementing entomological surveys and vector control interventions (Tajudeen et al. 2022; Al Neflai et al. 2022; Omosigho et al. 2023; Aborode et al. 2022). These measures are crucial in combating viral infections and promoting public health.

Additionally, the availability of trained personnel, rapid diagnostic facilities, and efficient surveillance systems is essential for effective control and prevention (Haselbeck et al. 2021). Multidisciplinary approaches, including enhanced diagnostics, improved surveillance and reporting, prognostic modelling, and education and public awareness campaigns, are also necessary to address the epidemiological control of these diseases in African countries.

Coordination between the human and veterinary health sectors under the "One Health" umbrella is crucial for the control and elimination of zoonotic diseases like rabies.

The COVID-19 pandemic has significantly impacted the control of other vaccine-preventable diseases (VPDs) in Africa. The pandemic has disrupted various cancer control activities, including prevention and screening efforts, leading to decreased access to cancer services and disruptions in research activities (Opara et al. 2022). Additionally, the pandemic has curtailed vaccine-preventable disease (VPD) surveillance activities, decreasing surveillance staff and changing health-seeking behaviours, affecting VPD surveillance efforts (Nakaganda et al. 2023). The pandemic has also affected the trend in the epidemiology of viral hemorrhagic fevers (VHFs) such as Lassa fever (LF) and yellow fever (YF), with an increase in LF cases and deaths and a continued burden of YF globally (Bigouette et al. 2022). To address these issues, it is recommended to strengthen health systems for cancer control, develop and implement evidence-based frameworks and comprehensive National

Cancer Control Plans, restore VPD surveillance to pre-pandemic levels, and leverage the infrastructure developed in response to COVID-19 to strengthen the health system for VPD control (Paintsil et al. 2023; Montcho et al. 2023a).

6.5 Conclusion

In conclusion, this chapter establishes that vaccine deployment to control viral diseases has risen in Africa in the last couple of years and thus benefits human health. Many VPDs have shown low morbidity and mortality rates due to vaccination measures, especially those commenced under EPI. However, there is still much to do: organisational relationships in the supply chain are strained, the funding is insufficient, and some people are still reluctant to be vaccinated. The re-emergence of some VPDs indicates the increasing potential of a renewed push to approach and optimise current vaccination and vaccine coverage. Furthermore, the recent COVID-19 crisis exposed the weakness in African Health Care systems, a situation that makes Africans extremely dependent on vaccines from developed countries, thereby magnifying the existing rift. Thus, countries must focus on infrastructure, acquiring manufacturing industries for vaccines, and countering public health misinformation campaigns to create a stronger vaccination system. The continent can enhance its mechanisms of averting viral diseases, protecting its population's health and embracing health equity across the continent by adopting multiple strategies involved in these approaches.

References

Abdul Rahman FK, Binti Wan Puteh SE, Bin Zainuddin MA (2024) E-dengue system insights: exploring the factors influencing dengue-related deaths in an urbanised state in a low-middle income country (LMIC). BMC Public Health 24:3055

Aborode AT, Corriero AC, Fajemisin EA, Hasan MM, Kazmi SK, Olajiga O (2022) Dengue and coronavirus disease (COVID-19) syndemic: double threat to an overburdened healthcare system in Africa. Int J Health Plann Manag 37:1851–1854

Adogo LY, Ogoh M (2019) Yellow fever in Nigeria: A review of the current situation. Afr J Clin Exper Microbiol 21:1–13

Africa WHO (2022) Vaccine-preventable disease outbreaks on the rise in Africa | Who | Regional Office for Africa [Online]. Available: https://www.afro.who.int/news/vaccine-preventable-disease-outbreaks-rise-africa. Accessed 23 March 2024

Ahmad S, Ahmad M, Zain-Ul-Abedin M, Channo A, Subhan A, Beig M, Irshad Z, Mujahid U, Khan A (2024) Zoonotic diseases: emerging threats to public Health and livestock production chapter history. Zoonosis, Unique Scientific Publishers, Faisalabad

Ajoke E, Solomon A, Ikhide E (2014) The role of dog trading and slaughter for meat in rabies epidemiology with special reference to Nigeria-a review

Akter R, Tasneem F, Das S, Soma MA, Georgakopoulos-Soares I, Juthi RT, Sazed SA (2024) Approaches of dengue control: vaccine strategies and future aspects. Front Immunol 15: 1362780

Al Neflai FM, Al Qarni NS, Al Gamdi AM, Arishi BM, Bin Assai NS, Al Abdale WM (2022) Effective strategies to Deal with pathogenic viruses and prevent their spread. Int J Bio-Med Inform e-Health 10:53–58

Alie MS, Abebe GF, Negesse Y, Adugna A, Girma D (2024) Vaccine hesitancy in context of Covid-19 in East Africa: systematic review and meta-analysis. BMC Public Health 24:2796

Amponsah-Dacosta E (2021) Hepatitis B virus infection and hepatocellular carcinoma in sub-Saharan Africa: Implications for elimination of viral hepatitis by 2030? World J Gastroenterol 27:6025–6038

Anoopkumar A, Aneesh EM (2022) A critical assessment of mosquito control and the influence of climate change on mosquito-borne disease epidemics. Environ Dev Sustain 24:8900–8929

Auta A, Adewuyi EO, Kureh GT, Onoviran N, Adeloye D (2018) Hepatitis B vaccination coverage among healthcare workers in Africa: a systematic review and meta-analysis. Vaccine 36(32 Pt B):4851–4860

Baba MM, Ikusemoran M (2017) Is the absence or intermittent Yf vaccination the major contributor to its persistent outbreaks in eastern Africa? Biosci Res Commun 492(4):548–557

Bardosh KL, Sambo M, Sikana L, Hampson K, Welburn SC (2014) Eliminating rabies in Tanzania? Local understandings and responses to mass dog vaccination in Kilombero and Ulanga districts. PLoS Negl Trop Dis 8:e2935

Bifani AM, Ong EZ, De Alwis R (2020) Vaccination and therapeutics: responding to the changing epidemiology of yellow fever. Curr Top Infect Dis 12:398–409

Bigouette JP, Callaghan AW, Donadel M, Porter AM, Rosencrans L, Lickness JS, Blough S, Li X, Perry RT, Williams AJ, Scobie HM, Dahl BA, Mcfarland J, Murrill CS (2022) Effects of COVID-19 on vaccine-preventable disease surveillance systems in the World Health Organization African Region, 2020. Emerg Infect Dis 28:S203–s207

Bon HB, Brouwers SA, Mote J, De Almeida S, Markle L, Sommariva S, Fol N (2023) Measuring behavioral and social drivers of COVID-19 vaccination in health workers in Eastern and Southern Africa. In: BMC Proceedings. Springer, p 14

Breakwell L, Tévi-Bénissan C, Childs L, Mihigo R, Tohme RA (2017) The status of hepatitis B control in the African region. Pan Afr Med J 27:17

Broban A, Tejiokem MC, Tiembré I, Druelles S, L'azou M (2018) Bolstering human rabies surveillance in Africa is crucial to eliminating canine-mediated rabies. PLoS Negl Trop Dis 12:e0006367

Butera N, De Sanjose S, Hoyt AM, Morgan K, Mcdonald MA, Senkomago V, Islam JY, Smith JS, Ramos S, Kim CJ (2018) Acceptability of two-versus three-dose human papillomavirus vaccination schedule among providers and mothers of adolescent girls: a mixed-methods study in five countries. Vaccine 36:453–460

Camargo S (1967) History of Aedes aegypti eradication in the Americas. Bull World Health Org 36(4):602–603

Cascella M, Rajnik M, Aleem A, Dulebohn SC, Di Napoli R (2023) Features, evaluation, and treatment of coronavirus (COVID-19). In: StatPearls [Internet]. StatPearls Publishing, Treasure Island

Chaves-Carballo E (2005) Carlos Finlay and yellow fever: triumph over adversity. Milit Med 170(10):881–885

Chen LH, Wilson ME (2020) Yellow fever control: current epidemiology and vaccination strategies. Trop Dis Travel Med Vacc 6

Concepcion F, Estivariz RL, Shimabukuro T (2021) Polio: epidemiology and prevention of vaccine-preventable diseases (14th edn). CDC Pink Book

Cooper LV, Bandyopadhyay AS, Gumede N, Mach O, Mkanda P, Ndoutabé M, Okiror SO, Ramirez-Gonzalez A, Touray K, Wanyoike S, Grassly NC, Blake IM (2022) Risk factors for the spread of vaccine-derived type 2 polioviruses after global withdrawal of trivalent oral poliovirus vaccine and the effects of outbreak responses with monovalent vaccine: a retrospective analysis of surveillance data for 51 countries in Africa. Lancet Infect Dis 22:284–294

Das A (1999) An economic analysis of different strategies of immunisation against hepatitis a virus in developed countries. Health Econ 8:29–36

Deng SQ, Yang X, Wei Y, Chen JT, Wang XJ, Peng HJ (2020) A review on dengue vaccine development. Vaccines (Basel) 8:63

Deressa W, Kayembe P, Neel AH, Mafuta E, Seme A, Alonge O (2020) Lessons learned from the polio eradication initiative in the Democratic Republic of Congo and Ethiopia: analysis of implementation barriers and strategies. BMC Public Health 20:1807

Dhama K, Nainu F, Frediansyah A, Yatoo MI, Mohapatra RK, Chakraborty S, Zhou H, Islam MR, Mamada SS, Kusuma HI (2023) Global emerging Omicron variant of SARS-CoV-2: impacts, challenges and strategies. J Infect Public Health 16:4–14

Dhawan M, Sharma A, Priyanka N, Thakur N, Rajkhowa TK, Choudhary OP (2022) Delta variant (B. 1.617. 2) of SARS-CoV-2: mutations, impact, challenges and possible solutions. Hum Vacc Immunother 18:2068883

Donaldson L, Alwan A, Frieden T, Goldstein S (2024) The long goodbye. In: Report (ed.). Independent Monitoring Board of the Global Polio Eradication Initiative

Ekezie W, Igein B, Varughese J, Butt A, Ukoha-Kalu BO, Ikhile I, Bosah G (2024) Vaccination communication strategies and uptake in Africa: a systematic review. Vaccine 12:1333

Ezezika O, Mengistu M, Opoku E, Farheen A, Chauhan A, Barrett K (2022) What are the barriers and facilitators to polio vaccination and eradication programs? A systematic review. PLoS Global Public Health 2:e0001283

Franka R, Smith TG, Dyer JL, Wu X, Niezgoda M, Rupprecht CE (2013) Current and future tools for global canine rabies elimination. Antiviral Res 100(1):220–225

Garske T, Van Kerkhove MD, Yactayo S, Ronveaux O, Lewis RF, Staples JE, Perea WA, Ferguson NM (2014) Yellow fever in Africa: estimating the burden of disease and impact of mass vaccination from outbreak and serological data. PLoS Med 11:e1001638

Gaythorpe KAM, Hamlet A, Jean K, Garkauskas Ramos D, Cibrelus L, Garske T, Ferguson NM (2020) The global burden of yellow fever. Elife 10:e64670

Haselbeck AH, Rietmann S, Tadesse BT, Kling K, Kaschubat-Dieudonné ME, Marks F, Wetzker W, Thöne-Reineke C (2021) Challenges to the fight against rabies-the landscape of policy and prevention strategies in Africa. Int J Environ Res Public Health 18

Hollinger FB, Bell B, Levy-Bruhl D, Shouval D, Wiersma S, Van Damme P (2007) Hepatitis A and B vaccination and public health. J Viral Hepat 14(Suppl 1):1–5

Hull HF, Ward NA, Hull BP, Milstien JB, Hull HF, De Quadros C (1994) Paralytic poliomyelitis: seasoned strategies, disappearing disease. Lancet 343:1331–1337

Jacobsen KH, Wiersma ST (2010) Hepatitis A virus seroprevalence by age and world region, 1990 and 2005. Vaccine 28:6653–6657

Kaare MT, Lembo T, Lembo T, Hampson K, Hampson K, Ernest EM, Estes AB, Mentzel C, Cleaveland S (2009) Rabies control in rural Africa: evaluating strategies for effective domestic dog vaccination. Vaccine 27(1):152–160

Kalthoum S, Guesmi K, Gharbi R, Baccar MN, Seghaier C, Zrelli M, Bahloul C (2021) Temporal and spatial distributions of animal and human rabies cases during 2012 and 2018, in Tunisia. Vet Med Sci 7:686–696

Kamal SM, Mahmoud SB, Sanaa M (2010) Viral hepatitis a to E in South Mediterranean countries. Mediterr J Hematol Infect Dis 2:e2010001

Kew MC (1996) Progress towards the comprehensive control of hepatitis B in Africa: a view from South Africa. Gut 38:S31–S36

Le Polain de Waroux O, Schellenberg JR, Manzi F, Mrisho M, Shirima K, Mshinda H, Alonso P, Tanner M, Schellenberg DM (2013) Timeliness and completeness of vaccination and risk factors for low and late vaccine uptake in young children living in rural southern Tanzania. Int Health 5:139–147

Lee JA, Kharel R, Naganathan S, Karim N, Aluisio AR, Levine AC (2022) Frameworks for global health collaboration in pandemic disease. R I Med J 2013(105):33–37

Lemoine M, Eholie SP, Lacombe K (2015) Reducing the neglected burden of viral hepatitis in Africa: strategies for a global approach. J Hepatol 62(2):469–476

Lone SA, Ahmad A (2020) COVID-19 pandemic–an African perspective. Emerg Microb Infect 9: 1300–1308

Margolis HS, Coleman PJ, Brown RE, Mast EE, Sheingold SH, Arevalo JA (1995) Prevention of hepatitis B virus transmission by immunisation. An economic analysis of current recommendations. JAMA 274(15):1201–1208

Mboussou F, Farham B, Nsasiirwe S, Atagbaza A, Oyaole D, Atuhebwe PL, Alegana V, Osei-Sarpong F, Bwaka A, Paluku G, Petu A, Efe-Aluta O, Kalu A, Bagayoko MM, Impouma B (2023) COVID-19 vaccination in the WHO African region: Progress made in 2022 and factors associated. Vaccines (Basel) 11

Mckay T, Robinson RS, Musungu S, Padi-Adjirackor NA, Angotti N (2024) The missing millions: uncovering the burden of COVID-19 cases and deaths in the African region. Popul Dev Rev 50: 7–58

Md Khairi LNH, Fahrni ML, Lazzarino AI (2022) The race for global equitable access to COVID-19 vaccines. Vaccines (Basel) 10

Medhat MA, El Kassas M (2020) COVID-19 in Egypt: uncovered figures or a different situation? J Glob Health 10

Memirie ST, Desalegn H, Naizgi M, Nigus M, Taddesse L, Tadesse Y, Tessema F, Zelalem M, Girma T (2020) Introduction of birth dose of hepatitis B virus vaccine to the immunisation program in Ethiopia: an economic evaluation. Cost Eff Resour Alloc 18:23

Miller N (2010) Recent progress in dengue vaccine research and development. Curr Opin Mol Ther 12:31–38

Mirza I, Ameda I-M, Ba AE, Traore C, Hagos MT, Gbaya AA, Schreiber B (2024) COVID-19 vaccination integration: efforts in 11 African countries to strengthen the primary health care system. Glob Health 12

Mkamba BS, Rutungwa E, Karimi PN, Ngenzi JL (2023) Factors that influence the availability of childhood vaccine in healthcare facilities at Tana River County, Kenya. J Pharma Pol Pract 16: 142

Mohanty A, Rohilla R, Zaman K, Hada V, Dhakal S, Shah A, Padhi BK, Al-Qaim ZH, Altawfiq KJA, Tirupathi R, Sah R, Al-Tawfiq JA (2023) Vaccine derived poliovirus (VDPV). Infez Med 31:174–185

Monath TP (2006) Yellow fever as an endemic/epidemic disease and priorities for vaccination. Braz J Infect Dis 99(5):341–347

Monath TP, Nasidi A (1993) Should yellow fever vaccine be included in the expanded program of immunisation in Africa? A cost-effectiveness analysis for Nigeria. Am J Trop Med Hygiene 48(2):274–299

Montcho Y, Nalwanga R, Azokpota P, Doumatè J, Lokonon B, Salako V, Wolkewitz M, Glele Kakaï RL (2023a) Assessing the impact of vaccination on the dynamics of COVID-19 in Africa: a mathematical modeling study. Vaccine 11:857

Montcho Y, Nalwanga R, Azokpota P, Doumatè JT, Lokonon BE, Salako VK, Wolkewitz M, Glèlè Kakaï R (2023b) Assessing the impact of vaccination on the dynamics of COVID-19 in Africa: A mathematical modeling study. Vaccines (Basel) 11

Mshelbwala PP, Weese JS, Sanni-Adeniyi OA, Chakma S, Okeme SS, Mamun AA, Rupprecht CE, Magalhães R (2021) Rabies epidemiology, prevention and control in Nigeria: Scoping progress towards elimination. PLoS Negl Trop Dis 15:e0009617

Nakaganda A, Lasebikan N, Garton EM, Kithaka B, Garanganga E, Livinski AA, Cira MK (2023) How Covid-19 exposed pre-existing roadblocks for cancer control in Africa: strategies, lessons and recommendations from the 2019-2020 Africa cancer research and control echo. Ecancermedicalscience 17:1516

Ndeffo-Mbah ML, Pandey A (2020) Global risk and elimination of yellow fever epidemics. J Infect Dis 221:2026–2034

Nichol A, Magnus D (2018) The one Health approach to zoonotic emerging infectious diseases. Am J Bioeth 18:1–2

Niyongabo F, Butoyi JM, Niyoyunguruza L, Esperance K, Coppieters Y (2024) Factors associated with correct vaccination among children aged 24 to 48 months hospitalised in the national hospitals of Bujumbura. medRxiv. 2024.03.18.24304508

Oghenebrume W, Muhammed Olanrewaju A, Christinah M, Yauba S, Obe Destiny B, Sidy N, Emmanuel AO, Terna N, Olalekan AU, Beate K (2023) COVID-19 vaccination implementation in 52 African countries: trajectory and implications for future pandemic preparedness. BMJ Glob Health 8:e013073

Olateju A, Peters MA, Osaghae I, Alonge O (2022) How service delivery implementation strategies can contribute to attaining universal health coverage: lessons from polio eradication using an implementation science approach. BMC Public Health 22:1271

Omosigho P, John OO, Olaleke N, Onyemaechi E, Singh A (2023) Dengue virus in Africa; what to know about the virus? J Appl Health Sci Med:23–29

Opara N, Nwagbara U, Hlongwana K (2022) The Covid-19 impact on the trends in yellow fever and Lassa fever infections in Nigeria. Infect Dis Reports 14:932–941

Osaghae I, Agrawal P, Olateju A, Alonge O (2022) Facilitators and barriers of infectious diseases surveillance activities: lessons from the global polio eradication initiative - a mixed-methods study. BMJ Open 12:e060885

Oyo-Ita A, Oduwole O, Arikpo D, Effa EE, Esu EB, Balakrishna Y, Chibuzor MT, Oringanje CM, Nwachukwu CE, Wiysonge CS (2023) Interventions for improving coverage of childhood immunisation in low-and middle-income countries. Cochrane Database Syst Rev 2023(2): CD008145

Ozer EA, Simons LM, Adewumi OM, Fowotade AA, Omoruyi EC, Adeniji JA, Olayinka OA, Dean TJ, Zayas J, Bhimalli PP (2022) Multiple expansions of globally uncommon SARS-CoV-2 lineages in Nigeria. Nat Commun 13:688

Paintsil E, Alimi Y, Abdulaziz M, Ogbuagu O, Ogunsola F, Kessy SJ, Horsney E, Lee C, Brundney K, Okwor T, Kabwe P, Waheed A, Vondran A, Bigirimana R, Ilesanmi O, Nsubuga DN, Raji T, Mankoula W, Ihekweazu C, Nkengasong J (2023) A continent-wide effort and solidarity at curbing COVID-19 pandemic: the Africa task force for novel coronavirus (AFTCOR) infection prevention and control technical working group's experience. BMC Public Health 23:893

Patel M, Cochi S (2017) Addressing the challenges and opportunities of the polio endgame: lessons for the future. J Infect Dis 216:S1–s8

Patterson AS (2018) Africa and global health governance: domestic politics and international structures. Johns Hopkins University Press, Baltimore

Pons-Salort M, Molodecky NA, O'reilly KM, Wadood MZ, Safdar RM, Etsano A, Vaz RG, Jafari H, Grassly NC, Blake IM (2016) Population immunity against serotype-2 poliomyelitis leading up to the global withdrawal of the oral poliovirus vaccine: Spatio-temporal modelling of surveillance data. PLoS Med 13:e1002140

Rachlin A, Patel JC, Burns CC, Jorba J, Tallis G, O'leary A, Wassilak SGF, Vertefeuille JF (2022) Progress toward polio eradication - worldwide, January 2020-April 2022. MMWR Morb Mortal Wkly Rep 71:650–655

Ramirez Gonzalez A, Farrell M, Menning L, Garon J, Everts H, Hampton LM, Dolan SB, Shendale S, Wanyoike S, Veira CL, Châtellier GMD, Kurji F, Rubin J, Boualam L, Chang Blanc D, Patel M (2017) Implementing the synchronized global switch from trivalent to bivalent Oral polio vaccines-lessons learned from the global perspective. J Infect Dis 216:S183–s192

Ripani A, Mérot J, Bouguedour R, Zrelli M (2017) Review of rabies situation and control in the North African region with a focus on Tunisia. Rev Sci Tech Int 36(3):831–838

Rocklöv J, Sjödin H, Wilder-Smith A (2020) Covid-19 outbreak on the Diamond Princess cruise ship: estimating the epidemic potential and effectiveness of public health countermeasures. J Travel Med 27:taaa030

Rotondo JC, Martini F, Maritati M, Mazziotta C, Di Mauro G, Lanzillotti C, Barp N, Gallerani A, Tognon M, Contini C (2021) SARS-CoV-2 infection: new molecular, phylogenetic, and pathogenetic insights. Efficacy of current vaccines and the potential risk of variants. Viruses 13:1687

Saidu Y, Ngenge BM, Nchinjoh SC, Amani A, Edwidge NN, Muteh NJ, Vouking MZ, Mbanga C, Agbor VN, Ousmane D (2024) Navigating vaccine procurement and financing challenges in Cameroon: insights and recommendations from a mixed-methods study (2015–2020). Public Health 237:261–269

Shapira G, Ahmed T, Drouard SHP, Amor Fernandez P, Kandpal E, Nzelu C, Wesseh CS, Mohamud NA, Smart F, Mwansambo C (2021) Disruptions in maternal and child health service utilisation during COVID-19: analysis from eight sub-Saharan African countries. Health Policy Plan 36:1140–1151

Sibanda M, Meyer JC, Godman B, Burnett RJ (2023) Low influenza vaccine uptake by healthcare workers caring for the elderly in South African old age homes and primary healthcare facilities. BMC Public Health 23:91

Sonderup MW, Spearman CW (2022) Global disparities in hepatitis B elimination—a focus on Africa. Vaccines 14:82

Spearman CW, Afihene MY, Ally R, Apica BS, Awuku YA, Cunha L, Dusheiko G, Gogela NA, Kassianides C, Kew M, Lam P, Lesi O, Lohouès-Kouacou M-J, Mbaye PS, Musabeyezu E, Musau B, Ojo O, Rwegasha J, Scholz B, Shewaye AB, Tzeuton C, Sonderup MW (2017) Hepatitis B in sub-Saharan Africa: strategies to achieve the 2030 elimination targets. Lancet Gastroenterol Hepatol 2(12):900–909

Tajudeen YA, Oladipo HJ, Oladunjoye IO, Yusuf RO, Sodiq H, Omotosho AO, Adesuyi DS, Yusuff SI, El-Sherbini MS (2022) Emerging arboviruses of public health concern in Africa: priorities for future research and control strategies. Challenges 13:60

Tambo E, Djuikoue IC, Tazemda GK, Fotsing MF, Zhou X-N (2021) Early stage risk communication and community engagement (RCCE) strategies and measures against the coronavirus disease 2019 (COVID-19) pandemic crisis. Glob Health J 5:44–50

Tegally H, San JE, Cotten M, Moir M, Tegomoh B, Mboowa G, Martin DP, Baxter C, Lambisia AW, Diallo A (2022) The evolving SARS-CoV-2 epidemic in Africa: insights from rapidly expanding genomic surveillance. Science 378:eabq5358

Thomas SJ (2023) Is new dengue vaccine efficacy data a relief or cause for concern? npj Vacc 8:55

Thomas SJ, Yoon I-K (2019) A review of Dengvaxia®: development to deployment. Hum Vacc Immunother 15:2295–2314

Tomori O (2002) Yellow fever in Africa: public health impact and prospects for control in the 21st century. Biol Res Nurs Dis Surveil 22(2):178–210

Unfried K, Priebe J (2024) Vaccine hesitancy and trust in sub-Saharan Africa. Sci Rep 14:10860

Uwishema O, Elebesunu EE, Bouaddi O, Kapoor A, Akhtar S, Effiong FB, Chaudhary A, Onyeaka H (2022) Poliomyelitis amidst the COVID-19 pandemic in Africa: efforts, challenges and recommendations. Clin Epidemiol Glob Health 16:101073

Vilches TN, Sah P, Abdollahi E, Moghadas SM, Galvani AP (2021) Importance of non-pharmaceutical interventions in the COVID-19 vaccination era: A case study of the Seychelles. J Glob Health 11:03104

Wariri O, Nkereuwem E, Erondu NA, Edem B, Nkereuwem OO, Idoko OT, Agogo E, Enegela JE, Sesay T, Conde IS (2021) A scorecard of progress towards measles elimination in 15 west African countries, 2001–19: a retrospective, multicountry analysis of national immunisation coverage and surveillance data. Lancet Glob Health 9:e280–e290

Wei CR, Kamande S, Lang'at GC (2023) Vaccine inequity: a threat to Africa's recovery from COVID-19. Trop Med Health 51:69

WHO (2010) Smallpox eradication programme - SEP (1966-1980) [Online]. Available: https://www.who.int/news-room/feature-stories/detail/the-smallpox-eradication-programme%2D%2D-sep-(1966-1980). Accessed 15 Oct. 2025

Wiysonge CS, Uthman OA, Ndumbe PM, Hussey GD (2012) Individual and contextual factors associated with low childhood immunisation coverage in sub-Saharan Africa: a multilevel analysis. PLoS One 7:e37905

Chapter 7
Rotaviruses and Noroviruses in Wastewater Across Africa

Natasha Potgieter, Leonard Kachienga, Mpumelelo Casper Rikhotso, Damien Jacobs, Afsatou Ndama Traore, and Akebe Luther King Abia

7.1 Introduction

7.1.1 Background on Rotaviruses and Noroviruses

Gastroenteritis cases alone account for approximately 1 billion morbidity cases annually, especially in children's diarrhea, estimated at half a million among children <5 years old. Most of these morbidity cases are rampant in Sub-Saharan Africa, South America, the Caribbean and South Asia, with over 100 persons in 100,000 population bearing the brunt of diarrheic morbidity (Omatola et al. 2024). Humans use water for several purposes, including industry, household, agriculture, aquaculture, recreation, and drinking (Dieter 2018). Water sources such as dams, lakes and rivers are subject to contamination by faecal pollution, originating from reservoirs of human (sewage and sewage plants) or animal (animal-based agriculture) (Nyairo et al. 2015). The Centres for Disease Control and Prevention reported that approximately 200,000 deaths of children worldwide are caused by gastroenteritis associated with viral pathogens (Omatola et al. 2024). The effect of gastroenteritis cases is limited in developed countries. However, it can sometimes result in high morbidity for young and elderly patients. Notwithstanding, the opposite is in developing countries; diarrheal diseases attributable to viral pathogens are a significant cause of death, particularly in infants (Shane et al. 2017).

N. Potgieter (✉) · L. Kachienga · M. C. Rikhotso · D. Jacobs · A. N. Traore
Department of Biochemistry and Microbiology, University of Venda, Thohoyandou, South Africa
e-mail: natasha.potgieter@univen.ac.za

A. L. K. Abia
Total Environment Research (TEN-R) Group, College of Health Sciences, University of KwaZulu-Natal, Durban, South Africa

Environmental Research Foundation, Westville, South Africa

J. A. Shenge, A. L. K. Abia (eds.), *Viral Diseases and One Health in Africa*,
https://doi.org/10.1007/978-3-032-09613-5_7

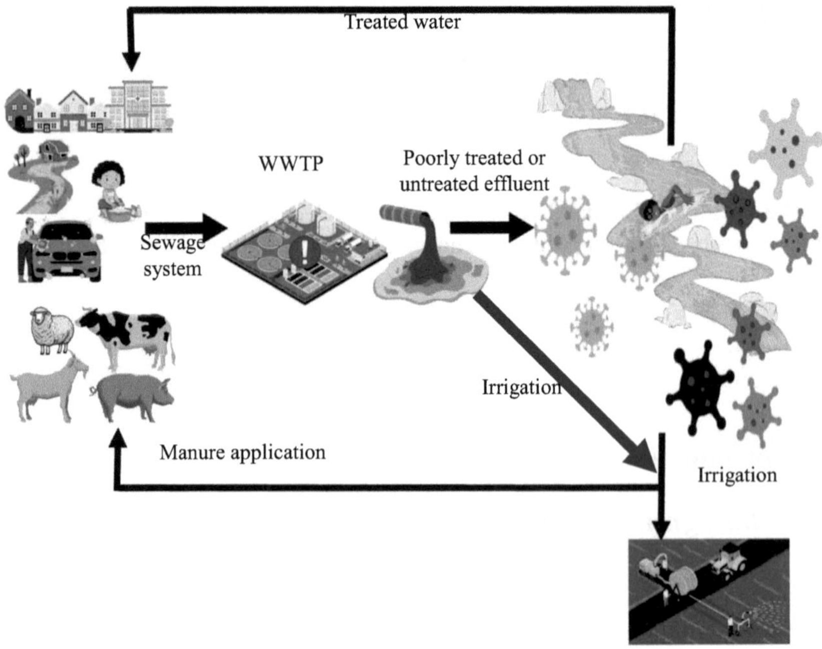

Fig. 7.1 The release of untreated/improperly treated wastewater from a wastewater treatment plant and back to the community. This may release viruses from effluents, causing downstream health, economic, and environmental challenges upon exposure to polluted water

According to Omatola et al. (2024), the epidemiology of rotavirus infection and the burden of the disease depend on the design and implementation of the oral Rotavirus and Norovirus vaccines currently in circulation globally, despite the widespread reports of the ineffectiveness of the vaccines in developing Sub-Saharan African countries. Despite the advancements to minimise their occurrence through the development of vaccines, Ghosh et al. (2018) reported that there are currently no licensed antivirals to treat or vaccines to prevent infection with enteropathogenic viruses. The factors that drive this phenomenon in these settings are malnutrition, poor access to healthcare, wasting, early cessation of breastfeeding or not breastfeeding, inadequate sanitation and hygiene, and not receiving any dose or the full dose of viral vaccine (e.g. oral Rotavirus or Norovirus vaccine) (Mero et al. 2021). Sewage leakage or insufficient wastewater effluent treatment enables the possibility of introducing waterborne pathogens, including waterborne enteric viruses (Fig. 7.1), making receiving water bodies unsuitable for use. These leakages or insufficient treatments thus lead to outbreaks of various enteric virus infections, like diarrhoea.

Norovirus- (NoV) and rotavirus (RoV)-associated acute gastroenteritis (AGE) are common in many countries, even those considered to be developed, such as the United Kingdom (UK) (Inns et al. 2017). Young children under 5 years are the most vulnerable, especially in developing countries, accounting for most hospitalisations and deaths linked to NoV and RoV, with rotavirus often associated with more severe cases of infection (Badur et al. 2019; Mans 2018; Inns et al. 2017). The greatest mortality among these children globally is linked to diarrhoea, with a death toll of approximately 10% annually (Anderson et al. 2010; Abdulazeez et al. 2020). According to Abdulazeez et al. (2020), viruses are the main etiologic agents of diarrhoea cases. The usual viral suspects are Rotaviruses (RV) and Norovirus (NV).

Rotaviruses are non-enveloped, icosahedral, double-stranded RNA viruses of a genus within the Reoviridae family (Dennehy 2015; Crawford et al. 2017). Rotaviruses lack envelopes and possess a genome of 11 double-stranded RNA (dsRNA) segments surrounded by a triplet of concentric capsid proteins, six non-structural proteins (NSP1-NSP6) and six structural viral proteins (VP1-VP4, VP6 and VP7) (Fig. 7.2a, b). NSP1 has been shown to play a role in genome replication and innate immune response antagonism, whereas NSP4 acts as a viral enterotoxin. RVs are currently classified into ten species or groups (A-J) based on differences in both genetic sequence and antigenicity of VP6. Globally, species A has been shown to have circulating strains with geographical variances. RoV B and C have been demonstrated to cause fewer infections, albeit still significant (LeClair and Budh 2023; Crawford et al. 2017).

The World Health Organization (WHO) has further recommended that most countries worldwide initiate vaccination programmes against rotaviruses in their national health programmes in the late 2000s (WHO 2009).

Noroviruses are equally the major cause of gastroenteritis in humans, with a mortality rate of approximately of over 100,000 in children under the age of five (Patel et al. 2009; Ayukekbong 2015; Alfajaro et al. 2017). Abdulazeez et al. (2020) reported that a NoV case was identified in Norwalk, Ohio, USA, in the early 1970s after an outbreak in children and staff in a school, and it was referred to as Norwalk infection. The name was only approved 30 years later, according to Mayo (2002). Children, the elderly and immunocompromised persons may experience more severe symptoms and/or extended duration of illness or even chronic diarrhoea. It is a positive-strand RNA, non-enveloped virus (Li et al. 2018). Ayukekbong et al. (2015) further opined that clinical judgment regarding association with diarrhoeal is difficult because of the asymptomatic Nov infections common within different populations.

Noroviruses are classified based on phylogenetic analysis of their capsid protein into ten (GI-GX) genogroups; human infections are associated with NoV genogroup GI, GII, GIV, GVIII, GX. They fall under the virus family *Caliciviridae*, which has three other genera: *Vesivirus*, *Sapovirus*, and *Lagovirus*. GI and GII have been associated with sporadic outbreaks and epidemics across all age groups. They are also the most studied in African wastewaters, with other genotypes being sparsely investigated, as shown in this chapter. Norovirus GII.4 strains, however, have been the cause of most outbreaks in the past decade, with epidemics occurring every 2–4 years (Mans et al. 2013). The genome consists of three open reading frames (ORFs). The first open reading frame encodes seven non-structural proteins as part of a polyprotein chain: [NSP1/2-p48], [NSP3-NTPase], [NSP4-p22], [NSP5-VPg], viral protease [NSP6-Pro, 3C-like] and an RNA-dependent RNA polymerase

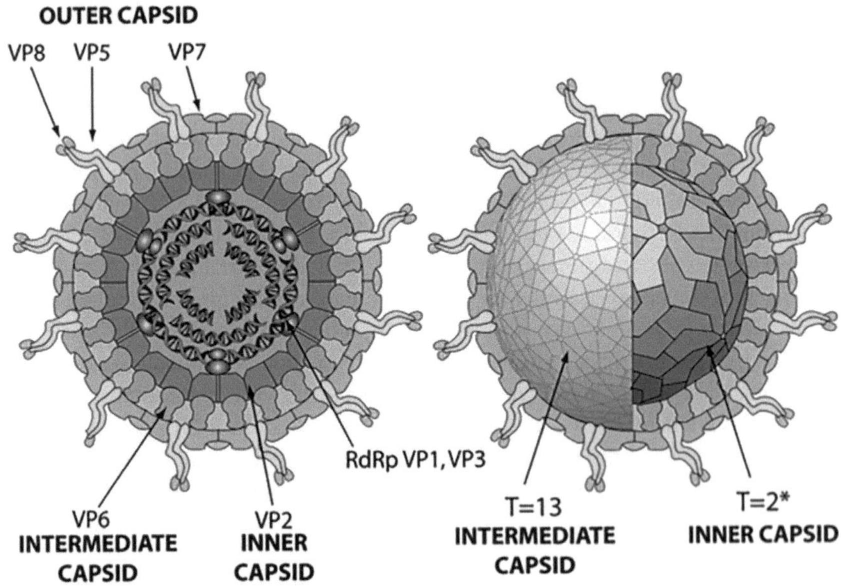

A

Genome	Gene	Product	Size (bp)	Function
	VP1	RNA polymerase	~3,302	RNA-dependent RNA polymerase
	VP2	Core shell	~2,690	Core capsid protein, forms inner capsid shell, scaffoids RNA
	VP3	RNA-capping methyltransferase	~2,591	Guanylyltransferase methyltransferase
	VP4	Protease-activated spike	~2,362	Caps viral mRNA
	NSP1	Interferon antagonist	~1,500	Viral attachment protein
	VP6	Intermediate capsid shell	~1,356	Antagonizes host interferon response, immune evasion
	NSP3	Translation regulator	~1,259	Hijacks host translation
	NSP2	Octameric NTPase	~1,059	Many onsumopotein, acontham competes with host mRNAs
	VP7	Outer-shell glycoprotein	1,062	Forms outer capsid
	NSP4	Enterotoxin	~751	Antigenic determinant (G type)
	NSP5/6	Phosphoprotein	~667	Viroplasm protein, regulates replication and packaging

B

Fig. 7.2 Schematic representation of the Rotavirus. (**a**) Rotavirus virion structure and genome composition (Source: https://upload.wikimedia.org/wikipedia/commons/c/cd/Rotavirus_virion_image.svg); (**b**) gene distribution within the genome, their sizes and functions

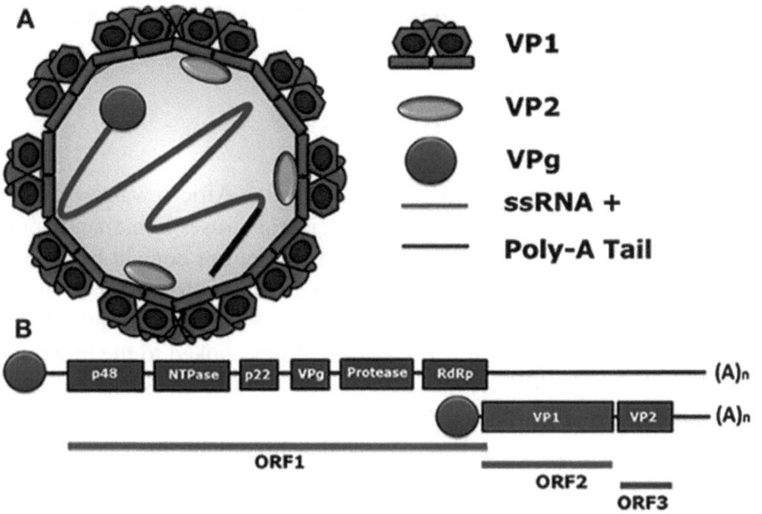

Fig. 7.3 Schematic representation of the Human Norovirus structure and genome composition (Campillay-Véliz et al. 2020)

[NS7-RdRp] (Glass et al. 2009). ORF 2 and 3 encode for VP1 (major capsid protein) and VP2 (minor capsid protein), respectively, and VP1 protein encodes for the shell (S) and protruding domains (P1/P2) as shown in Fig. 7.3.

The NoV has been detected in children below 5 years of age hospitalised with acute gastroenteritis (AGE) at the Queen Elizabeth Central Hospital (QECH) in Blantyre, Malawi, over ten years, between the late 1990s and 2000s. (Trainor et al. 2013). This prompted the health authorities to introduce the Rotavirus vaccine (Rotarix®) into the national childhood immunisation programme in 2012. In the far north of Malawi's borders, in Congo Brazzaville, diarrhoeal cases were higher among children below 5 years admitted to various healthcare facilities, with an annual mortality rate of 7.5% (Liu et al. 2015). Tate et al. (2012) further reported that severe cases of Rotavirus acute gastroenteritis are between 20% and 50% in young children worldwide. In 2008 alone, five countries accounted for more than half of the approximately half a million deaths from rotavirus diarrhoea; three countries were from Sub-Saharan Africa (Democratic Republic of Congo, Ethiopia and Nigeria) (Tate et al. 2012). Rotavirus and Norovirus in African wastewaters are poorly understood in terms of I) their extent, II) the methods used to isolate, detect and characterise them, and III) the challenges surrounding such methods. This chapter thus aims to inform the reader on those key aspects while touching on the discovery of the two viruses from some perspective.

7.2 Distribution of Rotaviruses and Noroviruses in African Wastewater

7.2.1 Prevalence in Wastewater Systems

Rotaviruses and Noroviruses are frequently detected in African wastewater systems, reflecting the widespread prevalence of these enteric viruses in human populations. Studies have shown that untreated and treated wastewater contain high concentrations of these pathogens, making wastewater a critical reservoir for environmental contamination and potential transmission (Mans et al. 2016; Chigor and Okoh 2012). The prevalence of rotaviruses in wastewater is closely linked to the high burden of diarrhoeal diseases, particularly in regions with limited access to sanitation and healthcare (Omatola et al. 2024). Similarly, Noroviruses, known for their role in gastroenteritis outbreaks, have been detected substantially in municipal sewage, particularly during peak gastroenteritis outbreaks (Trainor et al. 2013).

Africa is divided into North and Sub-Saharan Africa, with populations of 1.18 billion and 205 million, respectively, as of 2022. Sub-Saharan Africa is further subdivided into Western, Eastern, Middle and Southern Africa (The World Bank 2021). Globally, most water is dedicated to agricultural, industrial, and domestic uses. Literature has highlighted that water shortage is influenced by climate change and rapid population expansion (Nansubuga et al. 2016). Most research on these two viruses in wastewater occurs in Northern African countries (Egypt), followed by South Africa (Fig. 7.4). Tunisia, for example, is a country characterised by a dry climate and scarcity of water sources such as ground and surface water (blue water). This is reported to have a major impact on crops such as dates, figs, wheat, barley, and grapes that require more water than global averages; thus, repurposing wastewater is crucial in such countries (Chouchane et al. 2015).

Reports indicate that rotavirus detection in wastewater systems ranges from 20% to 50% in many African countries, with peaks occurring during the dry season due to increased human activity and wastewater generation (Tate et al. 2012). Norovirus detection rates are also substantial, often coinciding with community-level gastroenteritis outbreaks. Surveillance data from wastewater treatment plants across Africa suggest that both viruses are more prevalent in urban and peri-urban areas, where population density and inadequate sanitation infrastructure exacerbate the contamination (Omatola and Olaniran 2022). However, it should be noted that in many communities without centralised sewage systems, such data is often lacking, and statistics may only rely on hospital-reported cases. This paints an incomplete picture of the true prevalence of these viruses in most African countries.

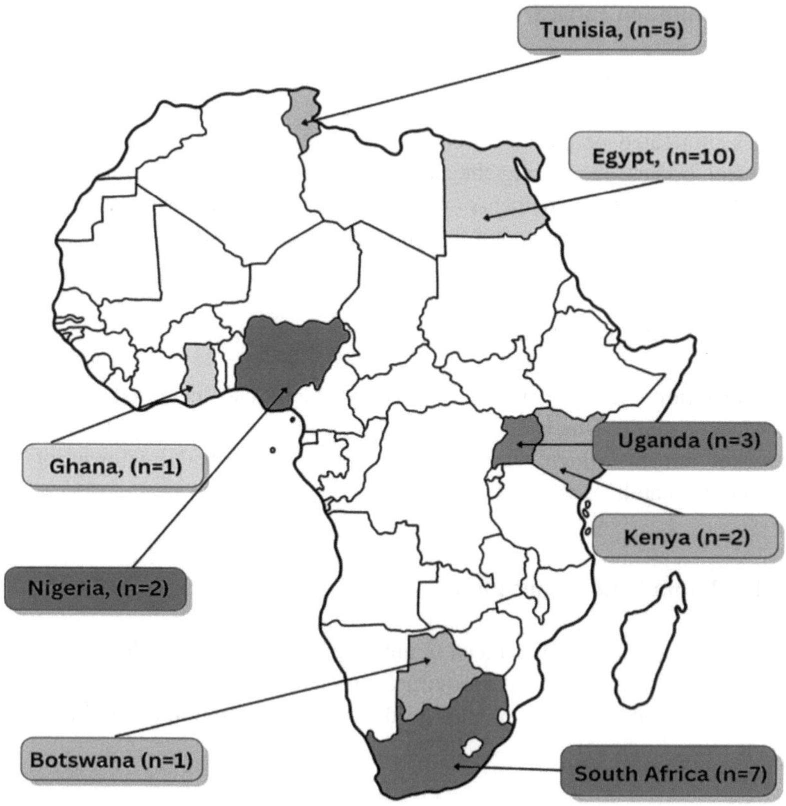

Fig. 7.4 The distribution of studies that detected Rotavirus and Norovirus in wastewater across Africa between 2013 and 2024

7.2.2 Factors Influencing the Prevalence of Rotaviruses and Noroviruses in Wastewater Systems

Several factors influence the distribution and persistence of Rotaviruses and Noroviruses in African wastewater systems.

7.2.2.1 Temperature and Climate

The warm climate across much of Africa supports the stability of enteric viruses in wastewater. Rotaviruses and Noroviruses exhibit higher persistence in moderate temperatures, which aligns with the climatic conditions in many African regions (Mero et al. 2021). Seasonal temperature variations also influence viral loads, with higher concentrations observed during cooler months in some areas due to enhanced virus stability (Pitkänen 2017).

7.2.2.2 Sanitation Infrastructure

Poor sanitation systems and inadequate wastewater treatment facilities significantly contribute to the prevalence of these viruses in wastewater. In many African countries, untreated or partially treated wastewater is discharged into rivers and other water bodies, facilitating the dissemination of viral pathogens (Chigor and Okoh 2012). Informal settlements and peri-urban areas are particularly vulnerable due to limited access to sanitation facilities (Mans et al. 2016).

7.2.2.3 Human Population Density

High population density in urban centres correlates with increased viral loads in wastewater systems. This is due to the higher volume of human waste entering the wastewater stream, which challenges the management and treatment of waste effectively (Omatola et al. 2024).

7.2.2.4 Rainfall and Water Flow

Heavy rainfall and flooding can lead to untreated wastewater overflow, contributing to the spread of rotaviruses and noroviruses in the environment. Conversely, during dry seasons, reduced water flow may lead to the concentration of viral particles in stagnant water bodies (Pang et al. 2004).

7.2.2.5 Socioeconomic Factors

Limited access to vaccines, poor hygiene practices, and malnutrition among vulnerable populations exacerbate the prevalence of enteric viruses. The lack of public awareness and education on sanitation practices further compounds the problem (Mero et al. 2021).

7.2.2.6 Wastewater Treatment Efficiency

The efficiency of wastewater treatment plants is crucial in determining the viral load in treated effluents. In many African countries, wastewater treatment infrastructure is outdated or poorly maintained, resulting in the incomplete removal of viral pathogens (Ibrahim et al. 2018). Advanced treatment processes, such as ultraviolet disinfection and membrane filtration, are rarely employed, leaving residual Rotaviruses and Noroviruses in treated wastewater (Villamizar-Gallardo et al. 2017).

7.3 Methodologies Used for Detection and Their Merits/Demerits

7.3.1 Cell Culture

According to Atabakhsh et al. (2021), the plaque assay is the most commonly used cell culture-based method to detect enteric viruses such as rotavirus and norovirus in wastewater systems, though they are time-consuming. This further leads to improper ways to reduce viral infectivity in wastewater reclamation systems significantly (Guarino et al. 1996). Cell culture is still the standard method for isolating viruses, but numerous cell lines are necessary for various cultivable viruses (Atabakhsh et al. 2021). In addition, researchers have not yet established an in vitro culture system for many enteric viruses. More sensitive non-culture-based methods, such as reverse transcription polymerase chain reaction (RT-PCR) and other recent advances in molecular detection methods, have provided high accuracy in detecting enteric viruses from wastewater systems (Hamza et al. 2011; Villamizar-Gallardo et al. 2017).

7.3.2 Immunological Detection

Determining the presence of rotavirus in wastewater systems is based on identifying protein antigens on the virus surface (VP6, VP7) (Atabakhsh et al. 2021). This has been made possible using an antigen detection method for most monitoring studies known as EIA (enzyme immunoassay), which uses rotavirus-specific antibodies to capture the antigen onto the wells of plates in proprietary kits (Javdani et al. 2012; Zafari et al. 2018). More than 85% of samples were detected with ELISA (enzyme-linked immunosorbent assay) in a study by Soltan et al. (2016). The advantages of this technique for detecting enteric viruses are its high sensitivity, specificity, and adaptability features to large sample volumes without the need for specialised equipment. Although serological methods are often utilised, they have the drawback of pretreating the sample to concentrate the viral content (Ruggeri et al. 2011; Javdani et al. 2012; Kargar et al. 2013).

7.3.3 Immunomagnetic Particles

This technique was developed to efficiently determine and concentrate multiple virus types, like RVA and HAdV, in water and wastewater samples. According to Ruggeri et al. (2011), using an antibody as the molecular receptor would ensure that the captured antigen corresponds to the intact infectious particles. Villamizar-Gallardo et al. (2017) further showed that the magnetic features of microparticles enable the

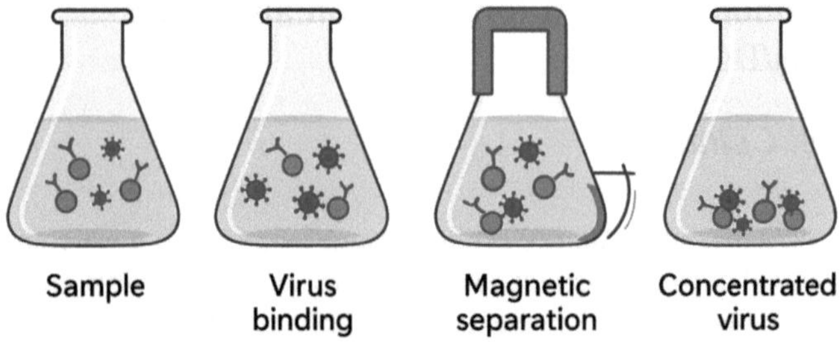

Fig. 7.5 Rotavirus concentrated with magnetofluorescent microparticles conjugated using an antigen-antibody reaction for RV detection

concentration and separation of the viral particles from the water, as shown in Fig. 7.5. This technique's advantage is its quantitative, rapid, and sensitive nature in capturing, separating, concentrating, and detecting infectious Rotavirus in water (Atabakhsh et al. 2021). The background interferences, such as PCR suppressors, are always eliminated. The only drawback of this technique is that it is costly and not user-friendly.

7.3.4 Microscopic Characterisation

This is a vital technique for detecting viruses in water and wastewater systems. It can be integrated with immuno methods to improve viral detection or localise viral antigens. It can also be used with transmission electron microscopy (TEM) and atomic force microscopy to confirm the presence of anti-RV antibodies connected to the magnetic microparticle surfaces and the surface of the bond viruses (Atabakhsh et al. 2021). The advantages of this technique are its simplicity, speed, good preservation of the three-dimensional structure of the viral structure and high resolution (Nakata et al. 1987). The only drawback is that quantification of the virus is time-consuming and expensive.

7.3.5 Molecular Methods

Polymerase chain reaction (PCR) has been introduced as the preferred molecular technique for RV counting, characterised by high sensitivity and potential detection of viruses that cannot be cultured (He et al. 2009; Chigor and Okoh 2012; Ibrahim et al. 2018). This is a faster and more reliable technique compared to culture techniques. This technique also assists in the quantitative determination of viruses and measures the viral particles. According to Pang et al. (2004), the sensitivity of enteric virus detection led to the use of real-time PCR (qPCR), which is mostly used in monoplex mode, where a single virus type can be quantified. Most qPCR methods available for genogrouping, such as the TaqMan and the SYBR green assays, target the VP6 gene (Atabakhsh et al. 2021). qPCR is preferable in terms of sensitivity when integrated with electron microscopy or immunological methods. The technique is extremely expensive and does not determine the infectivity of the viral particle detected.

7.3.6 Immunomagnetic Separation (IMS) Combined with Quantitative Reverse Transcription Polymerase Chain Reaction (RT-qPCR)

This method has been developed using reverse transcription polymerase chain reaction (IMS-RT-qPCR) to quantify and detect the rotavirus in water and wastewater samples (Atabakhsh et al. 2021). The sensitivity of this integrated technique is found to be one order of magnitude better than that of extracting RNA with commercial kits. It can also purify and detect RV seeded in 10^3-fold concentrated wastewater influents and other contaminated water samples. Yang et al. (2011) reported that this technique has shown higher reliability in detecting potentially infectious enteric viruses (Rotavirus and Norovirus) and presented proper and worthwhile outputs for evaluating the virus's health risks, which can hardly be cultured in vitro. Its detection rate is rapid, sensitive, and reliable, and it can detect Rota/Norovirus in extremely contaminated water. The only challenge is that it is specific to an assay.

7.3.7 Integrated Cell Culture RT-PCR (ICC- RT-PCR)

In this technique, cell culturing is done before the qPCR to enable replication and detection of the infectious Rotavirus, which may infect the cells and generate RNA. Due to its sensitivity, more than 42% of the RVs have been detected with ICC-RT-PCR, while only 21% and 12% of samples were positive with plaque counting or the RT-qPCR method (Li et al. 2010). The sensitivity of the ICC-RT-PCR method to detect RV, even at very low concentrations, has been evaluated. It is considered a fast and quantitative procedure to determine infectious RV in environmental waters, differentiating them from the inactivated RV. The disadvantage is that it is very expensive.

7.3.8 Next-Generation Sequencing (NGS)

This is an umbrella of several techniques developed some decades ago (Atabakhsh et al. 2021). NGS is a new technology used for DNA and RNA sequencing and variant/mutation detection that can sequence hundreds and thousands of genes or whole genomes quickly (Pitkänen 2017). This technique is widely accepted for parallel sequencing and has unique advantages in microbial ecology because of high throughput and capabilities of sequencing large numbers of different DNA (massively parallel) samples at once (Atabakhsh et al. 2021), unlike other sister techniques such as Sanger reaction which returns a single DNA sequence. Identifying transcripts can be done without prior knowledge of a particular gene or simultaneously taking alternative splicing and sequence variation into account (Damanka et al. 2019). The merits of this technique include offering an unlimited opportunity to examine samples. However, it has the characteristic of producing massive quantities of data, making data analysis procedures compulsory. This technique also creates an excess of one billion short reads per instrument run, which makes them useful for many biological applications. It further leads to massively parallel sequencing and single input of DNA/RNA. Finally, this technique can also perform simultaneous screening of multiple genes in multiple samples, quantitative and sensitive detection of genomic aberrations, and decreased sequencing costs per gene. The demerit is that it is expensive and has a time-consuming sample preparation protocol. The lack of bioinformatics skills also limits its use in many instances.

7.4 Gains in Detecting Rotaviruses and Noroviruses in Wastewater

7.4.1 Public Health Implications

Detecting Rotaviruses and Noroviruses in wastewater systems provides critical insights into the burden of these pathogens in communities, offering a non-invasive approach to monitoring population health. Wastewater surveillance serves as an early warning system for outbreaks of gastroenteritis caused by these viruses, enabling timely public health interventions. This is particularly significant in African settings, where outbreaks of diarrhoeal diseases remain a leading cause of morbidity and mortality, especially among children under five years old (Omatola et al. 2024).

By quantifying the viral load in wastewater, health authorities can identify hotspots of viral activity and assess the effectiveness of public health measures such as vaccination campaigns and sanitation improvements. Wastewater-based epidemiology (WBE) also allows for monitoring the success of rotavirus vaccination programs in Africa. For instance, countries that have introduced vaccines such as Rotarix® into their immunisation schedules have reduced severe diarrhoeal cases caused by Rotaviruses (Trainor et al. 2013; Tate et al. 2012). Similarly, Norovirus surveillance in wastewater provides valuable data on seasonal patterns, enabling more targeted public health responses during peak transmission periods (Mans et al. 2016).

Additionally, wastewater surveillance has significant implications for addressing inequities in healthcare access. In resource-limited settings, where clinical diagnostic facilities may be inadequate or inaccessible, wastewater detection provides a cost-effective method to estimate disease prevalence across communities (Chigor and Okoh 2012). It also facilitates tracking the emergence of new viral strains and variants, which is vital for guiding vaccine development and other preventive strategies.

7.4.2 Advancements in Research and Practice

Detecting Rotaviruses and Noroviruses in wastewater has driven advancements in virological research and environmental health practices. Innovations in molecular techniques, such as real-time PCR (RT-qPCR) and next-generation sequencing (NGS), have enhanced the sensitivity and accuracy of virus detection in wastewater, allowing for the identification of specific genotypes and variants (Atabakhsh et al. 2021; Pitkänen 2017). These advancements have improved our understanding of the genetic diversity and evolutionary dynamics of Rotaviruses and Noroviruses circulating in African settings.

The integration of advanced detection methods, such as immunomagnetic separation combined with RT-qPCR (IMS-RTqPCR), has facilitated the rapid and quantitative detection of viruses in highly contaminated wastewater samples. This technology has proven more reliable and sensitive than conventional culture-based methods, which are often time-consuming and less effective for detecting non-culturable or low-concentration viruses (Yang et al. 2011).

Furthermore, wastewater surveillance has fostered multidisciplinary collaboration among virologists, epidemiologists, environmental scientists, and public health practitioners. This collaboration has enabled the development of robust frameworks for WBE, which are increasingly being implemented in African countries to monitor enteric virus prevalence and assess the impact of public health interventions (Mans et al. 2016; Omatola et al. 2024).

Research advancements have also highlighted the role of environmental factors in virus survival and transmission, providing valuable data for designing interventions to improve wastewater treatment systems. Improved understanding of the resilience of Rotaviruses and Noroviruses in wastewater has informed the development of disinfection strategies, such as ultraviolet treatment and membrane filtration, to enhance the removal of viral pathogens (Ibrahim et al. 2018; Villamizar-Gallardo et al. 2017).

The gains in detecting Rotaviruses and Noroviruses in wastewater systems have paved the way for innovative public health solutions, contributing to disease prevention, health equity, and the advancement of global health security.

7.5 Challenges in Detection of Rotaviruses and Noroviruses in Wastewater Systems

Detecting Rotaviruses and Noroviruses in wastewater systems presents several challenges, particularly in resource-limited settings across Africa. One of the primary issues is the lack of standardised methods for viral detection. Although molecular techniques such as RT-qPCR have become the gold standard, their application is limited by high costs, the need for skilled personnel, and inadequate laboratory infrastructure (Atabakhsh et al. 2021).

The sensitivity of detection methods is another critical challenge. Low viral loads in wastewater and high levels of organic matter and chemical inhibitors often interfere with accurate virus quantification (Pang et al. 2004). These inhibitors reduce the efficiency of nucleic acid extraction and amplification, leading to false negatives or underestimation of viral prevalence.

Sample collection and concentration methods also affect detection reliability. The diversity of wastewater matrices requires robust concentration protocols, yet many commonly used techniques, such as ultracentrifugation or polyethylene glycol precipitation, are labour-intensive, time-consuming, and may not efficiently recover all virus particles (Hamza et al. 2011).

Another significant barrier is the high cost and maintenance of advanced detection tools, such as next-generation sequencing (NGS), which can identify viral variants but are often inaccessible in low-resource settings. Additionally, integrating multiple detection techniques, such as immunomagnetic separation with RT-qPCR, while improving sensitivity, adds complexity and expense (Yang et al. 2011).

Environmental conditions, including temperature, pH, and the presence of other microorganisms, also influence virus stability in wastewater, further complicating detection efforts. Inadequate disinfection and wastewater treatment practices exacerbate these challenges, as residual viral pathogens may persist in treated effluents and downstream water bodies (Chigor and Okoh 2012).

7.6 Knowledge Gaps and Future Directions

Limited data exist on the long-term epidemiology of Rotaviruses and Noroviruses in African wastewater systems. More comprehensive surveillance programs are needed to monitor viral prevalence, diversity, and seasonality, particularly in rural and peri-urban areas. Future research should also explore the correlation between wastewater viral loads and clinical cases to establish WBE as a reliable public health tool (Omatola et al. 2024).

7.6.1 Standardised Detection Methods

Developing affordable, robust, and user-friendly diagnostic tools for low-resource settings is a priority. Novel approaches, such as microfluidic devices and portable qPCR systems, could facilitate on-site wastewater testing. Additionally, establishing standardised protocols for sample collection, concentration, and analysis will enhance the comparability and reliability of results across studies (Villamizar-Gallardo et al. 2017). Protocols should account for the unique characteristics of wastewater matrices in different African settings.

7.6.2 Environmental Persistence and Transmission Dynamics

There is a need to better understand the environmental factors influencing the persistence and transmission of Rotaviruses and Noroviruses in wastewater systems. Studies on viral survival under varying temperatures, pH, and ultraviolet exposure conditions could inform the design of more effective wastewater treatment processes (Mans et al. 2016).

7.6.3 Integration of Advanced Technologies

Leveraging advanced molecular tools, such as metagenomics and NGS, can provide deeper insights into viral evolution, recombination, and emerging strains. Thus, wider implementation of NGS and other advanced molecular tools can enhance the detection of viral variants and provide valuable insights into the evolution and epidemiology of Rotaviruses and Noroviruses. However, efforts must be made to reduce the costs and technical barriers associated with these technologies to ensure widespread adoption in low-resource African research settings (Pitkänen 2017).

7.6.4 Capacity Building and Infrastructure Development

Investments in laboratory infrastructure, advanced detection technologies, and workforce training are essential to enhance the capacity for wastewater surveillance.

Portable and affordable diagnostic tools, such as microfluidic PCR systems, should be prioritised for resource-limited settings. Furthermore, enhancing the efficiency of wastewater treatment systems is essential to reducing the environmental dissemination of viral pathogens. Strategies such as adopting ultraviolet disinfection, advanced membrane filtration, and improved chlorination practices should be explored and implemented.

7.6.5 Public Health Impact of Treated Effluents

Further research is needed to assess the risks posed by treated wastewater released into the environment or used for irrigation. Quantifying the infectivity of viruses in treated effluents and evaluating their potential to cause disease outbreaks will help refine wastewater reuse policies and guidelines (Ibrahim et al. 2018). Therefore, WBE should be integrated with clinical surveillance programs to understand viral prevalence and transmission dynamics comprehensively. Data-sharing platforms and collaborations between researchers, health authorities, and policymakers will help translate findings into actionable public health interventions.

7.6.6 Vaccine Efficacy in Environmental Contexts

Expanding access to Rotavirus and Norovirus vaccines, particularly in underserved populations, is critical to reducing viral prevalence in wastewater. Public education campaigns on sanitation, hygiene, and the risks of untreated wastewater exposure can further mitigate transmission. However, despite widespread vaccination efforts for Rotavirus, the impact of vaccines on reducing viral loads in wastewater remains poorly understood. Investigating how vaccination campaigns influence wastewater virus prevalence and strain diversity could provide valuable insights into vaccine effectiveness and inform future immunisation strategies (Trainor et al. 2013).

7.6.7 Community Awareness and Engagement

Addressing knowledge gaps among communities regarding sanitation, hygiene, and the risks associated with wastewater contamination is critical. Public education campaigns and behavioural interventions could significantly reduce the transmission of enteric viruses, complementing technical advances in wastewater management.

7.6.8 *Collaboration and Funding Support*

Regional and international collaborations should be strengthened to support wastewater surveillance initiatives. Dedicated funding mechanisms are required to sustain research, capacity-building efforts, and the implementation of innovative technologies in African countries.

7.7 Conclusions and Recommendations

Rotaviruses and Noroviruses are widely distributed in African wastewater systems, reflecting the high burden of gastroenteritis caused by these pathogens. The prevalence of these viruses in wastewater is particularly significant in regions with inadequate sanitation, poor access to healthcare, and limited vaccination coverage. Environmental factors such as temperature, rainfall, and human population density influence the distribution and persistence of these viruses, with higher viral loads detected in urban and peri-urban wastewater systems.

Detection methodologies have advanced significantly, with molecular techniques such as RT-qPCR, next-generation sequencing (NGS), and immunomagnetic separation (IMS) providing high sensitivity and accuracy. However, challenges persist in high costs, technical complexity, and inhibitors in wastewater samples that compromise detection reliability. Though widely used, conventional methods like cell culture and plaque assays remain time-consuming and less sensitive than molecular approaches.

Wastewater-based epidemiology (WBE) offers a promising public health surveillance tool. Still, its potential is constrained by limited infrastructure, a lack of standardised protocols, and inadequate integration with clinical data. Moreover, gaps in understanding the environmental persistence of these viruses, their genetic diversity, and their public health implications further hinder progress.

References

Abdulazeez MS, Al-Shuwaikh AM, Latif II (2020) Detection and comparison of sapovirus, rotavirus and norovirus among infants and young children with acute gastroenteritis. Ann Trop Med Public Health 23:231–439

Alfajaro MM, Choi JS, Kim DS, Seo JY, Kim JY, Park JG, Soliman M, Baek YB, Cho EH, Kwon J, Kwon HJ (2017) Activation of COX-2/PGE2 promotes sapovirus replication via the inhibition of nitric oxide production. J Virol 91(3):10–1128

Anderson EJ (2010) Prevention and treatment of viral diarrhoea in pediatrics. Expert Rev Anti-Infect Ther 8(2):205–217

Atabakhsh P, Kargar M, Doosti A (2021) Detection and evaluation of rotavirus surveillance methods as viral indicator in the aquatic environments. Braz J Microbiol 52(2):811–820

Ayukekbong JA, Mesumbe HN, Oyero OG, Lindh M, Bergström T (2015) Role of noroviruses as aetiological agents of diarrhoea in developing countries. J Gen Virol 96(8):1983–1999
Badur S, Öztürk S, Pereira P, Abdel Ghany M, Khalaf M, Lagoubi Y, Ozudogru O, Hanif K, Saha D Systematic review of the rotavirus infection burden in the WHO-EMRO region. Hum Vaccin Immunother 15(11):2754–2768. https://doi.org/10.1080/21645515.2019.1603984
Campillay-Véliz CP, Carvajal JJ, Avellaneda AM, Escobar D, Covián C, Kalergis AM, Lay MK (2020) Human norovirus proteins: implications in the replicative cycle, pathogenesis, and the host immune response. Front Immunol 11:961
Chigor VN, Okoh AI (2012) Quantitative RT-PCR detection of hepatitis A virus, rotaviruses and enteroviruses in the Buffalo River and source water dams in the Eastern Cape Province of South Africa. Int J Environ Res Public Health 9(11):4017–4032
Chouchane H, Hoekstra AY, Krol MS, Mekonnen MM (2015) The water footprint of Tunisia from an economic perspective. Ecol Indic 52:311–319
Crawford SE, Ramani S, Tate JE, Parashar UD, Svensson L, Hagbom M, Franco MA, Greenberg HB, O'Ryan M, Kang G, Desselberger U (2017) Rotavirus infection. Nature Reviews Disease Primers 3(1):1–16
Damanka SA, Kwofie S, Dennis FE, Lartey BL, Agbemabiese CA, Doan YH, Adiku TK, Katayama K, Enweronu-Laryea CC, Armah GE (2019) Whole genome characterisation and evolutionary analysis of OP354-like P [8] rotavirus A strains isolated from Ghanaian children with diarrhoea. PLoS One 14(6):0218348
Dennehy PH (2015) Rotavirus infection: a disease of the past? Infect Dis Clin 29(4):617–635
Dieter CA (2018) Water availability and use science program: estimated use of water in the United States in 2015. Geological Survey
Ghosh S, Malik YS, Kobayashi N (2018) Therapeutics and immunoprophylaxis against noroviruses and rotaviruses: the past, present, and future. Curr Drug Metab 19(3):170–191
Glass RI, Parashar UD, Estes MK (2009) Norovirus gastroenteritis. N Engl J Med 361(18): 1776–1785
Guarino A, Casola A, Bruzzese E, Saini M, Nitsch L, Rubino A (1996) Human serum immunoglobulin counteracts rotaviral infection in Caco-2 cells. Pediatr Res 40(6):881–887
Hamza IA, Jurzik L, Überla K, Wilhelm M (2011) Methods to detect infectious human enteric viruses in environmental water samples. Int J Hyg Environ Health 214(6):424–436
He XQ, Cheng L, Zhang DY, Li W, Xie XM, Ma M, Wang ZJ (2009) First molecular detection of group A rotaviruses in drinking water sources in Beijing, China. Bull Environ Contam Toxicol 83:120–124
Ibrahim C, Hassen A, Pothier P, Mejri S, Hammami S (2018) Molecular detection and genotypic characterisation of enteric adenoviruses in a hospital wastewater. Environ Sci Pollut Res 25: 10977–10987
Inns T, Harris J, Vivancos R, Iturriza-Gomara M, O'Brien S (2017) Community-based surveillance of norovirus disease: a systematic review. BMC Infect Dis 17:1–10
Javdani N, Kargar M, Ghodsi M (2012) The assessment of efficiency of eliminating group A human rotaviruses in urban and hospitalised sewage refining system of Shiraz city. J Med Sci 22(3): 226–231
Kargar M, Javdani N, Najafi A, Tahamtan Y (2013) First molecular detection of group A rotavirus in urban and hospital sewage systems by nested-RT PCR in Shiraz, Iran. J Environ Health Sci Eng 11:1–6
LeClair CE, McConnell KA (2023) Rotavirus. In: StatPearls [Internet]. StatPearls Publishing
Li D, Gu AZ, Yang W, He M, Hu XH, Shi HC (2010) An integrated cell culture and reverse transcription quantitative PCR assay for detection of infectious rotaviruses in environmental waters. J Microbiol Methods 82(1):59–63
Li TF, Hosmillo M, Schwanke H, Shu T, Wang Z, Yin L, Curry S, Goodfellow IG, Zhou X (2018) Human norovirus NS3 has RNA helicase and chaperoning activities. J Virol 92(5):10–1128

Liu L, Oza S, Hogan D, Perin J, Rudan I, Lawn JE, Cousens S, Mathers C, Black RE (2015) Global, regional, and national causes of child mortality in 2000–13, with projections to inform post-2015 priorities: an updated systematic analysis. Lancet 385(9966):430–440

Mans J (2018) Longitudinal Seroprevalence study elucidates high norovirus burden in sub-Saharan Africa. J Infect Dis 218(5):676–678

Mans J, Netshikweta R, Magwalivha M, Van Zyl WB, Taylor MB (2013) Diverse norovirus genotypes identified in sewage-polluted river water in South Africa. Epidemiol Infect 141(2): 303–313

Mans J, Murray TY, Nadan S, Netshikweta R, Page NA, Taylor MB (2016) Norovirus diversity in children with gastroenteritis in South Africa from 2009 to 2013: GII. 4 variants and recombinant strains predominate. Epidemiology & Infection 144(5):907–916

Mayo MA (2002) Virus taxonomy-Houston 2002. Arch Virol 147(5):1071–1076

Mero S, Timonen S, Lääveri T, Løfberg S, Kirveskari J, Ursing J, Rombo L, Kofoed PE, Kantele A (2021) Prevalence of diarrhoeal pathogens among children under five years of age with and without diarrhoea in Guinea-Bissau. PLoS Negl Trop Dis 15(9):0009709

Nakata S, Petrie BL, Calomeni EP, Estes MK (1987) Electron microscopy procedure influences detection of rotaviruses. J Clin Microbiol 25(10):1902–1906

Nansubuga I, Banadda N, Verstraete W, Rabaey K (2016) A review of sustainable sanitation systems in Africa. Rev Environ Sci Biotechnol 15:465–478

Nyairo WN, Owuor PO, Kengara FO (2015) Effect of anthropogenic activities on the water quality of Amala and Nyangores tributaries of River Mara in Kenya. Environ Monit Assess 187:1–12

Omatola CA, Olaniran AO (2022) Genetic heterogeneity of group A rotaviruses: a review of the evolutionary dynamics and implication on vaccination. Expert Rev Anti-Infect Ther 20(12): 1587–1602

Omatola CA, Ogunsakin RE, Onoja AB, Okolo MLO, Abraham-Oyiguh J, Mofolorunsho KC, Akoh PQ, Adejo OP, Idakwo J, Okeme TO, Muhammed D (2024) Enteropathogenic viruses associated with acute gastroenteritis among African children under 5 years of age: A systematic review and meta-analysis. J Infect 88(6):106169

Pang XL, Lee B, Boroumand N, Leblanc B, Preiksaitis JK, Yu Ip CC (2004) Increased detection of rotavirus using a real-time reverse transcription-polymerase chain reaction (RT-PCR) assay in stool specimens from children with diarrhea. J Med Virol 72(3):496–501

Patel MM, Hall AJ, Vinjé J, Parashar UD (2009) Noroviruses: a comprehensive review. J Clin Virol 44(1):1–8

Pitkänen O (2017). Rotavirus whole genome sequencing with next-generation sequencing (Master's dissertation)

Ruggeri FM, Delogu R, Petouchoff T, Tcheremenskaia O, De Petris S, Fiore L, RotaNet-Italy Study Group (2011) Molecular characterisation of rotavirus strains from children with diarrhoea in Italy, 2007–2009. J Med Virol 83(9):1657–1668

Shane AL, Mody RK, Crump JA, Tarr PI, Steiner TS, Kotloff K, Langley JM, Wanke C, Warren CA, Cheng AC, Cantey J (2017) Infectious Diseases Society of America clinical practice guidelines for the diagnosis and management of infectious diarrhea. Clin Infect Dis 65(12): 45–80

Soltan MA, Tsai YL, Lee PYA, Tsai CF, Chang HFG, Wang HTT, Wilkes RP (2016) Comparison of electron microscopy, ELISA, real-time RT-PCR and insulated isothermal RT-PCR for the detection of Rotavirus group A (RVA) in feces of different animal species. J Virol Methods 235: 99–104

Tate JE, Burton AH, Boschi-Pinto C, Steele AD, Duque J, Parashar UD (2012) 2008 estimate of worldwide rotavirus-associated mortality in children younger than 5 years before the introduction of universal rotavirus vaccination programmes: a systematic review and meta-analysis. Lancet Infect Dis 12(2):136–141

The World Bank (2021) Population, total—Sub-Saharan Africa, The World Bank. [Available at: https://data.worldbank.org/indicator/SP.POP.TOTL?locations=ZG]. Accessed: 31 Jan 2025

Trainor E, Lopman B, Iturriza-Gomara M, Dove W, Ngwira B, Nakagomi O, Nakagomi T, Parashar U, Cunliffe N (2013) Detection and molecular characterisation of noroviruses in hospitalised children in Malawi, 1997–2007. J Med Virol 85(7):1299–1306

Villamizar-Gallardo RA, Osma JF, Ortíz OO (2017) New technique for direct fluoroimmunomagnetic detection of rotavirus in water samples. J Water Health 15(6):932–941

WHO (World Health Organization) (2009) Rotavirus vaccines: an update. Wkly Epidemiol Rec 84(51–52):533–537

Yang W, Gu AZ, Zeng SY, Li D, He M, Shi HC (2011) Development of a combined immunomagnetic separation and quantitative reverse transcription-PCR assay for sensitive detection of infectious rotavirus in water samples. J Microbiol Methods 84(3):447–453

Zafari E, Soleimanjahi H, Mohammadi A, Teimoori A, Mahravani H (2018) Molecular and biological characterisation of the human-bovine rotavirus-based reassortant rotavirus. Microb Pathog 121:65–69

Chapter 8
Environmental Reservoirs of Viral Infections in Africa

Akebe Luther King Abia, Therese Mulyangote, and Etando Ayukafangha

8.1 Introduction: Overview of Viral Disease Burden in Africa

Viruses have a long history in human (and animal) infections, demonstrated by the numerous pandemics they have caused since the time before Christ (430 BC) until recent years (Sampath et al. 2021). Although medicine has made significant strides in treating and preventing these infections through the discovery and use of several new drugs and vaccines, viral diseases still constitute a leading cause of morbidity and mortality globally (Baker et al. 2022; Li et al. 2024, 2025; Naghavi et al. 2024; Sirota et al. 2025). Furthermore, although medical advances have led to a global shift from infectious to non-communicable diseases, the progression is disparate, with the Sub-Saharan African region still significantly suffering from a high infectious disease burden, including those caused by viruses (Bloom 2025). Viruses that still have a significant adverse effect on public health in Africa include the Human Immunodeficiency Virus (HIV), Hepatitis Viruses (HBV and HCV), Measles Virus, SARS-CoV-2 (COVID-19), Arboviruses, Filoviruses, Lassa Fever Virus, Rabies Virus and many enteric viruses.

A. L. K. Abia (✉)
Total Environment Research (TEN-R) Group, College of Health Sciences, University of KwaZulu-Natal, Durban, South Africa

Environmental Research Foundation, Westville, South Africa

T. Mulyangote
Antimicrobial Research Unit, College of Health Sciences, University of KwaZulu-Natal, Durban, South Africa

Eswatini Medical Christian University, Mbabane, Eswatini

E. Ayukafangha
Antimicrobial Research Unit, College of Health Sciences, University of KwaZulu-Natal, Durban, South Africa

J. A. Shenge, A. L. K. Abia (eds.), *Viral Diseases and One Health in Africa*,
https://doi.org/10.1007/978-3-032-09613-5_8

HIV remains one of the most significant viral health burdens globally, with sub-Saharan Africa being the global epicentre of the epidemic, accounting for approximately two-thirds of the global HIV prevalence and associated deaths (UNAIDS 2025). According to the UNAIDS regional estimates, more than 26 million people were living with HIV in sub-Saharan Africa in 2024 (regional totals: ~21.1 million in eastern and southern Africa; ~5.2 million in western and central Africa) (UNAIDS 2025). Viral subtypes, including HIV-1 group M subtypes A, B, C, D, G and circulating recombinant forms, circulate widely across the region (Adhiambo et al. 2021).

Enteric viruses constitute a large group of viruses that are well-known for their role in gastrointestinal infections (Bishop and Kirkwood 2008). These viruses include rotaviruses, caliciviruses, adenoviruses, astroviruses, measles virus, reoviruses, polioviruses, coxsackieviruses, hepatitis A and E viruses, HIV and cytomegalovirus (Bishop and Kirkwood 2008) and are classified according to their mode of infection and how they cause disease. The intestinal tract, known for its nutrient-rich environment, ideal temperature, and actively dividing epithelial cells, represents a conducive setting for viral reproduction. Thus, a key consideration with this group of viruses within the African context is that they are shed through faeces and therefore have a marked environmental footprint, which favours their transmission and spread within the continent.

Chronic hepatitis B (HBV) and hepatitis C (HCV) infections represent a significant, yet underdiagnosed cause of liver disease and liver-related mortality in Africa. In 2022, the WHO regional office reported that over 90 million Africans lived with chronic HBV or HCV infection, accounting for approximately 125,000 hepatitis-attributable deaths in 2020 (WHO Regional Office for Africa 2022). HBV is highly endemic in many countries, with childhood infections, perinatal transmission and low diagnosis and treatment coverage contributing substantially to long-term disease burden (Sonderup and Spearman 2024; WHO Regional Office for Africa 2022).

Measles, a vaccine-preventable disease, continues to cause substantial mortality in Africa, particularly among unvaccinated children. Global modelling and surveillance data indicate a marked resurgence in measles incidence and estimated mortality following declines in routine immunisation coverage during the COVID-19 pandemic (Parums 2024). The Democratic Republic of Congo, Ethiopia, and Nigeria were the top three countries with the lowest immunisation coverage rates globally between 2019 and 2022 (Minta et al. 2023). Estimated measles deaths rose from approximately 95,000 in 2021 to 136,200 in 2022, with a high proportion of disruptive outbreaks occurring in African countries (Minta et al. 2023).

The incidence of Dengue is on the rise in Africa and is increasingly recognised as an emergent public-health concern in many countries (Xia and Dong 2025). Although varying annual dengue cases have been reported worldwide, there is a substantial and growing burden within the African continent (Mercy et al. 2024; Poongavanan et al. 2024). Despite the low mortality rates in well-resourced settings, this may not be the case in outbreaks with delayed recognition or limited clinical care, such as in Africa (Xia and Dong 2025). Other Arboviruses, such as the Yellow Fever Virus (WHO Africa, 2024), the Chikungunya virus (CDC 2025; ECDC 2025;

NICD 2025), the Zika virus (Baraka and Kweka 2016), and the Rift Valley fever virus (Ndishimye et al. 2024), continue to cause periodic outbreaks with localised mortality and sometimes broader public-health impact within the continent.

Filoviruses (Ebola and Marburg Viruses) have also been reported in Africa. Ebola virus (Zaire, Sudan, Bundibugyo species) has been the cause of multiple high-fatality outbreaks in West and Central Africa, with the largest reported outbreak being the one that occurred in West Africa between 2014 and 2016 (WHO 2025a). Marburg virus has similarly caused sporadic, deadly epidemics in East and Central Africa linked to cave or bat exposures (Semancik et al. 2024; Stephens et al. 2022). These outbreaks have been driven mainly by a combination of socioeconomic factors and deficiencies in health systems, among others (Stephens et al. 2022).

Other viral infections that have been reported in Africa over the years include COVID-19 caused by the SARS-CoV-2 virus (Africa CDC, 2021), Lassa fever, which is endemic to some West African countries and caused by the Lassa Fever virus (Aleke et al. 2023), rabies, with an estimated annual death toll of up to 25,000, is caused by the Rabies virus (Nyasulu et al. 2021).

8.2 Viruses in the Environment in Africa

The environment plays a pivotal role as a reservoir and vehicle for pathogenic microorganisms, including viruses. Water, soil, and air are among the environmental reservoirs that sustain and spread these viruses, making it easier for them to spread to people and animals. Although some of these viruses have animals as their primary hosts, human interference with the environment has resulted in some of these viruses infecting humans as an alternative to their natural host (da Silva et al. 2021). The environmental presence of viruses is particularly important within the African context, where the relationship between people and their natural environment is deeply intertwined, with traditional beliefs often emphasising a spiritual connection to nature and a holistic view of the world (Amanze 2024). This connection manifests in various ways, including the sacredness of certain natural features, the use of natural resources for sustenance and cultural practices, and a strong emphasis on maintaining a harmonious balance with the environment (Awoyemi et al. 2024; Mpofu 2021). These connections, which once posed minimal risk in a pristine environment, now represent a massive challenge in an era of astronomically increasing environmental pollution with diverse pollutants, particularly microbial ones, including viruses. Thus, in present-day Africa, a gross lack of sanitation increases the risk of exposure to these pathogenic viruses. Therefore, the following section focuses on water, soil and air as environmental reservoirs in Africa. It is, however, essential to know that the role of wildlife as reservoirs of viral infections is not ignored but rather considered as zoonotic in the context of this chapter.

8.2.1 Water as an Environmental Reservoir

Water plays a critical role as a reservoir for enteric viruses in Africa, especially in contexts of limited sanitation infrastructure (Okoh et al. 2010). Human enteroviruses, including hepatitis A virus (HAV), hepatitis E virus (HEV), noroviruses, poliovirus, and rotaviruses, often contaminate surface water and groundwater via human and animal faecal discharge (e.g. through deficient treatment systems or agricultural runoff) (Gall et al. 2015; Nwachcuku and Gerba 2004; Nwachuku et al. 2005; WHO 2025b). For instance, HAV can survive for months in both fresh and salt water, owing to its stability at varying temperatures and pH levels. Therefore, the transmission of enteric viruses to humans poses significant challenges in underdeveloped countries, including those in Africa, where it is believed that 80–90% of untreated or poorly treated sewage is discharged into rivers, streams, and various aquatic ecosystems, polluting the surrounding environment (Upfold et al. 2021). African countries, especially in the Sub-Saharan region, are particularly at risk for infectious diseases due to high population density and lack of proper sanitation facilities, with an estimated 55% of urban residents currently living in informal settlements (Upfold et al. 2021; van de Vossenberg et al. 2021). In rural and peri-urban communities, seasonal rainfall and flooding events can increase viral load in surface waters (Levy et al. 2018) due to overflow from sewer systems (Perry et al. 2024) and open defecation (Fagunwa et al. 2025). Viruses such as Rift Valley fever virus (RVFV) may also indirectly be linked to water reservoirs through mosquito breeding sites associated with stagnant water bodies (Anyamba et al. 2010).

Another major issue associated with the presence of viruses in African aquatic ecosystems is that most African countries rely on surface water as their primary source for drinking water production. With suboptimal treatment, viruses from polluted rivers could pass through the drinking water system, ending up in households. For example, a study conducted in South Africa in 2005 examined human adenoviruses in treated drinking water (Van Heerden et al. 2005). Furthermore, viruses in the environment can infiltrate and end up in wells and boreholes. In Benin, West Africa, scientists reported the presence of adenoviruses and rotaviruses in water samples collected from wells and boreholes, and attributed this to the presence of latrines in proximity to the water sources (Verheyen et al. 2009).

The presence of viruses in the water environment in Africa has led to wastewater-based epidemiology (WBE) being increasingly employed as a surveillance tool for viral diseases on the continent. During the COVID-19 pandemic, some countries like South Africa implemented WBE systems to detect SARS-CoV-2 RNA in wastewater, often preceding clinical case detection and enabling early public health responses (Johnson et al. 2021; Street et al. 2021; WHO Africa 2022). Similarly, in Zambia, SARS-CoV-2 RNA was detected in wastewater with temporal trends that mirrored clinical incidence, reinforcing WBE's utility in early warning systems (Shempela et al. 2024).

8.2.2 Soil as an Environmental Reservoir

Soil can act as a long-term reservoir for various enteric viruses, particularly in contexts where contaminated sludge or wastewater is applied to land. Experimental studies have shown that some viruses can persist in moist, cool soil for extended periods, sometimes several months, whereas survival is significantly shorter in warmer or drier conditions (Vasickova and Kovarcik 2013), depending on the soil type. The transition between moist and drying conditions leads to distinct inactivation mechanisms, moisture-related degradation of viral RNA and desiccation-related capsid damage (Yeagert and O'brien 1979). It has been shown that clay-rich soils tend to bind and preserve viral particles more effectively than sandy or organic soils (Guardabassi et al. 2003; Vasickova and Kovarcik 2013). For example, poliovirus survived up to 110–130 days in loamy soil at 3–10 °C, compared to only 40–90 days at higher temperatures (Vasickova and Kovarcik 2013); another study detected viable poliovirus in winter soil for up to 96 days, but only up to 11 days during summer (Tierney et al. 1977). Furthermore, enteric viruses such as HAV, adenoviruses, and enteroviruses can adsorb to soil particles and remain infectious (Gerba and Pepper 2019).

Viral persistence in the soil is therefore a cause for concern, given the low level of environmental sanitation in most African countries. Over 70% of individuals in Eastern and Southern Africa, equating to 340 million people, still lack access to fundamental sanitation services, 19% (98 million people) of whom engage in open defecation (UNICEF, n.d.). Furthermore, most wastewater treatment plants in most of these countries do not function properly, resulting in the discharge of effluent water containing viruses (Osuolale and Okoh 2017). The application of such inadequately treated wastewater sludge as fertiliser can introduce viral pathogens into soils, increasing the risk of contamination of crops and subsequent human exposure (Ali et al. 2023). Soil also plays a role in the ecology of zoonotic viruses such as RVFV, which persists in mosquito eggs embedded in moist soils until flooding triggers hatching and subsequent transmission cycles (Linthicum et al. 1985).

8.2.3 Air as an Environmental (Aerosol) Reservoir

Airborne transmission of viruses is a well-recognised public health concern. It is a significant pathway for respiratory viruses such as influenza, measles, SARS-CoV-2, and respiratory syncytial virus (RSV) (Setti et al. 2020). *Bioaerosols*, comprising bacteria, pollen, fungi, and viruses, are suspended in the air via wind, dust storms, or surface turbulence. In sub-Saharan Africa, dust-driven bioaerosols have been linked to meningococcal meningitis outbreaks (among other respiratory infections), illustrating the potential for airborne viral disease spread via environmental particles (Smets et al. 2016). For example, the role of air in spreading zoonotic viruses, such as avian influenza from poultry farms, has been documented in Egypt (Mahmoud et al. 2024; Saad et al. 2024). While direct evidence of viral infection via Sahara dust or urban dust remains limited, studies from other regions suggest the potential for viruses to be carried over long distances attached to dust particles (Nagy et al. 2025; Smets et al. 2016). Moreover, respiratory viruses, including influenza and SARS-CoV-2, can remain viable in aerosol particles for minutes to hours, particularly within enclosed or poorly ventilated settings; such modes of transmission are relevant in healthcare settings across Africa (Alsved et al. 2023; Kalisa et al. 2019; Santarpia et al. 2022; Thuresson et al. 2022).

Table 8.1 is a summary of some studies reporting on the presence of viruses in the environment in Africa.

8.3 Public Health Significance of Viruses in the Environment in Africa

From the studies reviewed in the previous sections of this chapter, it is evident that environmental reservoirs, particularly water, soil, and air, play a crucial role in the persistence, transmission, and epidemiology of viral pathogens in Africa. The continent's diverse climatic zones (Wright et al. 2024), rapid urbanisation (Juma et al. 2020), inadequate sanitation infrastructure (Hlongwa et al. 2024), weak healthcare systems (Oleribe et al. 2019) and a high prevalence of immunocompromising conditions such as HIV/AIDS (Boutayeb 2010) amplify the risks posed by environmental viral contamination.

As noted earlier, the African aquatic ecosystem is a reservoir for numerous diverse enteric viruses originating from the discharge of untreated or poorly treated wastewater from WWTPs and surface runoff from areas without proper sanitation facilities. Therefore, climate change-associated events, such as extreme flooding on the one hand, would exacerbate the risk by mobilising pathogens from human waste into drinking water sources. Populations could be exposed to these viruses by drinking poorly treated water in urban areas or using the polluted surface water sources directly, as in informal settlements and slums without access to potable water. A study in South Africa used quantitative microbial risk assessment to estimate the risk of infection from exposure to polluted river water and reported varying rates depending on the land use around the river (Abia et al. 2016). The authors further demonstrated that any disturbances in the river system due to events like flooding increased the risk of infection by over 50% in some cases. Although this study was based on bacterial pathogens, it shows that exposure to such water sources containing viruses is a health hazard for surrounding populations. Furthermore, people in areas without proper sanitation systems use the same rivers for the disposal of their waste. This creates a cycle of transmission leading to outbreaks of acute gastroenteritis, hepatitis, and other waterborne diseases.

Another important aspect is that flooding will amplify outbreaks, which could also lead to cross-border spread via shared water bodies and movement of people.

Table 8.1 Examples of viruses detected in the environment in Africa

Virus	Disease	Environmental reservoir(s)	Countries reported	References
Adenovirus	Gastroenteritis, respiratory, urinary tract, and eye infections	Surface water, wastewater, drinking water	South Africa, Benin, Ethiopia	Ali et al. (2023), Okoh et al. (2010), Van Heerden et al. (2005), Verheyen et al. (2009)
Rotavirus	Severe diarrhoea in children	River water, drinking water, sewage effluent	Benin, Egypt, Kenya, Nigeria	Kiulia et al. (2010), Magdy RIZK and Kamal ALLAYEH (2020), Motayo et al. (2018), Verheyen et al. (2009)
Norovirus	Gastroenteritis	Irrigation water, soil, manure, vegetables, wastewater	Burkina Faso, Ghana	Silverman et al. (2013) and Traore et al. (2024)
Hepatitis A virus (HAV)	Hepatitis A	Treated wastewater, river water, dam water, drinking water	Kenya, Tunisia, South Africa, Chad	Gharbi-Khelifi et al. (2011), Guerrero-Latorre et al. (2011), Kiulia et al. (2010), Ouardani et al. (2016), Rachida and Taylor (2020), Sibanda and Okoh (2013), Taylor et al. (2001)
Hepatitis E Virus	Liver disease	Drinking water	Chad	Guerrero-Latorre et al. (2011)
Enteroviruses (incl. poliovirus)	Poliomyelitis, meningitis	River water, Dam water, treated wastewater, drinking water	Nigeria, Tunisia, South Africa	Bislava et al. (2024), Chigor and Okoh (2012), Ehlers et al. (2005), Ibrahim et al. (2023), Sibanda and Okoh (2013)
Rift Valley fever virus (RVFV)	Hemorrhagic fever, encephalitis	Water (mosquito breeding), soil (egg persistence)	Kenya, South Africa, Mauritania	Linthicum et al. (1985)
Astroviruses	diarrhoea	River and dam water	South Africa	Taylor et al. (2001)
Influenza viruses	Influenza	Air, surfaces (cages, tables), water	Egypt	Mahmoud et al. (2024)
SARS-CoV-2	COVID-19	Air	South Africa, Lesotho	Katende et al. (2022), Roy et al. (2025)
Avian influenza viruses (H5N1, H5N8)	Avian influenza	Air (poultry farm aerosols)	Egypt	Saad et al. (2024)

For example, in 2008, a large cholera outbreak occurred in Mozambique following an extreme flooding event, leading to the mass displacement of over 184,000 people (Sidley 2008). The following year (2009), South Africa experienced a cholera outbreak reported to be imported from Zimbabwe. While flooding was not the direct cause of the outbreak's start, it contributed to the spread and severity of the outbreak (NICD 2009). It can therefore be assumed that such events could lead to the transport of virally polluted water across borders with severe adverse effects on neighbouring populations.

On the other hand, extreme droughts in different areas will reduce personal and household hygiene, leading to the outbreak of WASH (water, sanitation, and hygiene)-related infections. Poor WASH practices have been linked with increased gastrointestinal infections, placing a significant threat to public health in Africa (Okesanya et al. 2024). This will lead to increased viral disease burden, especially in refugee and informal settlements with poor sanitation.

The lack of proper waste disposal infrastructure forces many communities in Africa to practice open defecation, which introduces viral pathogens into the soil. Also, as observed in Table 8.1, numerous viruses have been identified in African treated effluents from WWTPs and in rivers. Using such water for irrigation also introduces viruses into the soil. Given the ability of viruses to persist in soil, this enables direct human exposure through handling and consumption of contaminated produce from such farms, creating a food safety risk and a potential for foodborne disease outbreaks. In rural and informal settings without access to clean water, children are at a higher risk of transferring soil-borne viruses from the environment into their mouths, which can lead to illness. The polluted soil could also increase occupational exposure for farmers and waste handlers. Finally, these polluted soils could enable delayed outbreaks even after initial contamination.

Rapid urbanisation in most African cities could favour a high transmission potential in densely populated informal settlements. Thus, overcrowded urban environments, poorly ventilated public transport, and high patient density in healthcare facilities could facilitate airborne spread. Seasonal dust events, such as the Harmattan winds, may exacerbate respiratory vulnerability by damaging mucosal barriers. With poor healthcare infrastructure, this could increase nosocomial disease outbreaks in healthcare facilities with inadequate ventilation. This is particularly favoured by the high HIV burden on the continent, which weakens the immune system and makes the affected population vulnerable to airborne viral infection.

8.4 Conclusion and Recommendations

The environment plays a vital role as a reservoir and transmission route of viruses in Africa. The interplay between water, soil, and air reservoirs is critical. Such interconnected pathways heighten the complexity of controlling viral spread in African settings, especially given the dynamic climatic scenarios. As such, climate adaptation strategies must account for environmental persistence and mobilisation of viruses during extreme weather events. The weakened health systems and inability to rapidly diagnose viral infections could exacerbate shedding and spread through environmental matrices within communities. It should, however, be noted that although the current chapter has focused on water, soil and air, the environmental reservoirs of viral infections in Africa are complex and multifaceted, involving wildlife, aquatic systems, and human-animal interaction. Therefore, there is a need to integrate One Health surveillance systems, which are essential to monitor viral presence across environmental settings and their interaction with humans and animals. Also, it is crucial to implement wastewater-based epidemiology in African countries as an early warning system for outbreaks. Investing in sanitation and water treatment can reduce environmental viral loads. Likely, the current literature on the environmental dimension of viruses in Africa is underreported, given the lack of literature on many aspects. Much emphasis has been placed on the water environment, while soil and water remain uninvestigated. Thus, increasing funding in this niche would lead to increased capacity building in environmental virology within the continent and provide solid evidence that would inform the implementation of strategic actions to curb the spread of viral infections through the environment.

References

Abia ALK, Ubomba-Jaswa E, Genthe B, Momba MNB (2016) Quantitative microbial risk assessment (QMRA) shows increased public health risk associated with exposure to river water under conditions of riverbed sediment resuspension. Sci Total Environ 566–567:1143–1151. https://doi.org/10.1016/j.scitotenv.2016.05.155

Adhiambo M, Makwaga O, Adungo F, Kimani H, Mulama DH, Korir JC, Mwau M (2021) Human immunodeficiency virus (Hiv) type 1 genetic diversity in hiv positive individuals on antiretroviral therapy in a cross-sectional study conducted in Teso, Western Kenya. Pan Afr Med J 38. https://doi.org/10.11604/pamj.2021.38.335.26357

Africa CDC (2021) Africa Centres for Disease Control and Prevention. Research and Development Priorities for COVID-19 in Africa

Aleke CO, Mong EU, Obande-Ogbuinya EN, Omaka-Amari LN, Ngwakwe PC, Nashwan AJ (2023) Re-emergence of Lassa fever outbreaks in Africa with ongoing threat from COVID-19. J Med Surg Public Health 1:100005. https://doi.org/10.1016/j.glmedi.2023.100005

Ali AS, Gari SR, Goodson ML, Walsh CL, Dessie BK, Ambelu A (2023) Contamination in the wastewater irrigation system and its health threat to wastewater-based farming households. Environ Health Insights 17. https://doi.org/10.1177/11786302231181307

Alsved M, Nyström K, Thuresson S, Nygren D, Patzi-Churqui M, Hussein T, Fraenkel CJ, Medstrand P, Löndahl J (2023) Infectivity of exhaled SARS-CoV-2 aerosols is sufficient to transmit COVID-19 within minutes. Sci Rep 13. https://doi.org/10.1038/s41598-023-47829-8

Amanze JN (2024) African approaches to the protection and conservation of the environment: the role of African traditional religions. Religion and Development 2:445–462. https://doi.org/10.30965/27507955-20230031

Anyamba A, Linthicum KJ, Small J, Britch SC, Pak E, De La Rocque S, Formenty P, Hightower AW, Breiman RF, Chretien JP, Tucker CJ, Schnabel D, Sang R, Haagsma K, Latham M, Lewandowski HB, Magdi SO, Mohamed MA, Nguku PM, Reynes JM, Swanepoel R (2010) Prediction, assessment of the Rift Valley fever activity in east and southern Africa 2006-2008 and possible vector control strategies. Am J Trop Med Hyg. https://doi.org/10.4269/ajtmh.2010.09-0289

Awoyemi AG, Ibáñez-Rueda N, Guardiola J, Ibáñez-Álamo JD (2024) Human-nature interactions in the Afrotropics: Experiential and cognitive connections among urban residents in southern Nigeria. Ecol Econ. https://doi.org/10.1016/j.ecolecon.2024.108105

Baker RE, Mahmud AS, Miller IF, Rajeev M, Rasambainarivo F, Rice BL, Takahashi S, Tatem AJ, Wagner CE, Wang L-F, Wesolowski A, Metcalf CJE (2022) Infectious disease in an era of global change. Nat Rev Microbiol 20:193–205. https://doi.org/10.1038/s41579-021-00639-z

Baraka V, Kweka EJ (2016) The threat of Zika virus in Sub-Saharan Africa—the need to remain vigilant. Front Public Health 4. https://doi.org/10.3389/fpubh.2016.00110

Bishop RF, Kirkwood CD (2008) Enteric viruses. In: Encyclopedia of virology. Elsevier, pp 116–123. https://doi.org/10.1016/B978-012374410-4.00386-1

Bislava SB, Daja A, Oderinde BS, Uzairu SM (2024) Prevalence of vaccine-derived poliovirus in sewage waters in Maiduguri, Borno State, Nigeria. Inf Med 32:90–98. https://doi.org/10.53854/liim-3201-12

Bloom K (2025) The disparate burden of infectious diseases. Gene Ther 32:1–3. https://doi.org/10.1038/s41434-024-00501-w

Boutayeb A (2010) The impact of infectious diseases on the development of Africa. In: Handbook of disease burdens and quality of life measures. Springer, New York, pp 1171–1188. https://doi.org/10.1007/978-0-387-78665-0_66

CDC (2025) Center for Disease Prevention and Control. Areas at Risk for Chikungunya [WWW Document]. https://www.cdc.gov/chikungunya/data-maps/index.html. Accessed 8 Dec 2025

Chigor V, Okoh A (2012) Quantitative RT-PCR detection of hepatitis A virus, rotaviruses and enteroviruses in the Buffalo River and source water dams in the Eastern Cape Province of South Africa. Int J Environ Res Public Health 9:4017–4032. https://doi.org/10.3390/ijerph9114017

da Silva PG, Mesquita JR, de São José Nascimento M, Ferreira VAM (2021) Viral, host and environmental factors that favor anthropozoonotic spillover of coronaviruses: An opinionated review, focusing on SARS-CoV, MERS-CoV and SARS-CoV-2. Sci Total Environ. https://doi.org/10.1016/j.scitotenv.2020.141483

ECDC (2025) European Centre for Disease Prevention and Control. Chikungunya virus disease worldwide overview. Situation update, July 2025 [WWW Document]. https://www.ecdc.europa.eu/en/chikungunya-monthly. Accessed 8 Dec 2025

Ehlers MM, Grabow WOK, Pavlov DN (2005) Detection of enteroviruses in untreated and treated drinking water supplies in South Africa. Water Res 39:2253–2258. https://doi.org/10.1016/j.watres.2005.04.014

Fagunwa OE, Mthiyane T, Fagunwa A, Olayemi KI, Alozie A, Onyeaka H, Akinsemolu A, Ojo A (2025) Priority regions for eliminating open defecation in Africa: implications for antimicrobial resistance. Environ Dev Sustain 27:2675–2699. https://doi.org/10.1007/s10668-023-03992-6

Gall AM, Mariñas BJ, Lu Y, Shisler JL (2015) Waterborne viruses: a barrier to safe drinking water. PLoS Pathog. https://doi.org/10.1371/journal.ppat.1004867

Gerba CP, Pepper IL (2019) Microbial contaminants. In: Environmental and pollution science. Elsevier, pp 191–217. https://doi.org/10.1016/B978-0-12-814719-1.00013-6

Gharbi-Khelifi H, Ben N, Abid S, Sdiri K, Harrath R, Beji A, Bhiri L, Billaudel S, Ferre V, Aouni M (2011) Characterization of outbreak hepatitis a isolates in five Tunisian childcare centers. Braz J Microbiol 42:1204–1212

Guardabassi, L., Dalsgaard, A., Sobsey, M., 2003. Sustainable urban renewal and wastewater treatment occurence and survival of viruses in composted human faeces

Guerrero-Latorre L, Carratala A, Rodriguez-Manzano J, Calgua B, Hundesa A, Girones R (2011) Occurrence of water-borne enteric viruses in two settlements based in Eastern Chad: Analysis of hepatitis E virus, hepatitis A virus and human adenovirus in water sources. J Water Health 9:515–524. https://doi.org/10.2166/wh.2011.126

Hlongwa N, Nkomo SL, Desai SA (2024) Barriers to water, sanitation, and hygiene in Sub-Saharan Africa: a mini review. J Water Sanit Hyg Dev. https://doi.org/10.2166/washdev.2024.266

Ibrahim C, Hammami S, Khelifi N, Hassen A (2023) Detection of enteroviruses and SARS-CoV-2 in Tunisian wastewater. Food Environ Virol 15:224–235. https://doi.org/10.1007/s12560-023-09557-0

Johnson R, Muller CJF, Ghoor S, Louw J, Archer E, Surujlal-Naicker S, Berkowitz N, Volschenk M, Bröcker LHL, Wolfaardt G, van der Walt M, Mutshembele AM, Malema S, Gelderblom HC, Mdhluli M, Gray G, Mathee A, Street RA (2021) Qualitative and quantitative detection of SARS-CoV-2 RNA in untreated wastewater in Western Cape Province, South Africa. S Afr Med J 111:198–202. https://doi.org/10.7196/SAMJ.2021.V111I3.15154

Juma K, Juma A, Shumba C, Otieno P, Asiki G (2020) Non-communicable diseases and urbanization in African cities: a narrative review. In: Public health in developing countries—challenges and opportunities. IntechOpen. https://doi.org/10.5772/intechopen.89507

Kalisa E, Archer S, Nagato E, Bizuru E, Lee K, Tang N, Pointing S, Hayakawa K, Lacap-Bugler D (2019) Chemical and biological components of urban aerosols in Africa: current status and knowledge gaps. Int J Environ Res Public Health. https://doi.org/10.3390/ijerph16060941

Katende B, Fernández LG, Muhairwe J, Glass TR, Ayakaka I, Labhardt ND, Ruhwald M, de Vos M, Bresser M, Reither K (2022) Diagnosis of SARS-CoV-2 infection from breath—a proof-of-concept study. IJID Regions 5:163–164. https://doi.org/10.1016/j.ijregi.2022.10.007

Kiulia NM, Netshikweta R, Page NA, Van Zyl WB, Kiraithe MM, Nyachieo A, Mwenda JM, Taylor MB (2010) The detection of enteric viruses in selected urban and rural river water and sewage in Kenya, with special reference to rotaviruses. J Appl Microbiol 109:818–828. https://doi.org/10.1111/j.1365-2672.2010.04710.x

Levy K, Smith SM, Carlton EJ (2018) Climate change impacts on waterborne diseases: moving toward designing interventions. Curr Environ Health Rep. https://doi.org/10.1007/s40572-018-0199-7

Li XC, Zhang YY, Zhang QY, Liu JS, Ran JJ, Han LF, Zhang XX (2024) Global burden of viral infectious diseases of poverty based on Global Burden of Diseases Study 2021. Infect Dis Poverty 13. https://doi.org/10.1186/s40249-024-01234-z

Li D, Chen M, Li W, Xu X, Li Q (2025) Global burden of viral skin diseases from 1990 to 2021: a systematic analysis for the global burden of disease study 2021. Front Public Health 13. https://doi.org/10.3389/fpubh.2025.1464372

Linthicum KJ, Davies FG, Kairo A, Bailey CL (1985) Rift Valley fever virus (family Bunyaviridae, genus Phlebovirus). Isolations from Diptera collected during an inter-epizootic period in Kenya. J Hyg 95:197–209. https://doi.org/10.1017/S0022172400062434

Magdy Rizk N, Kamal Allayeh A (2020) Genotyping of Rotaviruses in River Nile in Giza, Egypt. Iran J Public Health

Mahmoud SH, Gomaa M, El Taweel A, Moatasim Y, Kamel MN, El Sayes M, Abo Shama NM, Badra R, Mahmoud M, McKenzie PP, Webby RJ, Kandeil A, Ali MA, El-Shesheny R, Kayali G (2024) Transmission dynamics of avian influenza viruses in Egyptian poultry markets. NPJ Viruses 2. https://doi.org/10.1038/s44298-024-00035-3

Mercy K, Youm E, Aliddeki D, Faria NR, Kebede Y, Ndembi N (2024) The looming threat of dengue fever: the Africa context. Open Forum Infect Dis 11. https://doi.org/10.1093/ofid/ofae362

Minta AA, Ferrari M, Antoni S, Portnoy A, Sbarra A, Lambert B, Hatcher C, Hsu CH, Ho LL, Steulet C, Gacic-Dobo M, Rota PA, Mulders MN, Bose AS, Caro WP, O'Connor P, Crowcroft NS (2023) Progress toward measles elimination—worldwide, 2000–2022. MMWR Morb Mortal Wkly Rep 72:1262–1268. https://doi.org/10.15585/mmwr.mm7246a3

Motayo BO, Faneye A, Adeniji JA (2018) Molecular characterization of group A rotavirus in sewage effluent from Nigeria. Int J Infect Dis 73:366. https://doi.org/10.1016/j.ijid.2018.04.4243

Mpofu B (2021) Pursuing fullness of life through harmony with nature: towards an African response to environmental destruction and climate change in southern Africa. HTS Teologiese Studies/Theological Studies 77. https://doi.org/10.4102/hts.v77i4.6574

Naghavi M, Mestrovic T, Gray A, Gershberg Hayoon A, Swetschinski LR, Robles Aguilar G, Davis Weaver N, Ikuta KS, Chung È, Wool EE, Han C, Araki DT, Albertson SB, Bender R, Bertolacci G, Browne AJ, Cooper BS, Cunningham MW, Dolecek C, Doxey M, Dunachie SJ, Ghoba S, Haines-Woodhouse G, Hay SI, Hsu RL, Iregbu KC, Kyu HH, Ledesma JR, Ma J, Moore CE, Mosser JF, Mougin V, Naghavi P, Novotney A, Rosenthal VD, Sartorius B, Stergachis A, Troeger C, Vongpradith A, Walters MK, Wunrow HY, Murray CJ, Naghavi M, Mestrovic T, Gray A, Gershberg Hayoon A, Swetschinski L, Davis Weaver N, Ikuta K, Chung E, Wool E, Han C, Araki D, Albertson S, Bender R, Bertolacci G, Cunningham M, Doxey M, Ghoba S, Hay S, Kyu H, Ledesma J, Ma J, Mosser J, Mougin V, Novotney A, Troeger C, Vongpradith A, Wunrow H, Murray C, Naghavi M, Mestrovic T, Hay S, Kyu H, Mosser J, Sartorius B, Murray C, Chung E, Stergachis A, Stergachis A, Chung E, Mestrovic T, Robles Aguilar G, Cooper B, Dolecek C, Ikuta K, Bender R, Browne A, Doxey M, Dunachie S, Walters M, Dunachie S, Iregbu K, Ledesma J, Moore C, Naghavi P, Rosenthal V (2024) Global burden associated with 85 pathogens in 2019: a systematic analysis for the Global Burden of Disease Study 2019. Lancet Infect Dis 24:868–895. https://doi.org/10.1016/S1473-3099(24)00158-0

Nagy A, Černíková L, Sedlák K (2025) Genetic data and meteorological conditions: unravelling the windborne transmission of H5N1 high-pathogenicity avian influenza between commercial poultry outbreaks. https://doi.org/10.1101/2025.02.12.637829

Ndishimye P, Umuhoza T, Umutoni B, Zakham F, Ndayambaje M, Hewins B, Ngabo Gasana M, Ostadgavahi AT, Sganzerla G, Ndayisenga F, Kelvin D, Udahemuka JC (2024) Rift valley fever outbreaks in the East African Community: insights from ProMed data (2010–2024). Front Public Health 12. https://doi.org/10.3389/fpubh.2024.1298594

NICD (2009) Cholera outbreak. Commun Dis Commun 8

NICD (2025) National Institute for Communicable Disease of South Africa. Chikungunya Cases Rise: South African Travellers Urged to Take Care [WWW Document]. https://www.nicd.ac.za/chikungunya-cases-rise-south-african-travelers-urged-to-take-care/. Accessed 8 Dec 2025

Nwachcuku N, Gerba CP (2004) Emerging waterborne pathogens: can we kill them all? Curr Opin Biotechnol. https://doi.org/10.1016/j.copbio.2004.04.010

Nwachuku N, Gerba CP, Oswald A, Mashadi FD (2005) Comparative inactivation of adenovirus serotypes by UV light disinfection. Appl Environ Microbiol 71:5633–5636. https://doi.org/10.1128/AEM.71.9.5633-5636.2005

Nyasulu PS, Weyer J, Tschopp R, Mihret A, Aseffa A, Nuvor SV, Tamuzi JL, Nyakarahuka L, Helegbe GK, Ntinginya NE, Gebreyesus MT, Doumbia S, Busse R, Drosten C (2021) Rabies mortality and morbidity associated with animal bites in Africa: A case for integrated rabies disease surveillance, prevention and control: a scoping review. BMJ Open. https://doi.org/10.1136/bmjopen-2020-048551

Okesanya OJ, Eshun G, Ukoaka BM, Manirambona E, Olabode ON, Adesola RO, Okon II, Jamil S, Singh A, Lucero-Prisno DE, Ali HM, Chowdhury ABMA (2024) Water, sanitation, and hygiene (WASH) practices in Africa: exploring the effects on public health and sustainable development plans. Trop Med Health. https://doi.org/10.1186/s41182-024-00614-3

Okoh AI, Sibanda T, Gusha SS (2010) Inadequately treated wastewater as a source of human enteric viruses in the environment. Int J Environ Res Public Health 7:2620–2637. https://doi.org/10.3390/ijerph7062620

Oleribe OO, Momoh J, Uzochukwu BSC, Mbofana F, Adebiyi A, Barbera T, Williams R, Taylor-Robinson SD (2019) Identifying key challenges facing healthcare systems in Africa and potential solutions. Int J Gen Med 12:395–403. https://doi.org/10.2147/IJGM.S223882

Osuolale O, Okoh A (2017) Human enteric bacteria and viruses in five wastewater treatment plants in the Eastern Cape, South Africa. J Infect Public Health 10:541–547. https://doi.org/10.1016/j.jiph.2016.11.012

Ouardani I, Turki S, Aouni M, Romalde JL (2016) Detection and molecular characterization of hepatitis A virus from Tunisian wastewater treatment plants with different secondary treatments. Appl Environ Microbiol 82:3834–3845. https://doi.org/10.1128/AEM.00619-16

Parums DV (2024) A review of the resurgence of measles, a vaccine-preventable disease, as current concerns contrast with past hopes for Measles elimination. Med Sci Monit. https://doi.org/10.12659/MSM.944436

Perry WB, Ahmadian R, Munday M, Jones O, Ormerod SJ, Durance I (2024) Addressing the challenges of combined sewer overflows. Environ Pollut. https://doi.org/10.1016/j.envpol.2023.123225

Poongavanan J, Lourenço J, Tsui JLH, Colizza V, Ramphal Y, Baxter C, Kraemer MUG, Dunaiski M, de Oliveira T, Tegally H (2024) Dengue virus importation risks in Africa: a modelling study. Lancet Planet Health 8:e1043–e1054. https://doi.org/10.1016/S2542-5196(24)00272-9

Rachida S, Taylor MB (2020) Potentially infectious novel hepatitis a virus strains detected in selected treated wastewater discharge sources, South Africa. Viruses 12. https://doi.org/10.3390/v12121468

Roy CJ, Barer MR, Ueckermann V, Beddingfield B, Cordier D, Fourie B, Vincent R, Dibobo S, Van Reenen T, Jensen P, De Kock O, De Kock E, Nardell E (2025) Human source severe acute respiratory syndrome coronavirus 2 aerosol transmission to remote sentinel hamsters. Open Forum Infect Dis 12. https://doi.org/10.1093/ofid/ofaf196

Saad N, Esaki M, Kojima I, Khalil AM, Osuga S, Shahein MA, Okuya K, Ozawa M, Alhatlani BY (2024) Phylogenetic characterization of novel reassortant 2.3.4.4b H5N8 highly pathogenic avian influenza viruses isolated from domestic ducks in Egypt during the winter season 2021–2022. Viruses 16. https://doi.org/10.3390/v16111655

Sampath S, Khedr A, Qamar S, Tekin A, Singh R, Green R, Kashyap R (2021) Pandemics throughout the history. Cureus. https://doi.org/10.7759/cureus.18136

Santarpia JL, Herrera VL, Rivera DN, Ratnesar-Shumate S, Reid SP, Ackerman DN, Denton PW, Martens JWS, Fang Y, Conoan N, Callahan MV, Lawler JV, Brett-Major DM, Lowe JJ (2022) The size and culturability of patient-generated SARS-CoV-2 aerosol. J Expo Sci Environ Epidemiol 32:706–711. https://doi.org/10.1038/s41370-021-00376-8

Semancik CS, Cooper CL, Postler TS, Price M, Yun H, Zaric M, Kuteesa M, Malkevich N, Kilianski A, Gupta SB, Francis SC (2024) Prevalence of human filovirus infections in sub-Saharan Africa: A systematic review and meta-analysis protocol. Syst Rev 13. https://doi.org/10.1186/s13643-024-02626-w

Setti L, Passarini F, De Gennaro G, Barbieri P, Perrone MG, Borelli M, Palmisani J, Di Gilio A, Torboli V, Fontana F, Clemente L, Pallavicini A, Ruscio M, Piscitelli P, Miani A (2020) SARS-Cov-2RNA found on particulate matter of Bergamo in Northern Italy: first evidence. Environ Res 188. https://doi.org/10.1016/j.envres.2020.109754

Shempela DM, Muleya W, Mudenda S, Daka V, Sikalima J, Kamayani M, Sandala D, Chipango C, Muzala K, Musonda K, Chizimu JY, Mulenga C, Kapona O, Kwenda G, Kasanga M, Njuguna M, Cham F, Simwaka B, Morrison L, Muma JB, Saasa N, Sichinga K, Simulundu E, Chilengi R (2024) Wastewater surveillance of SARS-CoV-2 in Zambia: an early warning tool. Int J Mol Sci 25. https://doi.org/10.3390/ijms25168839

Sibanda T, Okoh AI (2013) Real-time PCR quantitative assessment of hepatitis A virus, rotaviruses and enteroviruses in the Tyume River located in the Eastern Cape Province, South Africa. Water SA 39:295–304. https://doi.org/10.4314/wsa.v39i2.14

Sidley P (2008) Floods in southern Africa result in cholera outbreak and displacement. BMJ 336: 471.2-471. https://doi.org/10.1136/bmj.39503.700903.DB

Silverman AI, Nelson KL, Akrong MO, Amoah P, Drechsel P (2013) Quantification of human norovirus GII, human adenovirus, and fecal indicator organisms in wastewater used for irrigation in Accra, Ghana. J Water Health 11:473–488. https://doi.org/10.2166/wh.2013.025

Sirota SB, Doxey MC, Dominguez RMV, Bender RG, Vongpradith A, Albertson SB, Novotney A, Burkart K, Carter A, Abdi P, Abdoun M, Abebe AM, Abegaz KH, Aboagye RG, Abolhassani H, Abreu LG, Abualruz H, Abu-Gharbieh E, Aburuz S, Adane MM, Addo IY, Adekanmbi V, Adnani QES, Adzigbli LA, Afzal MS, Afzal S, Ahinkorah BO, Ahmad S, Ahmed A, Ahmed H, Ahmed SA, Akinosoglou K, Akkaif MA, Al Awaidy S, Alalalmeh SO, Albashtawy M, AlBataineh MT, Al-Gheethi AAS, Alhalaiqa FN, Alhassan RK, Ali A, Ali L, Ali MU, Ali SS, Ali W, Almazan JU, Alqahtani JS, Alrawashdeh A, Al-Rifai RH, Alshahrani NZ, Altartoor K, Al-Tawfiq JA, Alvis-Guzman N, Al-Worafi YM, Aly H, Aly S, Alzoubi KH, Al-Zyoud WA, Amhare AF, Amu H, Amusa GA, Anil A, Anvari S, Anyabolo EE, Arabloo J, Arafat M, Areda D, Aregawi BB, Aremu A, Athari SS, Aujayeb A, Aynalem ZB, Azadnajafabad S, Azzam AY, Badar M, Taghanaki PB, Bahramian S, Baig AA, Bajcetic M, Balakrishnan S, Banach M, Bardhan M, Barqawi HJ, Bastan MM, Batra K, Batra R, Behnoush AH, Beiranvand M, Belete AG, Belete MA, Beloukas A, Beran A, Bhardwaj P, Bhargava A, Bhat AN, Bhuiyan MA, Bitra VR, Bodunrin AO, Bogale EK, Boppana SH, Borhany H, Bouaoud S, Brown CS, Buonsenso D, Bustanji Y, Cámera LA, Castañeda-Orjuela CA, Cegolon L, Cenderadewi M, Chakraborty S, Chattu VK, Cheng ETW, Chichagi F, Ching PR, Chopra H, Choudhari SG, Christopher DJ, Chu DT, Chukwu IS, Chung E, Corlateanu A, Cruz-Martins N, Dadana S, Dadras O, Dahiru T, Dai X, Das JK, Dash NR, Dashti M, Dashtkoohi M, De la Hoz FP, Debopadhaya S, Demessa BH, Demis AB, Devanbu VGC, Devegowda D, Dhama K, Dhulipala VR, Diaz D, Diaz MJ, Do TC, Do THP, Dodangeh M, Dorostkar F, Dsouza AC, Dsouza HL, Duraisamy S, Durojaiye OC, Dziedzic AM, Ed-Dra A, Ekholuenetale M, Ekundayo TC, El Sayed I, El-Dahiyat F, Elhadi M, Elshaer M, Eslami M, Eze UA, Fagbamigbe AF, Faramarzi A, Fasina FO, Ferreira N, Fischer F, Fitriana I, Flor LS, Gaihre S, Gajdács M, Galehdar N, Ganiyani MA, Gebregergis MW, Gebrehiwot M, Gebremeskel TG, Getahun GK, Getie M, Ghadiri K, Ghasemzadeh A, Ghorbani M, Goldust M, Golechha M, Goleij P, Gorini G, Goyal A, Guan SY, Guarducci G, Gudeta MD, Gupta R, Gupta S, Gupta VB, Gupta VK, Hadei M, Hadi NR, Haj-Mirzaian A, Halwani R, Hamidi S, Hammoud A, Hanifi N, Hanna F, Haq ZA, Haque MR, Mahmudul Hasan SM, Hasani H, Hasnain MS, Hassankhani H, Haubold J, Hayat K, Hegazi OE, Hezam K, Holla R, Hoogar P, Horita N, Hostiuc M, Huynh HH, Ibitoye SE, Ilesanmi OS, Ilic IM, Ilic MD, Imam MT, Isa MA, Islam MR, Islam SMS, Ismail NE, Iwagami M, Vinothini J, Jafarzadeh A, Jaggi K, Jairoun AA, Jakovljevic M, Jamshidi E, Jayaram S, Jeswani BM, Jha RP, Jose J, Joseph N, Joshua CE, Jozwiak JJ, Vaishali K, Kabir Z, Kandel H, Kanmodi KK, Kant S, Kantar RS, Karaye IM, Behnagh AK, Kaur N, Khajuria H, Khalaji A, Khamesipour F, Khan G, Nuruzzaman Khan M, Khan M, Khan MJ, Kim MS, Kimokoti RW, Kochhar S, Korshunov VA, Kosen S, Krishan K, Krishna H, Krishnamoorthy V, Defo BK, Kuddus MA, Kuddus M, Kuitunen I, Kulimbet M, Kumar D, Kurmi OP, Simhachalam Kutikuppala LV, Lahariya C, Lal DK, Lasrado S, Latifinaibin K, Le HH, Le NHH, Le TTT, Le TDT, Lee SW, Lee WC, Li MC, Li P, Lim SS, Liu G, Liu R, Liu W, Liu, Xiaofeng, Liu, Xuefeng, Lorenzovici L, Luo L, Majeed A, Rad EM, Malhotra K, Malik I, Manilal A, Mehta B, Meto TM, Mekonnen MM, Meles HN, Memish ZA, Mendez-Lopez MA, Meo SA, Merati M, Mestrovic T, Mettananda S, Minh LHN, Mirrakhimov EM, Misra AK, Mohamed AI, Mohamed NS, Mohammed, Mesud, Mohammed, Mustapha, Mokdad AH, Monasta L, Moni MA, Moodi Ghalibaf AA, Moore CE, Morawska L, Motappa R, Mougin V, Mousavi P, Mustafa G, Naghavi P, Naik GR, Nainu F, Najafi MS, Najdaghi S, Najmuldeen HHR, Nargus S, Davani DN, Naser M, Natto ZS, Nayak BP, Nejadghaderi SA, Nguyen DH, Nguyen HTH, Nguyen VT, Nikolouzakis TK, Noman EA, Nri-Ezedi CA, Nuñez-Samudio V, Nwatah VE, Odetokun IA, Okekunle AP, Okonji OC, Okwute PG, Olanipekun TO, Olufadewa II, Olusanya BO, Omer GL, Onyedibe KI, Ordak M, Orish VN, Ortiz-Prado E, Otstavnov N, Ouyahia A, Mahesh Padukudru PA, Padubidri JR, Pandey A, Pantazopoulos I, Pardhan S, Parija PP, Parikh RR, Park S, Parthasarathi A,

Pasovic M, Pathan AR, Patil S, Pawar S, Peprah P, Perianayagam A, Perumal D, Petcu IR, Pham HN, Pham HT, Philip AK, Pigott DM, Piracha ZZ, Poddighe D, Polibin RV, Postma MJ, Pourbabaki R, Prates EJS, Puvvula J, Qazi AS, Qian G, Rafferty Q, Rahim F, Rahimi M, Rahimi-Movaghar V, Rahman MO, Rahman M, Rahman MA, Rahmanian M, Rahmanian N, Rahmanian V, Rahmati M, Rajput P, Ramadan MM, Ramasamy SK, Ramesh PS, Rao IR, Rao M, Rao SJ, Rashedi S, Rashidi MM, Rathish D, Ravikumar N, Rawaf S, Redwan EMM, Reyes LFF, Rezaei, Nazila, Rezaei, Nima, Rezahosseini O, Rizvi SMD, Rodriguez JAB, Ronfani L, Roudashti S, Roy P, de Andrade Ruela G, Saddik BA, Saeb MR, Saeed U, Saeedi P, Safari M, Saheb Sharif-Askari F, Saheb Sharif-Askari N, Sahebkar A, Sahu M, Sakshaug JW, Salam N, Salami AA, Saleh MA, Sallam M, Samodra YL, Sanjeev RK, Santric-Milicevic MM, Saravanan A, Sartorius B, Sathyanarayan A, Saulam J, Saxena S, Saya GK, Schaarschmidt BM, Schumacher AE, Sedighi M, Sendekie AK, Senthilkumaran S, Sethi Y, Seyed-Alinaghi SA, Shafie M, Shahid S, Shaikh MA, Sham S, Shamshirgaran MA, Shanawaz M, Shannawaz M, Sharifan A, Sharifi-Rad J, Shastry RP, Sheikh A, Shigematsu M, Shiri R, Shittu A, Shiue I, Shorofi SA, Siddig EE, Simpson CR, Singh JA, Singh P, Singh S, Sinto R, Solanki R, Soliman SSM, Suleman M, Suliankatchi Abdulkader RS, Swain CK, Szarpak L, Tabatabaei SM, Tabish M, Taha ZMA, Taiba J, Talaat IM, Tamuzi JL, Taye BT, Tefera YM, Temsah MH, Terefa DR, Thakur R, Thapar R, Thirunavukkarasu S, Tichopad A, Ticoalu JHV, Tovani-Palone MR, Tran NM, Tran NH, Duc NTM, Tsegay GM, Tumurkhuu M, Udoakang AJ, Upadhyay E, Vahabi SM, Vaithinathan AG, Valizadeh R, Vasankari TJ, Vinayak M, Waqas M, Weldetinsaa HL, Wickramasinghe ND, Yadollahpour A, Yaghoubi S, Yezli S, Yin D, Yon DK, Yonemoto N, Yu Y, Zakham F, Zandieh GGZ, Zare I, Zarimeidani F, Zastrozhin M, Zhai C, Zhang H, Zhang ZJ, Zhao Y, Zhou J, Zia H, Zielinska M, Zoladl M, Zyoud SH, Aravkin AY, Kassebaum NJ, Naghavi M, Vos T, Hay SI, Murray CJL, Kyu HH (2025) Global, regional, and national burden of upper respiratory infections and otitis media, 1990–2021: a systematic analysis from the Global Burden of Disease Study 2021. Lancet Infect Dis 25:36–51. https://doi.org/10.1016/S1473-3099(24)00430-4

Smets W, Moretti S, Denys S, Lebeer S (2016) Airborne bacteria in the atmosphere: Presence, purpose, and potential. Atmos Environ. https://doi.org/10.1016/j.atmosenv.2016.05.038

Sonderup MW, Spearman CW (2024) HBV elimination in Africa-Current status and challenges. Clin Liver Dis (Hoboken). https://doi.org/10.1097/CLD.0000000000000166

Stephens PR, Sundaram M, Ferreira S, Gottdenker N, Nipa KF, Schatz AM, Schmidt JP, Drake JM (2022) Drivers of African Filovirus (Ebola and Marburg) outbreaks. Vector-Borne and Zoonotic Diseases 22:478–490. https://doi.org/10.1089/vbz.2022.0020

Street R, Mathee A, Mangwana N, Dias S, Sharma JR, Ramharack P, Louw J, Reddy T, Brocker L, Surujlal-Naicker S, Berkowitz N, Malema MS, Nkambule S, Webster C, Mahlangeni N, Gelderblom H, Mdhluli M, Gray G, Muller C, Johnson R (2021) Spatial and temporal trends of SARS-CoV-2 RNA from wastewater treatment plants over 6 weeks in Cape Town, South Africa. Int J Environ Res Public Health 18. https://doi.org/10.3390/ijerph182212085

Taylor MB, Cox N, Vrey MA, Grabow WOK (2001) The occurrence of hepatitis A and astroviruses in selected river and dam waters in South Africa. Wat Res

Thuresson S, Fraenkel CJ, Sasinovich S, Soldemyr J, Widell A, Medstrand P, Alsved M, Löndahl J (2022) Airborne severe acute respiratory syndrome coronavirus 2 (SARS-CoV-2) in hospitals: effects of aerosol-generating procedures, HEPA-filtration units, patient viral load, and physical distance. Clin Infect Dis 75:E89–E96. https://doi.org/10.1093/cid/ciac161

Tierney JT, Sullivan R, Larkin EP, Branch V (1977) Persistence of poliovirus 1 in soil and on vegetables grown in Soil previously flooded with inoculated sewage sludge or effluent. Appl Environ Microbiol 23:109–113

Traore KA, Fawa Djingtouin A, Sanou M, Ouoba JB, Ouoba LB, Roques P, Barro N (2024) Detection of norovirus in fresh fruits, vegetables, wastewater and manure from irrigated farms in Ouagadougou, Burkina Faso. Afr J Microbiol Res 18:153–160. https://doi.org/10.5897/AJMR2024.9759

UNAIDS (2025) Fact sheet 2025: Global and regional HIV statistics (Fact sheet). UNAIDS

UNICEF (n.d.) United Nations Children's Fund. Sanitation and Hygiene

Upfold NS, Luke GA, Knox C (2021) Occurrence of human enteric viruses in water sources and shellfish: a focus on Africa. Food Environ Virol. https://doi.org/10.1007/s12560-020-09456-8

van de Vossenberg J, Hoiting Y, Kamara AK, Tetteh MK, Simaika JP, Lutterodt G, Komakech H, Kulabako R, Nyenje PM, Foppen JW (2021) Double-stranded DNA virus assemblages in groundwater in three informal urban settlements in sub-Saharan Africa differ from each other. ACS Environ Sci Technol Water 1:1992–2000. https://doi.org/10.1021/acsestwater.0c00306

Van Heerden J, Ehlers MM, Heim A, Grabow WOK (2005) Prevalence, quantification and typing of adenoviruses detected in river and treated drinking water in South Africa. J Appl Microbiol 99:234–242. https://doi.org/10.1111/j.1365-2672.2005.02617.x

Vasickova P, Kovarcik K (2013) Natural persistence of food- and waterborne viruses. In: Viruses in food and water: risks, surveillance and control. Elsevier Ltd., pp 179–204. https://doi.org/10.1533/9780857098870.3.179

Verheyen J, Timmen-Wego M, Laudien R, Boussaad I, Sen S, Koc A, Uesbeck A, Mazou F, Pfister H (2009) Detection of adenoviruses and rotaviruses in drinking water sources used in rural areas of Benin, west africa. Appl Environ Microbiol 75:2798–2801. https://doi.org/10.1128/AEM.01807-08

WHO (2025a) Ebola disease [WWW Document]. https://www.who.int/health-topics/ebola#tab=tab_1. Accessed 8 Dec 2025

WHO (2025b) Hepatitis A [WWW Document]. https://www.who.int/news-room/fact-sheets/detail/hepatitis-a. Accessed 8 Nov 2025

WHO Africa (2022) How wastewater surveillance is helping the COVID-19 fight [WWW Document]. https://www.afro.who.int/news/how-wastewater-surveillance-helping-covid-19-fight?utm_source=chatgpt.com. Accessed 8 Nov 2025

WHO Regional Office for Africa (2022) WHO Regional Office for Africa. (2022, July 27). 91 million Africans infected with Hepatitis B or C (News release)

Wright CY, Kapwata T, Naidoo N, Asante KP, Arku RE, Cissé G, Simane B, Atuyambe L, Berhane K (2024) Climate change and human health in Africa in relation to opportunities to strengthen mitigating potential and adaptive capacity: strategies to inform an African "Brains Trust". Ann Glob Health. https://doi.org/10.5334/aogh.4260

Xia H, Dong X (2025) The global, regional, and national burden trends of dengue among adults aged 20–49 from 1990 to 2021. Sci Rep 15. https://doi.org/10.1038/s41598-025-10824-2

Yeagert JG, O'brien RT (1979) Structural changes associated with Poliovirus inactivation in soil. Appl Environ Microbiol 38:702–709. https://doi.org/10.1128/aem.38.4.702-709.1979

Chapter 9
Vector-Borne Viral Diseases as Neglected Risks to Public Health

Juliet Adamma Shenge and Mimidoo Naomi Shenge

9.1 Introduction

A vector is an organism which transmits diseases or parasites from one animal or plant to another. Vectors act as vehicles for transmitting infectious diseases and, in most cases, remain natural hosts or reservoirs for such pathogens. Most arthropod-borne or arboviral diseases are known as vector-borne diseases due to the involvement of these insects or rodent reservoirs that spread the pathogens (Wang 2024). The viral families implicated in the emergence of vector-borne diseases include RNA viruses in the Flaviviridae, Bunyaviridae and Togaviridae families.

Disease vectors are numerous, including mosquitoes, flies, lice, fleas, ticks and rodents. For instance, mosquitoes such as *Aedes aegypti* and other *Aedes spp* are known for transmitting yellow fever, Zika, dengue, and a host of others (Shenge and Opayele 2020). According to Swei et al. (2020), about 90% of vectors of diseases belong to acari (ticks and mites) and diptera (flies), hard ticks (family Ixodidae), and mosquitoes (family Culicidae), which are a major cause of over 75% of emerging vector-borne zoonotic diseases (Swei et al. 2020).

Transmission of infectious diseases by vectors may be either active or passive (direct or indirect involvement of the vector (WHO 2024). In recent years, there has been a surge in the outbreak of arboviral diseases, blamed mostly on changing environments and other climatic factors that alter the lifecycle of the pathogen-carrying animals in the wild and in suburban settings (WHO 2024). This has become a global trend as outbreaks are often reported in different geographical zones. In the USA, for instance, there has been an increasing number of tick-borne diseases. The

J. A. Shenge (✉)
Virology Research Laboratory, Biological Sciences, Dominican University Ibadan, Ibadan, Nigeria

M. N. Shenge
Department of Public Health, College of Health Sciences, Bowen University, Iwo, Nigeria

J. A. Shenge, A. L. K. Abia (eds.), *Viral Diseases and One Health in Africa*,
https://doi.org/10.1007/978-3-032-09613-5_9

vector, a black-legged tick (*Ixodes scapularis*), known for transmitting Lyme disease, rabies, Bourbon virus, Heartland virus, Colorado tick fever, Powassan virus disease, anaplasmosis, Rocky Mountain spotted fever, and babesiosis, has been reported in recent years across the country, especially in the Northeast. Most tick diseases present with similar symptoms, which may include fever, rash, aches and pains (CDC 2024).

Some of the most common vector-borne diseases reported in Africa include West Nile, dengue fever, chikungunya fever, Rift Valley fever, and yellow fever (Chauhan et al. 2020). Given the tropical climate in Africa and the high density of forest zones in mostly West, East, and Southern Africa, the expected increase in arboviral infections poses a serious public health threat (Chauhan et al. 2020).

9.2 Dengue Haemorrhagic Fever

Dengue is a common mosquito-borne disease that typically occurs in tropical and sub-tropical regions worldwide. Dengue fever has been a neglected tropical viral disease that is highly underreported in Africa due to inadequate diagnostics and surveillance. Outbreaks of dengue have been reported in other countries and regions, including the Caribbean, and pockets of infections are equally common in temperate areas, such as North America and other temperate zones. Dengue has been reported in Northern Africa, Eritrea, Ethiopia, and adjoining countries. A study carried out between 2005 and 2015 in Eritrea recorded the first dengue outbreak in the Agordet district in 2005 and the second in the Massawa district (Chauhan 2020; Usman et al. 2016). There has been an increase in the occurrence of dengue in West Africa. According to the European Center for Disease Prevention and Control, as of February 2025, 640,349 dengue cases have been reported, with about 159 dengue-related deaths from 48 countries, including countries in Africa, America, Southeast Asia and Western Pacific regions, but no autochthonous cases in mainland Europe (ECDC 2025).

The dengue virus that causes dengue fever (DF) and dengue haemorrhagic fever (DHF) is a single-stranded positive-sense RNA virus consisting of four notable serotypes (DENV-1, DENV-2, DENV-3, DENV-4). It belongs to the family Flaviviridae of the genus *Flavivirus,* and the *Aedes aegypti* and *Aedes albopictus* mosquitoes are the known primary and secondary vectors for the transmission of the virus, respectively (Whitehorn and Farrar 2010). During mosquito bites, the virus is injected into the bloodstream.

Symptoms of dengue fever are similar to those of malaria and other febrile illnesses. However, as the infection progresses and at a severe stage, haemorrhage may occur, leading to dengue haemorrhagic fever or dengue shock syndrome. Symptoms include high fever, flu-like symptoms, headache, myalgia, nausea, vomiting, pain behind the eyes, swollen glands, rashes and typical bone or joint pain. Dengue shock syndrome (DSS) occurs as a result of damaged or leaky blood vessels, resulting in a low count of clot-forming cells, internal bleeding or haemorrhagic episodes, circulatory shock, multiple organ failure and death (Parveen et al. 2023).

Dengue fever is a preventable disease, and most importantly by getting vaccinated. However, the availability of dengue vaccines in low- and middle-income countries is a huge concern. Going by the transmission pattern and pathogenesis of dengue virus, one health approach to prevention may be achieved by avoiding mosquito bites, using mosquito-treated nets, mosquito repellent, and protective clothing. Environmentally, destroying mosquito habitats to reduce their number, reducing stagnant water bodies, keeping bushes and lawns low, and picking water-collecting containers around houses will make the breeding sites for mosquitoes non-conducive.

9.3 Chikungunya Fever

Chikungunya is another neglected mosquito-borne viral disease that is common in tropical areas. This disease is spread to people by infected mosquito bites and can be introduced to new areas by infected travellers (CDC 2024). Symptoms of chikungunya disease are similar to those of dengue. These include fever, joint pain, swelling, headache, muscle pain, and rash, which are typical of the disease. There is no specific medication for treating Chikungunya; however, a vaccine is available in some regions (CDC 2024).

9.4 Zika Viral Disease

The emergence of the Zika virus in 2015, especially in South and Central America, created a broad awareness about this mosquito-borne viral infection. Subsequently, in the years following, widespread Zika virus transmission was reported in other parts of the globe. Zika virus disease is typically marked by a congenital Zika syndrome that results in neurological defects in babies or the occurrence of foetal death among infected pregnant women (Swei et al. 2020). The involvement of an arthropod intermediate vector (in this case, blood-feeding or haematophagous mosquito) makes most vector-borne viral diseases, including Zika, a serious threat to public health, as these vectors spread over a large space, get introduced to and adapt in a new environment.

Human pathogens transmitted by mosquitoes are increasing, which points to growing ecological challenges and evolutionary characteristics of viral pathogens involved in the emergence of diseases. In a way, this opens a new horizon or research gaps to understand the evolutionary processes that trigger or support the increased emergence of vector-borne viral pathogens around the globe.

9.5 Drivers of Vector-Borne Viral Disease Outbreaks

9.5.1 Land Use

Several factors have been considered as drivers for the increased rate of outbreaks of vector-borne diseases. Studies have shown that vector-borne diseases are becoming a global threat as their emergence increases (WHO 2024). One crucial potential driver is land use change, which accounts for about 26% of vector-borne diseases (Swei et al. 2020). Notable indicators range from deforestation, use of harmful chemicals, including pesticides and herbicides, unconventional agricultural practices and degradation activities that affect the structure and function of the ecosystem.

9.5.2 Globalization

The world is connected mainly through global travel and services, especially international trade and commerce. As the nations interact and people mix, pathogens are easier to spread. Globalization is a notable driver for the transmission of diseases, including vector-borne zoonotic diseases, accounting for about 11% of vector-borne zoonotic diseases (Swei et al. 2020).

9.5.3 Ecological Shifts and Climate Change

Increased emergence of vector-borne diseases has also been attributed to ecological shifts or changes in climatic factors such as temperature, rainfall, and relative humidity that may result in extreme weather conditions and influence the abundance and adaptation of vectors in any given environment (WHO 2024). Disease burden or outbreaks may be influenced by changing weather or ecological shifts, as seen in the case of Rift Valley fever, which increases during longer periods of heavy rainfall, which in turn makes the environment conducive as breeding sites for the vectors (Shenge and Opayele 2020; WHO 2024). Ecological changes influence vector abundance and survival in any environment, accounting for 10% of vector-borne zoonotic diseases, according to a study by Swei et al. (2020).

9.6 Detection of Vector-Borne Viral Diseases

Most arboviral infections can be detected in the laboratory using basic virological tests, which include tissue culture techniques, serological and immunological tests, including antibody detection such as immunoglobulin G and M (IgG and IgM) antibodies, and nucleic acid tests (NAT). Clinically, symptoms in an individual may not be enough to diagnose or differentiate a particular arboviral infection, as many other viral infections may have similar symptoms. However, clinical or subclinical features may provide a lead as to which test will be most appropriate for proper diagnosis.

Nucleic acid tests (NAT) are essential for confirmation of infection, as they are more sensitive and can detect early infection in any population. Where serological tests cannot detect early infection or relevant markers of disease such as IgG or IgM, NAT may be able to detect it faster. Using NAT to confirm samples (NAT-reactive samples) negative by serology (blood screening) will ensure the safety of blood for transfusion (Yang et al. 2025). This essential quality control system must be implemented to ensure comprehensive surveillance of emerging and re-emerging vector-borne diseases globally. This has implications for public health and control of arboviral infection.

9.7 Recommendation and Future Direction

- There is a need to prevent viral zoonotic vector-borne diseases that affect animals and can be transmitted to humans by adopting implementation and interventional strategies on vector control, as well as socio-cultural or behavioural modifications to reduce infection in endemic areas.
- A comprehensive surveillance system should be set up for emerging transfusion-transmitted arboviruses, including Dengue, Zika, and Chikungunya, which are serious public health concerns. Hence, it has become imperative to include blood screening for these arboviruses (dengue, zika and Chikungunya) before transfusion.
- One major way to ensure proper blood screening and detection of early warning signs is to set up reference molecular laboratories for arbovirus repositories in every region and across borders for adequate control.
- Education and awareness creation in communities about exposure, the nature of disease-carrying insects and rodents, transmission patterns, and prevention will contribute to reducing human infection.
- Strengthening research collaboration and surveillance among global partners, along with stakeholders' involvement in neglected tropical diseases, is urgently recommended to abate the dangers of vector-borne diseases across Africa and beyond.

9.8 Conclusion

Vector-borne viral diseases are neglected risks to public health, as they can potentially result in a pandemic. Hence, paying attention to the environment and human behaviour becomes paramount in controlling vector-borne diseases since the presence, abundance, and life cycle of these pathogen-carrying vectors are repeatedly influenced by the environment and human activity.

References

Center for Disease Control and Prevention, USA (2024) Chikungunya virus. Accessed 17 Mar 2025

Chauhan RP, Dessie ZG, Noreddin A, El Zowalaty ME (2020) Systematic review of important viral diseases in Africa in light of the 'one health' concept. Pathogens 9(4):301

European Center for Disease Prevention and Control (2025) Dengue worldwide overview. www.ecdc.europa.eu. Accessed 17 Mar 2025

Parveen S, Riaz Z, Saeed S, Ishaque U, Sultana M, Faiz Z et al (2023) Dengue hemorrhagic fever: a growing global menace. J Water Health 21(11):1632–1650

Shenge JA, Opayele AV (2020) The impact and control of emerging and re-emerging viral diseases in the environment: an African perspective. In: Abia Lutherking Akebe, Guy Lanza (eds) Current microbiological research in Africa. Selected Applications in Sustainable Environmental Management, pp 185–202

Swei A, Couper LI, Coffey LL, Kapan D, Bennett S (2020) Patterns, drivers and challenges of vector-borne disease emergence. Vector-Borne Zoonotic Dis 20(3):159–170

Usman A, Ball JD, Rojas DP, Berhane A, Ghebrat Y, Mebrahtu G, Gebresellasie A et al (2016) dengue fever outbreaks in Eritrea, 2005–2015: a case for strengthening surveillance, control and reporting. Glob Health Res Policy 1:17

Wang P (2024) Vector-borne viral diseases. Section of Infectious Diseases, Yale University School of Medicine, New Haven. Accessed 7 Feb 2025. https://onlinelibrary.witey.com

Whitehorn J, Farrar J (2010) Dengue. Br Med Bull 95:161–173

World Health Organization (2024) Rift Valley Fever. https://www.who.int

Yan Y, Liu X, Lu S, Chang L, Dong J, Ji H, Sun H, Wang L (2025) Two-year surveillance of Dengue, Zika and Chikungunya viruses among Chinese blood donors-Guangxi and Yunnan PLADs, China, 2022–2023. China CDC Wkly 7(11):357–362. https://doi.org/10.46234/ccdcw2025.058

Chapter 10
Viral Disease Burden in Plants: Implications for Crop Yield and Food Security in Africa

Stephen Ejike Eze

10.1 Introduction

In Africa, agriculture is more than just an economic activity; it is a lifeline for millions. However, this critical sector faces persistent threats from viral diseases that significantly compromise crop yields, threatening the food security of the continent. Viral pathogens such as Cassava Mosaic Virus (CMV) and Maize Streak Virus (MSV) are among the most devastating, leading to substantial reductions in the production of staple crops like cassava and maise. These crops are vital for the survival of many communities, and their decline exacerbates the already severe problem of food insecurity across the continent (Keesing et al. 2010). As emphasised by the One Health framework, the interconnectedness of human, animal, and environmental health underscores the need for a collaborative approach to disease management (Gibbs 2014). This chapter explores the role of sustainable agricultural practices, enhanced disease surveillance, and holistic health strategies in ensuring food security in Africa.

10.2 The Impact of Viral Diseases on Crop Yields and Food Security

Viral diseases have long been recognised as a significant threat to agricultural productivity in Africa. Unlike bacterial or fungal pathogens, viruses cannot be managed by chemical treatments once they have infected a plant, making them particularly challenging to control. The losses incurred due to these diseases are significant, reducing food availability, increasing poverty, and heightening

S. E. Eze (✉)
University of Ibadan, Ibadan, Nigeria

J. A. Shenge, A. L. K. Abia (eds.), *Viral Diseases and One Health in Africa*,
https://doi.org/10.1007/978-3-032-09613-5_10

vulnerability to food insecurity. Among the myriad viral diseases affecting crops in Africa, Cassava Mosaic Virus (CMV) and Maize Streak Virus (MSV) stand out due to their widespread impact on two of the continent's most important staple crops.

Cassava is a primary energy source for over 600 million people in sub-Saharan Africa (Waidi 2023). This virus, spread primarily by the whitefly (*Bemisia tabaci*), causes Cassava Mosaic Disease (CMD), which is characterised by symptoms such as leaf curling, chlorosis, and reduced plant vigour. In severe cases, CMD can cause yield losses of up to 90%, leading to substantial food shortages in regions where cassava is a staple food (Alabi et al. 2015). The economic implications of CMD are equally severe. In Nigeria, for example, CMD has been estimated to cause annual losses of up to $1.25 billion, affecting subsistence farmers and commercial producers (Patil and Fauquet 2009). These losses not only reduce the availability of food but also diminish household incomes, exacerbating poverty and limiting the ability of communities to invest in education, healthcare, and other essential services.

Maise is another cornerstone of African agriculture, providing millions of people with a critical source of calories and nutrients. The Maize Streak Virus (MSV), transmitted by leafhoppers, is one of Africa's most significant viral threats to maise production. It is one of the most predominant viral diseases of maise in sub-Saharan Africa (Chikoti and Tembo 2022). Its symptoms include yellow streaks on leaves, leading to chlorosis and reduced photosynthesis, which can drastically lower yields. Yield loss in heavily infected fields can be up to 100%, further compromising food availability and affordability of the crop, which is a staple food for millions and also plays a critical role in the region's economy (Benjamin et al. 2024).

The impact of MSV is particularly devastating in regions where maise is not only a food crop but also a cash crop. In countries like Kenya, Uganda, and Tanzania, MSV outbreaks can decimate entire harvests, leading to food shortages and increasing maise product prices. This has a ripple effect on food security, as maise is a staple in the diets of many African communities. The reduction in maise availability can lead to increased reliance on less nutritious or less accessible food sources, contributing to malnutrition and other health problems (Macfadyen et al. 2018).

These viral diseases reduce the quantity of food available and impact its quality. Infected crops are often less nutritious, which can lead to a rise in malnutrition, particularly among vulnerable populations such as children and older people (Alabi et al. 2011). The cumulative effect of these diseases, therefore, extends beyond immediate food shortages and famines to long-term health implications, making the issue of food security even more pressing.

10.3 Health Implications of Food Insecurity

The health implications of food insecurity caused by plant viral diseases are profound and multifaceted. When food security is compromised, the health of vulnerable populations, particularly children, pregnant women, and older people, is at significant risk.

10.3.1 Malnutrition and Undernutrition

Malnutrition and undernutrition are among the most immediate health consequences of food insecurity. The loss of staple crops like cassava and maise can lead to insufficient caloric intake, resulting in wasting, stunting, and underweight in children. Malnutrition weakens the immune system, making individuals more susceptible to infectious diseases and reducing their ability to recover. In adults, malnutrition can lead to chronic health problems, reduced productivity, and increased mortality rates (Black et al. 2013).

10.3.2 Micronutrient Deficiencies

Viral disease-induced food insecurity can also lead to micronutrient deficiencies, which have serious health implications (Macfagdyen et al. 2018). For example, a diet lacking in maise and cassava can result in deficiencies in essential nutrients such as vitamin A, iron, and zinc. Vitamin A deficiency can cause blindness and increase the risk of severe infections, particularly in children. Iron deficiency is a leading cause of anaemia, which can impair cognitive and physical development and increase the risk of complications during pregnancy (Jones 2020).

10.3.3 Mental Health Issues

The stress and uncertainty associated with food insecurity can also have significant mental health impacts. Studies have shown that food insecurity is associated with higher levels of anxiety, depression, and other mental health disorders. In communities where agriculture is the primary livelihood, the loss of crops due to viral diseases can lead to a sense of hopelessness and despair, exacerbating mental health challenges (Hadley and Patil 2006). These mental health issues can further undermine individuals' ability to work and care for their families, creating a vicious cycle of poverty and food insecurity.

10.3.4 Reproductive Health Complications

Food insecurity can also have serious implications for reproductive health. Malnutrition and micronutrient deficiencies during pregnancy can lead to complications such as low birth weight, preterm birth, and increased risk of maternal and infant mortality (Roba et al. 2022). In regions where viral diseases in plants lead to widespread food shortages, pregnant women may not have access to the nutrients they need for a healthy pregnancy, putting both their lives and the lives of their infants at risk.

10.4 The One Health Approach: A Holistic Response

The One Health framework offers a comprehensive approach to tackling the multifaceted challenges of viral agricultural diseases. By recognising the interconnectedness of human, animal, and environmental health, One Health advocates for integrated efforts in disease management, which are essential for building resilient food systems (Okello et al. 2011).

One Health promotes the idea that the health of crops, livestock, and humans is intrinsically linked. For instance, viral diseases in crops can lead to reduced food availability, which in turn can cause malnutrition and increased susceptibility to diseases in humans. Moreover, livestock, which often rely on these staple crops for feed, can also suffer, leading to a cascade of health issues across species (Gibbs 2014). Therefore, addressing viral diseases in crops is not just an agricultural issue but a public health priority.

10.4.1 Sustainable Agricultural Practices

One of the One Health framework's key strategies is promoting sustainable agricultural practices. These practices include crop rotation, intercropping, and the use of disease-resistant crop varieties (Pretty 2008). Crop rotation and intercropping can help break the life cycles of pathogens and reduce the incidence of viral diseases. For example, rotating maise with legumes or other non-host crops can reduce the spread of MSV (Anderson et al. 2004).

The development and dissemination of disease-resistant crop varieties also play a crucial role. Biotechnology and traditional breeding methods have created cassava and maise varieties that are more resistant to CMV and MSV (Sheat and Winter 2023). However, these varieties must be made accessible to smallholder farmers, who are often the most affected by crop diseases. Additionally, educating farmers on best disease prevention and management practices is essential for these interventions' long-term sustainability (Thresh and Cooter 2005).

10.4.2 Enhanced Disease Surveillance

Effective disease management requires robust surveillance systems that can detect and respond to outbreaks early. The One Health framework emphasises the need for integrated surveillance systems that simultaneously monitor the health of crops, animals, and humans (Buregyeya et al. 2020). Such systems can help identify emerging threats and allow for rapid response measures to be implemented before widespread damage occurs.

In many parts of Africa, however, surveillance systems are underdeveloped. Investments in infrastructure, technology, and training are needed to build the capacity for effective disease monitoring. Mobile technology and remote sensing tools offer promising avenues for improving surveillance, particularly in remote and rural areas (Gogoi et al. 2018). By providing real-time data on disease outbreaks, these technologies can help farmers and authorities take timely action to mitigate the impact of viral diseases.

10.5 Conclusion: Building Resilient Food Systems in Africa

The threat of viral diseases to Africa's food security is a complex and urgent challenge that demands a comprehensive response. The One Health framework offers a valuable perspective by highlighting the interconnectedness of human, animal, and environmental health. By advocating for sustainable agricultural practices, enhanced disease surveillance, and integrated health strategies, this approach aims to build resilient food systems that can withstand the pressures of viral diseases and secure the future of food security in Africa.

The fight against viral diseases in crops is not just an agricultural battle—it is a fight for the health and well-being of millions across the continent. It is pertinent to ensure resilient food systems through collaborative efforts and innovative solutions to safeguard Africa's agricultural future and the health of its people.

References

Alabi OJ, Kumar PL, Naidu RA (2011) Cassava mosaic disease: a curse to food security in Sub-Saharan Africa. American Phytopathological Society Features. https://doi.org/10.1094/APSnetFeature-2011-0701

Alabi OJ, Mulenga R, Legg J (2015) In: Tennant P, G. F (eds) Cassava mosaic December 2015: virus diseases of tropical and subtropical crops. (chapter 5); CAB International, Wallingford

Anderson PK, Cunningham AA, Patel NG, Morales FJ, Epstein PR, Daszak P (2004) Emerging infectious diseases of plants: pathogen pollution, climate change and agrotechnology drivers. Trend Ecol Evol 19(10):535–544

Benjamin J, Oyedokun DO, Oziegbe EV, Oni J, Ogundare EO, Ujah GO, Adebayo A (2024) Cereal production in Africa: the threat of current plant pathogens in changing climate—a review. Discov Agric 2:33. https://doi.org/10.1007/s44279-024-00040-3

Black RE, Victoria CG, Walker SP, Bhutta ZA, Christian P, Onis M, Ezzati M, Grantham-Mcgregor, Katz J, Martorell R, Uauy R (2013) Maternal and child undernutrition and overweight in low-income and middle-income countries. Lancet 382(9890):427–451

Buregyeya E, Atusingwize E, Nsamba P, Musoke D, Naigaga I, Kabasa JD, Amuguni H, Bazeyo W (2020) Operationalising the one health approach in Uganda: challenges and opportunities. J Epidemiol Global Health 10(4):250–257

Chikoti P, Tembo M (2022) Expansion and impact of cassava brown streak and cassava mosaic diseases in Africa: a review. Front Sustain Food Syst 6:1076364. https://doi.org/10.3389/fsufs.2022.1076364

Gibbs EP (2014) The evolution of one health: a decade of progress and challenges for the future. Vet Rec 174(4):85–91

Gogoi NK, Deka B, Bora LC (2018) Remote sensing and its use in detection and monitoring plant diseases: a review. Agric Rev. https://doi.org/10.18805/ag.R-1835

Hadley C, Patil C (2006) Food insecurity in rural Tanzania is associated with maternal anxiety and depression. Am J Hum Biol 18:359–368

Jones RA (2020) Disease pandemics and major epidemics arising from new encounters between indigenous viruses and introduced crops. Viruses 4(12):1388. https://doi.org/10.3390/v12121388

Keesing F, Belden L, Daszak P, Dobson A, Harvell C, Holt R, Hudson P, Joles A, Jones K, Mitchell C, Myers S, Bogicj T (2010) Impacts of biodiversity on the emergence and transmission of infectious diseases. Nature 468(7324):647–652

Macfadyen S, Paull C, Boykin LM, De Barro P, Maruthi MN, Otim M, Kalyebi A, Vassão DG, Sseruwagi P, Tay WT, Delatte H, Seguni Z, Colvin J, Omongo CA (2018) Cassava whitefly, *Bemisia tabaci* (Gennadius) (Hemiptera: Aleyrodidae) in East African farming landscapes: a review of the factors determining abundance. Bull Entomol Res 108(5):565–582

Okello AL, Gibbs EP, Vandersmissen A, Welburn SC (2011) One health and the neglected zoonoses: turning rhetoric into reality. Vet Rec 169(11):281–285

Patil BL, Fauquet CM (2009) Review: cassava mosaic geminiviruses: actual knowledge and perspectives. Mol Plant Pathol 10:685–701

Pretty J (2008) Agricultural sustainability: concepts, principles and evidence. Philos Trans R Soc B or Philos Trans R Soc Lond B Biol Sci 363(1491):447–465

Roba KT, Hassen TA, Wilfong T, Legese N, Darsene H, Zewdu G, Negese T, Yifru B, Mohammed E, Raru TB (2022) Association of undernutrition and female infertility in East Africa: findings from multi-country demographic and health surveys. Front Glob Womens Health 15(3):1049404. https://doi.org/10.3389/fgwh.2022.1049404

Sheat S, Winter S (2023) Developing broad-spectrum resistance in cassava against viruses causing the cassava mosaic and the cassava brown streak diseases. Front Plant Sci. https://doi.org/10.3389/fpls.2023.1042701

Tembo M, Adediji AO, Bouvaine S, Chikoti PC, Seal SE, Silva G (2020) A quick and sensitive diagnostic tool for detection of Maize streak virus. Sci Rep 10(1):19633

Thresh JM, Cooter RJ (2005) Strategies for controlling cassava mosaic virus disease in Africa. Plant Pathol 54(5):587–614

Waidi GA (2023) Cassava production in Africa: a panel analysis of drivers and trends. Heliyon 9(9):e19939. https://doi.org/10.1016/j.heliyon.2023.e19939

Chapter 11
Antiviral Resistance in Africa: Prevalence, Challenges and Mitigation Measures

Akebe Luther king Abia

11.1 Introduction

Antimicrobial resistance (AMR) is one of the biggest challenges faced by humans in modern times (Ahmed et al. 2024). AMR occurs when microorganisms, such as bacteria, viruses, fungi, or parasites, mutate or adapt in ways that render treatments ineffective, making infections more challenging to treat, increasing the risk of spread, severe illness, and death (Salam et al. 2023).

While AMR arises naturally, the overuse and misuse of antimicrobials in humans, animals, and plants greatly accelerate its development (Ahmed et al. 2024). For example, antibiotics are often inappropriately used for viral infections or in unnecessary situations in human health, contributing to resistance (Australian Government 2022). The World Bank estimates that over half of the antimicrobials used in humans globally are misused and that one-third (over 50 million) of antibiotics prescribed in the USA annually by doctors are unnecessary (World Bank 2017). Furthermore, the rapid growth of the world population has led to increased demand for animal proteins, resulting in intensified production of food animals. Such farming practices lead to the substantial use of antimicrobials on farms for growth promotion and disease prevention, leading to resistance in livestock that can spread to humans (FAO 2025). However, most pharmaceuticals consumed by humans and animals are excreted in partially metabolised or unmetabolised form and end up in the environment through wastewater treatment plants or manure application (Abia et al. 2023). These excreted antimicrobial residues and those from pharmaceutical manufacturing

A. L. k. Abia (✉)
Total Environment Research (TEN-R) Group, College of Health Sciences, University of KwaZulu-Natal, Durban, South Africa

Environmental Research Foundation, Westville, South Africa
e-mail: AbiaAkebeL@ukzn.ac.za

J. A. Shenge, A. L. K. Abia (eds.), *Viral Diseases and One Health in Africa*,
https://doi.org/10.1007/978-3-032-09613-5_11

pollute water and soil, serving as reservoirs for stressors that can trigger resistance in environmental microorganisms (FAO 2025).

The increased rates of AMR in humans, animals and the environment not only impact public health, but also have rippling effects with severe economic implications. In 2019 alone, AMR directly caused 1.27 million deaths and contributed to nearly five million deaths globally (WHO 2023). It is estimated that around 1.14 million AMR-linked deaths occur worldwide (Wellcome 2024). The estimated AMR-associated economic loss is projected to be approximately 3.8% of global GDP annually by 2050 (World Bank 2024). Also, the Food and Agriculture Organization (FAO) of the United Nations warns that without appropriate action, AMR in agriculture could produce US$3.4 trillion losses in GDP within a decade (FAO 2025).

It should, however, be noted that although AMR is a global concern, its occurrence and impacts are not without disparities, as the burden is mainly felt in low- and middle-income countries, especially in Africa. Furthermore, while the focus has been on bacterial infections, AMR in viruses remains under-investigated, hence, underreported.

11.2 Antimicrobial Resistance in Viruses—Antiviral Resistance

11.2.1 Overview of Antiviral Resistance

Research on AMR is increasing worldwide due to the need to address it and protect humans, animals, and the environment. However, while AMR is well-recognised as a global health threat, the focus weighs heavily on bacteria and research on AMR in viruses is indeed less developed compared to bacterial AMR. This is mainly driven by the challenge of studying viruses themselves, due to their small sizes, rapid evolution, and diverse interactions with hosts. These challenges include difficulties in viral detection (Carrillo-Tripp et al. 2015; Cobbin et al. 2021; Sanjuán et al. 2021; Wang 2020), understanding complex evolutionary dynamics (Sanjuán et al. 2021; Wu and Peng 2024), accurately predicting viral behaviour (Kawasaki et al. 2025), culturing viruses (Wadell 1983), setting up experimental systems to study viruses (Nagyová and Subr 2007), the complex virus-host interaction (Hoenen and Groseth 2022) and the unclear epidemiological role of viruses on their host's health and disease (Herrington et al. 2015), among others.

Despite these challenges, this relative lack of attention to viral AMR is a significant concern, as viral infections pose a substantial burden on human, animal and plant health, and the emergence of antiviral resistance can severely limit treatment options.

11.2.2 Mechanisms of Antiviral Resistance

Antiviral resistance arises when viruses acquire genetic mutations or undergo recombination events that reduce the effectiveness of antiviral drugs. Resistance can be driven by selective pressure from widespread antiviral use, incomplete treatment courses, and the high mutation rates of many viruses, particularly RNA viruses. These mutations can affect drug targets, making them less susceptible to inhibition, or they can lead to increased production of viral proteins that overwhelm the drug's impact. In some cases, viruses can also develop mechanisms to actively expel the drug from infected cells (Vere Hodge and Field 2011). Thus, antiviral resistance mechanisms are diverse, and often virus- and drug-specific. For example, RNA viruses, such as HIV and influenza, have high mutation rates because their RNA-dependent RNA polymerase or reverse transcriptase enzymes lack the "proof-reading" or error-correcting mechanisms found in DNA polymerases. This high rate of mutation leads to the rapid generation of new genetic variants. When these mutations occur in genes targeted by antiviral drugs, they can alter the viral protein, preventing the drug from binding or inhibiting its function. This results in drug-resistant strains that can proliferate, rendering the treatment ineffective. In contrast, DNA viruses (like herpesviruses) have much lower mutation rates, as their replication machinery is more stable and includes proofreading mechanisms (Domingo and Holland 1997; Smyk et al. 2022; Yeo et al. 2020). The general mechanisms of viral resistance are summarised in Table 11.1, with examples.

11.3 Antiviral Resistance in Africa

The state of antiviral resistance in Africa has become a growing public health concern, particularly in the treatment of major viral diseases like HIV, influenza, and hepatitis, among others. While significant progress has been made in expanding access to antiviral therapies, this has been accompanied by the emergence and spread of drug-resistant viruses (Nsonga et al. 2024). The past few decades show a complex picture of both successes and emerging challenges.

11.3.1 HIV Drug Resistance

HIV is still a significant public health burden in Africa. Although there was a widespread rollout of antiretroviral therapy (ART) since the early 2000s that saved millions of lives, this intervention was also followed by an increased selective pressure for the development of resistance (WHO 2025a, b), making HIV drug resistance in Africa a complex and evolving challenge, with regional variations in prevalence. The Middle and East African regions have historically shown a higher

Table 11.1 Mechanisms of antiviral resistance

Mechanism of resistance	Description	Examples	References
Target site mutations	Mutations in viral enzymes reduce drug binding	HIV reverse transcriptase mutations → NRTI/ NNRTI resistance; Influenza neuraminidase H275Y mutation → oseltamivir resistance; HBV polymerase YMDD mutation → lamivudine resistance	Asahchop et al. (2012), Clavel and Hance (2004), McColl and Chen (2010), Okomo-Adhiambo et al. (2010), Preston et al. (1988)
Efflux pumps / drug expulsion	Upregulation of host efflux transporters lowers intracellular drug concentrations	HIV protease inhibitors affected by P-glycoprotein (ABCB1) efflux; HCV protease inhibitors show altered efficacy with transporter activity	Ghoshal et al. (2023), Karthika et al. (2022), Sankatsing et al. (2004), Shafer (2002), Zhang et al. (2014)
Enzymatic drug modification	Viral or host enzymes alter or fail to activate the drug	Cytomegalovirus (CMV) UL97 kinase mutations → ganciclovir resistance; Herpes Simplex Virus thymidine kinase mutations → acyclovir resistance	Andrei et al. (2007)
Reduced drug uptake	Alterations in viral/ host proteins reduce entry or activation	HSV TK-deficient strains fail to phosphorylate acyclovir; Influenza M2 mutations reduce amantadine uptake	Bacon et al. (2003)
Compensatory mutations	Secondary/tertiary mutations restore viral fitness while keeping resistance	HIV protease compensatory mutations (A431V, L449F) restore fitness; HBV polymerase compensatory mutations	Molla et al. (1996)
Gene amplification or Overexpression of target site	Increased expression of viral target enzyme overwhelms inhibitor	CMV UL97 gene amplification confers higher-level ganciclovir resistance	Andrei et al. (2007)
Horizontal gene transfer/ reassortment	Resistance spreads via recombination or genome segment exchange.	Influenza reassortment spreads resistance genes; HBV recombination events cause polymerase resistance	Okomo-Adhiambo et al. (2010)

prevalence of transmitted drug resistance compared to Southern and West Africa (Stadeli and Richman 2013). Despite an overall drop in resistance rates, non-nucleoside reverse transcriptase inhibitor (NNRTI) resistance found in regimens like efavirenz has been a significant concern in several countries, with rates exceeding 10% in some East African countries (de waal et al. 2018; Stadeli and Richman 2013; WHO 2021). This significantly impacts the effectiveness of older first-line antiretroviral therapy (ART) regimens.

Thus, to combat HIV resistance in Africa, many countries have transitioned to the WHO-recommended integrase-based inhibitors, like dolutegravir (DTG), which have a higher genetic barrier to resistance (WHO Africa 2019). However, maintaining treatment quality, ensuring drug adherence, and implementing comprehensive surveillance programs are crucial to prevent the emergence and spread of resistance, especially with the increasing use of pre-exposure prophylaxis (PrEP) and the "treat all" strategy (WHO 2021; WHO Africa 2019). For example, while DTG-based resistance is expected to be low, recent surveillance in South Africa has shown an increase in INSTI resistance, necessitating continued monitoring (NICD 2024). Also, as with previous drugs, resistance to the current recommendations could be increased due to low adherence to treatment regimens as a result of shortages in drug supply, inadequate follow-up of patients, and limited healthcare resources (Azia et al. 2016; WHO 2025a, b). With these limitations, it is projected that the resistance could increase to about 50% of all cases in South Africa by 2035 (Loosli et al. 2025).

11.3.2 Influenza Drug Resistance

Influenza remains a significant public health challenge in Africa, causing severe illness and death, particularly among high-risk groups like the elderly, pregnant women, and individuals with HIV (Wolter et al. 2025). While influenza seasons typically occur from April to October in Southern Hemisphere countries like South Africa, prevalence and activity levels vary annually. In South Africa, for example, approximately 14% of inpatients with lower respiratory tract infection and 25% of patients with influenza-like illness (ILI) test positive for influenza during the season (Blumberg et al. 2017).

Despite the significant impact of Influenza infection on public health in Africa, influenza resistance is generally low within the continent for currently circulating strains, particularly to neuraminidase inhibitors, though genetic drift can affect vaccine effectiveness (NICD n.d.). The shift to more potent neuraminidase inhibitors like oseltamivir, zanamivir, peramivir, and laninamivir was fuelled by the almost 100% resistance observed against adamantane (an M2 inhibitor), resulting in the WHO guarding against its use (Hussain et al. 2017; Oh et al. 2023). However, surveillance confirmed the spread of oseltamivir-resistant influenza A(H1N1) viruses in Southern Africa, specifically South Africa (Besselaar et al. 2008) and Senegal (Dia et al. 2013), during the 2008 winter season, linked to the H275Y mutation in the neuraminidase (NA) protein that confers high-level resistance to oseltamivir. This emergence was a significant public health concern, as oseltamivir was the most widely used antiviral drug for influenza at the time. This occurrence suggests that continued surveillance is crucial to monitor viral evolution and to ensure that vaccine strains and treatment recommendations remain effective against emerging resistance in the region. In line with this, African countries are contributing to the WHO Global Influenza Surveillance and Response System (GISRS) through FluNet/FluID, which collects and analyses data on influenza virus circulation and antiviral resistance (WHO 2025a, b). This participation helps the WHO provide timely guidance on influenza prevention and control, including vaccine recommendations and antiviral use. It also strengthens the global capacity for early detection of potential pandemic threats. Such initiatives could have contributed to rapid interventions, hence the low level of resistance observed in influenza within the continent.

11.3.3 Hepatitis Drug Resistance

Hepatitis drug resistance is a significant public health challenge in Africa, particularly for the highly prevalent Hepatitis B Virus (HBV), affecting both drug-exposed and non-exposed populations (Mokaya et al. 2018). This is often driven by the extensive use of lamivudine (3TC) for HIV co-treatment (Mathew et al. 2023; Mokaya et al. 2018). Resistance mutations are common, especially in HIV/HBV coinfected populations, leading to treatment failure and potential long-term complications like cirrhosis and liver cancer (Phinius et al. 2024). Hepatitis B and C resistance has been reported in many countries across the continent, such as in Nigeria (Anejo-Okopi et al. 2022), South Africa (Maepa et al. 2022; Mokaya et al. 2020), Mozambique (Mathew et al. 2023), Botswana (Phinius et al. 2024), Gabon (Abe et al. 2023) and Uganda (Lumley et al. 2025). However, the lack of data regarding the circulating genotypes and drug resistance mutations limits the full understanding of the level of hepatitis virus antiviral resistance in Africa.

The overall picture is that while significant strides have been made in treating viral infections in Africa (Table 11.2), the emergence of antiviral resistance poses a major threat to the progress made so far. Although not yet reported, there are growing concerns that future resistance may arise to other viral infections, such as monkeypox (Bapolisi et al. 2024; Pipitò et al. 2025) and SARS-COV-2 and other respiratory viral infections (Batool et al. 2025; Nooruzzaman et al. 2024), as these have already been reported in other parts of the world.

11.4 Challenges Associated with Antiviral Resistance in Africa

The overall picture is that while significant strides have been made in treating viral infections in Africa, the emergence of antiviral resistance poses a major threat to these gains. The main challenges are broadly discussed below.

Table 11.2 Antiviral resistance milestones in Africa (2000–2025)

Virus	Year/ period	Event/development	Country/region highlight	Reference
HIV	Early 2010s	NNRTI pretreatment resistance (PDR) ≥10% detected in several African countries	Mozambique, Kenya, Nigeria, Tanzania, South Africa, Guinea-Bissau, Malawi	Beck et al. (2020), Chimukangara et al. (2019), Rutstein et al. (2019), WHO (2017), Wilhelmson et al. (2018)
	2015–2019	WHO recommends dolutegravir (DTG) as first-line therapy (phased roll-out)	Global, with evidence base from Sub-Saharan Africa	Bangalee et al. (2022), WHO (2016, 2019), Zaniewski et al. (2024)
	Late 2010s–2020s	DTG resistance observed at treatment failure; modelling predicts growth to the 2030s	South Africa, regional	Mahomed et al. (2020), Malinga et al. (2023), Naidoo et al. (2025)
HBV	2005–2015	Lamivudine (3TC) resistance is widely reported	Global, especially Sub-Saharan Africa	Meijer et al. (2014)
	2015–2024	WHO guidelines recommend tenofovir or entecavir as preferred therapy; dual tenofovir-based treatment is recommended where monotherapy fails	Africa-wide	Easterbrook et al. (2024), Spearman (2024)
HCV	Late 2010s	Recognition of NS5A resistance-associated substitutions (RAS)	Egypt	Ahmed et al. (2021), Ramadan et al. (2018)
	2018–present	Rollout of pan-genotypic DAAs; Egypt national elimination program	Egypt (flagship program), Rwanda	Coalision for Global Hepatitis Elimination (2022), Cooke et al. (2019), Cousins (2024), El Behery et al. (2025), Umutesi et al. (2019), Waked et al. (2020), WHO (2018)
Influenza	Early 2000s–mid 2000s	Adamantane resistance becomes widespread	Africa-wide	Ndihokubwayo et al. (2013)
	Ongoing (2020s)	Antiviral resistance surveillance (neuraminidase inhibitors, incl. H275Y)	Africa-wide	Blumberg et al. (2025), Boivin (2013), Meijer et al. (2014), Patel et al. (2024), Zambon (2013)

(continued)

Table 11.2 (continued)

Virus	Year/ period	Event/development	Country/region highlight	Reference
Mpox	2023–2024	Tecovirimat (F13L) resistance mutations reported, but not specifically in Africa.	DRC	Ali et al. (2025), Pipitò et al. (2025), Srivastava et al. (2024)
	2024	DRC randomised controlled trial: tecovirimat showed no clinical benefit vs placebo		

11.4.1 Limited Surveillance

A lack of robust laboratory testing and data systems across many African countries hinders the ability to track and respond to drug resistance accurately (Beesham et al. 2022). The "blind spot" in the surveillance of antimicrobial resistance as a whole, and antiviral resistance, in particular, in Africa is a critical issue. It means that health officials and policymakers do not have the data needed to understand the true scope of the problem. This can lead to delays in updating treatment guidelines, a misallocation of resources, and a continued rise in untreatable infections. The situation varies by country, with some having more developed surveillance systems than others.

The surveillance "blind spot" is particularly pronounced in Gabon and Central Africa for diseases like viral hepatitis (HBV and HCV). Research in Gabon has revealed that while the prevalence of these viruses is high, there is a lack of sufficient data to understand the prevalent viral genotypes and any associated resistance-related mutations (Abe et al. 2023). This limited information makes it difficult to design and implement effective direct-acting antiviral therapies, as resistance can compromise their efficacy.

A similar example is the challenge faced by South Africa with HIV drug resistance despite the significant progress made nationwide. Surveys conducted by the National Institute for Communicable Diseases (NICD) and National Health Laboratory Service (NHLS) have shown that the prevalence of drug resistance is declining, which is a promising sign (NICD 2024). However, they also found a significant drop in the proportion of specimens with detectable drug levels, suggesting that treatment failure is often due to sub-optimal adherence rather than outright drug resistance. This highlights that surveillance data is only part of the story; other interventions must complement to ensure patient care.

Broadly speaking, within the African context, a major study by the Mapping Antimicrobial Resistance and Antimicrobial Use Partnership (MAAP) across 14 African countries underscored the severity of this issue. The study found that across these countries, fewer than 2% of health facilities were equipped to test for bacterial infections, and a mere 12% of drug resistance records were linked to patient information (Africa CDC, 2025). Although this data relates to bacterial infections, the situation could be even worse for viruses, given that the latter are more complex to deal with within most African routine laboratories (Ashenafi et al. 2024). This stark finding demonstrates a widespread systemic failure to monitor and track resistance, making it nearly impossible to mount a data-driven, effective response.

11.4.2 Low Adherence to Treatment Regimens

Suboptimal treatment adherence is a major driver of antiviral resistance in Africa. When patients fail to take their medications as prescribed, whether due to drug shortages, side effects, or a lack of understanding, this creates an opportunity for viruses to replicate and mutate, at times leading to the evolution of drug-resistant strains that can no longer be killed with existing drugs and that can pass such traits on to other viruses (Azia et al. 2016; Bijker et al. 2017; Gumede et al. 2023; Peltzer et al. 2010).

A sub-Saharan study in Botswana on adult combination antiretroviral therapy highlighted that, despite high rates of virologic suppression and adherence among patients who remained in care, loss to follow-up and high mortality rates were significant problems (Wester et al. 2009). Patients who stopped taking their medication often did so within the first six months of treatment, which provides a key window for the development of resistance. Addressing this requires robust patient retention strategies, including consistent follow-up and support.

Similarly, in South Africa, a study on HIV drug resistance found that a significant portion of patients with detectable viral loads lacked any detectable drug levels in their system (NICD 2024). This finding strongly suggests that treatment failure is due to sub-optimal adherence rather than a failure of the drugs themselves. This issue is often compounded by limited healthcare access in rural areas and a lack of resources for patient counselling and education on the importance of consistent medication use.

11.4.3 Pretreatment Resistance

This is a significant and growing problem in Africa, where individuals are infected with a drug-resistant virus from the very beginning, even before they start their first-line antiretroviral therapy. This is often the case with older HIV medications, which have a lower genetic barrier to resistance (Melku et al. 2022). This phenomenon is particularly concerning as it compromises the effectiveness of standard treatment regimens and necessitates the use of more complex and expensive second-line therapies.

For example, a study on pretreatment HIV-1 drug resistance among South African women who acquired HIV during a prospective study found high levels of resistance mutations (Beesham et al. 2022). This is a major concern because it threatens to undermine the UNAIDS 95-95-95 targets, one of which is the goal of achieving viral suppression in 95% of individuals on treatment (UNAIDS, 2025). The study found a steady increase in the prevalence of pretreatment resistance, especially to NRTIs, from 2001 onwards (Beesham et al. 2022). The lack of access to resistance testing in many African countries makes it difficult to detect this issue early.

This is not a country-specific challenge, as the WHO has reported that in some African countries, up to 26% of people initiating treatment are infected with a virus carrying resistance to first-line antiretroviral drugs. The level of HIV drug resistance is even higher in infants born to mothers with HIV, approaching 70% in some cases, partly due to the widespread use of NNRTI-based regimens, which are more susceptible to resistance mutations (Melku et al. 2022).

11.4.4 Socioeconomic Factors

Poverty, lack of access to consistent healthcare, and geographical disparities between urban and rural areas are all linked to higher rates of antiviral resistance in Africa (Nsonga et al. 2024). These socioeconomic factors create an environment where successful treatment is hindered, and drug-resistant viruses are more likely to emerge and spread.

A study on predicting HIV drug resistance in sub-Saharan Africa found a strong link between lower socioeconomic status (SES) indicators and increased rates of resistance to HIV drugs (HIVDR). Countries with lower SES, as measured by unemployment and median household income, tended to have higher levels of HIVDR (Nsonga et al. 2024). This is because lower-income individuals often face more significant barriers to consistent treatment access and adherence. The study also highlighted the role of geographical disparities, noting that healthcare services and patient engagement in care are often affected by the differences between urban and rural areas. A lack of resources and infrastructure in rural and remote areas poses a challenge to effective treatment. This disparity can lead to inconsistent drug supply, limited access to viral load testing, and fewer healthcare workers with the specialised knowledge to manage complex cases of drug resistance. Patients in these areas may have to travel long distances, miss appointments, and eventually interrupt their treatment, increasing the risk of resistance. This was also the case with the Botswanan study, which highlighted that while virologic suppression and adherence rates were on par with resource-rich settings, loss to follow-up and high mortality rates, especially within the first six months of treatment, remain a significant problem. This suggests that even in a country with a relatively strong health system, challenges in patient retention and ongoing care can contribute to treatment failure, which in turn can lead to the development of drug resistance (Wester et al. 2009).

11.4.5 Lack of (or Insufficient) Investment in Healthcare

The lack of investment is a primary driver of antiviral resistance in Africa, as it starves public health systems of the resources needed for effective prevention, surveillance, and treatment. This leads to drug shortages, outdated infrastructure, and a shortage of trained personnel, all of which contribute to the emergence and spread of resistant viruses (Africa CDC, 2025). There is an urgent need for African governments to prioritise and invest in strengthening laboratory infrastructure, routine testing, and digital systems to monitor and address antiviral resistance. Without these actions, the effectiveness of current and future antiviral treatments could be jeopardised (Africa CDC, 2025). For example, while South Africa has a more advanced healthcare system than many of its neighbours, a lack of investment still affects rural and remote areas (Ogbodu et al. 2025). Drug shortages and a lack of specialised infrastructure in these regions mean that patients may not have consistent access to their medications or the necessary viral load testing to monitor treatment efficacy. This inconsistent supply chain is a direct result of underinvestment and leads to treatment interruptions, providing a clear pathway for viruses to develop resistance.

11.5 Strategies to Mitigate Antiviral Resistance in Africa

Although Africa as a continent has shown remarkable achievements in addressing viral infections and antiviral resistance, a lot still needs to be done to prevent a retrograde to previous challenges. Implementing and strengthening certain key strategies, as discussed below, can help African countries combat antiviral resistance and protect the gains made in public health.

11.5.1 Integrated Surveillance

This involves implementing and strengthening national surveillance programs to monitor the emergence and spread of drug resistance. It is essential for informing treatment decisions and guiding public health policy. A lack of robust laboratory testing and data systems makes it challenging to track resistance accurately. Integrated surveillance programs, such as those recommended by the WHO, provide a systematic way to collect data on resistance patterns. This helps health authorities identify which drug regimens are failing and when to switch to new ones. The National HIV Drug Resistance Surveillance in South Africa, conducted by the NICD, is a clear example (NICD 2024). The surveys track resistance among adults with viral non-suppression and provide valuable data on the effectiveness of different ART regimens. Adopting such proactive monitoring would allow African countries to rely on a data-driven approach to adapting national treatment guidelines.

11.5.2 Ensuring Quality Antiviral Treatment Delivery

Monitoring and improving the quality of drug delivery is a core recommendation from the WHO to minimise the emergence and spread of resistant viruses. This includes ensuring consistent drug supply, proper patient counselling, and access to care. High-quality drug delivery reduces opportunities for the viruses to develop resistance. This is because consistent, uninterrupted treatment maintains viral suppression, preventing the virus from replicating and mutating. Conversely, a lack of investment can lead to drug shortages, creating treatment interruptions and driving resistance.

11.5.3 Patient Retention and Adherence

Ensuring that people living with viral infections like HIV, for example, stay on treatment and maintain adherence is critical. Poor patient retention and drug stock-outs are significant risk factors for resistance. Antiviral drugs are most effective when taken consistently. When patients are lost to follow-up or face drug shortages, their viral load can rebound, providing a fertile ground for the development of resistance. Lessons from Botswana show that while adherence rates can be high among patients who remain in care, loss to follow-up and high mortality rates in the initial months of treatment remain a significant problem. These patient drop-offs create a major gap in the treatment cascade and contribute to the spread of resistant strains (Wester et al. 2009).

11.5.4 Treatment Failure Monitoring

Monitoring for treatment failure is crucial for the early detection of drug resistance and prompt intervention, especially in vulnerable populations like children and adolescents. Early detection of rising viral loads allows clinicians to switch a patient's regimen before a fully resistant virus emerges. Without this monitoring, a patient could unknowingly be on a failing regimen for years, accumulating more resistance mutations. For example, the WHO reports a high level of HIV drug resistance in infants born to HIV-positive mothers (Melku et al. 2022). Thus, early and consistent monitoring for treatment failure in this young demographic is essential to ensure they receive a successful long-term treatment plan.

11.5.5 Creating and Maintaining Strategic Partnerships

Active engagement with ministries of health, research institutions, and other stakeholders, locally and internationally, is needed to develop and implement effective national antiviral drug resistance strategic plans. No single organisation can tackle this problem alone. Partnerships facilitate the sharing of data, resources, and best practices. They also help to secure the funding and political will needed to implement large-scale interventions. This is the backbone of the One Health Concept that calls for effective communication between all sectors (Collignon and McEwen 2019). The MAAP study, supported by the UK's Fleming Fund and the US CDC, is a prime example. This international partnership allowed for a large-scale assessment of drug resistance across 14 African countries and produced data that can now be used to inform national and regional policies (Africa CDC, 2025).

11.6 Conclusion

Over the recent decades, antiviral resistance in Africa has emerged as a major public health crisis, threatening to undermine significant progress in the treatment of diseases like HIV, hepatitis, and influenza. The situation is complex, marked by both successes and critical challenges, including limited surveillance, suboptimal treatment adherence, pretreatment resistance, and socioeconomic factors. Addressing these challenges calls for a multifaceted approach involving integrated surveillance, ensuring quality drug delivery, improving patient retention and adherence to treatment, and establishing strategic local and international partnerships.

References

Abe H, Ushijima Y, Bikangui R, Ondo GN, Pemba CM, Zadeh VR, Mpingabo PI, Ueda H, Agnandji ST, Lell B, Yasuda J (2023) Genetic diversity of hepatitis B and C viruses revealed by continuous surveillance from 2015 to 2021 in Gabon, Central Africa. Microorganisms 11. https://doi.org/10.3390/microorganisms11082046

Abia A, Baloyi T, Traore A, Potgieter N (2023) The African wastewater resistome: identifying knowledge gaps to inform future research directions. Antibiotics 12:805. https://doi.org/10.3390/antibiotics12050805

Africa CDC (2025) New study reveals widespread drug resistance across 14 African Countries [WWW Document]. https://africacdc.org/news-item/new-study-reveals-widespread-drug-resistance-across-14-african-countries/#:~:text=Supported%20by%20the%20UK's%20Fleming,testing%2C%20and%20stronger%20digital%20systems. Accessed 24. Aug 2025

Ahmed HR, Waly NGFM, Abd El-Baky RM, Yahia R, Hetta HF, Elsayed AM, Ibrahem RA (2021) Distribution of naturally occurring NS5B resistance-associated substitutions in Egyptian patients with chronic Hepatitis C. PLoS One 16. https://doi.org/10.1371/journal.pone.0249770

Ahmed SK, Hussein S, Qurbani K, Ibrahim RH, Fareeq A, Mahmood KA, Mohamed MG (2024) Antimicrobial resistance: Impacts, challenges, and future prospects. J Med Surg Public Health 2: 100081. https://doi.org/10.1016/j.glmedi.2024.100081

Ali et al (2025) Tecovirimat for Clade I MPXV Infection in the Democratic Republic of Congo. N Engl J Med 392:1484–1496. https://doi.org/10.1056/NEJMoa2412439

Andrei G, Fiten P, Froeyen M, De Clercq E, Opdenakker G, Snoeck R (2007) DNA polymerase mutations in drug-resistant herpes simplex virus mutants determine in vivo neurovirulence and drug-enzyme interactions. Antivir Ther 12:719–732

Anejo-Okopi J, Okeke E, Davwar PM, Onwuamah C, Onywera H, Omaiye P, Duguru M, Okojokwu OJ, Ujah OI, Jonathan B, George CA, Crown RS, Yakubu FB, Sokei JO, Okoli LC, Audu O, Inzaule SC, Abah IO, Agaba P, Agbaji OO, Sagay AS, Hawkins C (2022) Molecular detection of hepatitis B virus genotype E with immune escape mutations in chronic hepatitis B patients on long-term antiviral therapy in Jos, Nigeria. Afr J Lab Med 11. https://doi.org/10.4102/ajlm.v11i1.1677

Asahchop EL, Wainberg MA, Sloan RD, Tremblay CL (2012) Antiviral drug resistance and the need for development of new HIV-1 reverse transcriptase inhibitors. Antimicrob Agents Chemother. https://doi.org/10.1128/AAC.00591-12

Ashenafi A, Sule O, Peter T, Mashate S, Otieno O, Kebede A, Oio J, Kao K, Carter J, Whistler T, Ndlovu N, Kebede Y (2024) Diagnostics for detection and surveillance of priority epidemic-prone diseases in Africa: an assessment of testing capacity and laboratory strengthening needs. Front Public Health 12. https://doi.org/10.3389/fpubh.2024.1438334

Australian Government (2022) Antimicrobial resistance. What causes AMR? [WWW Document]. https://www.amr.gov.au/about-amr/what-causes-amr. Accessed 20 Aug 2025

Azia IN, Mukumbang FC, Van Wyk B (2016) Barriers to adherence to antiretroviral treatment in a regional hospital in Vredenburg, Western Cape, South Africa. South Afr J HIV Med 17. https://doi.org/10.4102/sajhivmed.v17i1.476

Bacon TH, Levin MJ, Leary JJ, Sarisky RT, Sutton D (2003) Herpes simplex virus resistance to acyclovir and penciclovir after two decades of antiviral therapy. Clin Microbiol Rev. https://doi.org/10.1128/CMR.16.1.114-128.2003

Bangalee A, Hanley S, Bangalee V (2022) Dolutegravir as first-line antiretroviral therapy in South Africa: Beware the one-size-fits-all approach. S Afr Med J. https://doi.org/10.7196/SAMJ.2022.v112i10.16596

Bapolisi WA, Krasemann S, Wayengera M, Kirenga B, Bahizire E, Malembaka EB, Siewe Fodjo JN, Colebunders R, Katoto PD (2024) Mpox outbreak—tecovirimat resistance, management approaches, and challenges in HIV-endemic regions. Lancet Infect Dis. https://doi.org/10.1016/S1473-3099(24)00591-7

Batool S, Chokkakula S, Jeong JH, Baek YH, Song MS (2025) SARS-CoV-2 drug resistance and therapeutic approaches. Heliyon. https://doi.org/10.1016/j.heliyon.2025.e41980

Beck IA, Levine M, McGrath CJ, Bii S, Milne RS, Kingoo JM, So I, Andersen N, Dross S, Coombs RW, Kiarie J, Chohan B, Sakr SR, Chung MH, Frenkel LM (2020) Pre-treatment HIV-drug resistance associated with virologic outcome of first-line NNRTI-antiretroviral therapy: A cohort study in Kenya. EClinicalMedicine 18. https://doi.org/10.1016/j.eclinm.2019.100239

Beesham I, Parikh UM, Mellors JW, Davey DLJ, Heffron R, Palanee-Phillips T, Bosman SL, Beksinska M, Smit J, Ahmed K, Makkan H, Selepe P, Louw C, Kotze P, Justus Hofmeyr G, Singata-Madliki M, Nursing G, Rees H, Baeten JM, Wallis C (2022) High levels of pretreatment HIV-1 drug resistance mutations among South African women who acquired HIV during a prospective study. J Acquir Immune Defic Syndr

Besselaar TG, Naidoo D, Buys A, Gregory V, McAnerney J, Manamela JM, Blumberg L, Schoub BD (2008) Widespread oseltamivir resistance in influenza A viruses (H1N1), South Africa. Emerg Infect Dis 14:1809–1810. https://doi.org/10.3201/eid1411.080958

Bijker R, Jiamsakul A, Kityo C, Kiertiburanakul S, Siwale M, Phanuphak P, Akanmu S, Chaiwarith R, Wit FW, Sim BLH, Boender TS, Ditangco R, De Wit TFR, Sohn AH, Hamers RL (2017) Adherence to antiretroviral therapy for HIV in sub-Saharan Africa and Asia: A comparative analysis of two regional cohorts. J Int AIDS Soc 20. https://doi.org/10.7448/IAS.20.1.21218

Blumberg L, Cohen C, Dawood H, Hellferscee O, Karstaedt A, Mccarthy K, Madhi S, Mcmorrow M, Moyes J, Nel J, Puren A, Variava E, Ramkrishna W, Reubenson G, Tempia S, Treurnicht F, Walaza S (2017) Influenza. NICD Recommendations for the diagnosis, prevention, management and public health response. Influenza Guidelines 25_05_2017

Blumberg L, Cohen C, Dawood H, Madhi, S., Karstaedt, A., Mccarthy, K., Moyes, J., Nel, J., Puren, A., Ramkrishna, W., Reubenson, G., Treurnicht, F., Variava, E., Von Gottberg, A., Wolter, N., Zar, H.J (2025) Influenza: NICD recommendations for the diagnosis, management, prevention and public health response

Boivin G (2013) Detection and management of antiviral resistance for influenza viruses. Influenza Other Respir Viruses. https://doi.org/10.1111/irv.12176

Carrillo-Tripp J, Bonning BC, Miller WA (2015) Challenges associated with research on RNA viruses of insects. Curr Opin Insect Sci. https://doi.org/10.1016/j.cois.2014.11.002

Chimukangara B, Lessells RJ, Rhee SY, Giandhari J, Kharsany ABM, Naidoo K, Lewis L, Cawood C, Khanyile D, Ayalew KA, Diallo K, Samuel R, Hunt G, Vandormael A, Stray-Pedersen B, Gordon M, Makadzange T, Kiepiela P, Ramjee G, Ledwaba J, Kalimashe M, Morris L, Parikh UM, Mellors JW, Shafer RW, Katzenstein D, Moodley P, Gupta RK, Pillay D, Abdool Karim SS, de Oliveira T (2019) Trends in pretreatment HIV-1 drug resistance in antiretroviral therapy-naive adults in South Africa, 2000–2016: a pooled sequence analysis. EClinicalMedicine 9:26–34. https://doi.org/10.1016/j.eclinm.2019.03.006

Clavel F, Hance AJ (2004) HIV drug resistance. N Engl J Med 350:1023

Coalision for Global Hepatitis Elimination (2022) National hepatitis elimination profiles released for two of the world's most advanced HCV elimination programs: Egypt and Rwanda [WWW Document]. https://www.globalhep.org/news-blogs/national-hepatitis-elimination-profiles-released-two-worlds-most-advanced-hcv#:~:text=The%20Egyptian%20Presidential%20Initiative%2C%20100,on%20National%20Hepatitis%20Elimination%20Profiles. Accessed 23 Aug 2025

Cobbin JC, Charon J, Harvey E, Holmes EC, Mahar JE (2021) Current challenges to virus discovery by meta-transcriptomics. Curr Opin Virol. https://doi.org/10.1016/j.coviro.2021.09.007

Collignon P, McEwen S (2019) One health—its importance in helping to better control antimicrobial resistance. Trop Med Infect Dis 4:22. https://doi.org/10.3390/tropicalmed4010022

Cooke GS, Andrieux-Meyer I, Applegate TL, Atun R, Burry JR, Cheinquer H, Dusheiko G, Feld JJ, Gore C, Griswold MG, Hamid S, Hellard ME, Hou JL, Howell J, Jia J, Kravchenko N, Lazarus JV, Lemoine M, Lesi OA, Maistat L, McMahon BJ, Razavi H, Roberts TR, Simmons B, Sonderup MW, Spearman CW, Taylor BE, Thomas DL, Waked I, Ward JW, Wiktor SZ, Abdo A, Aggarwal R, Aghemo A, Al-Judaibi B, Al Mahtab M, Altaf A, Ameen Z, Asselah T, Baatarkkhuu O, Barber E, Barnes E, Boulet P, Burrows L, Butsashvili M, Chan E, Chow C, Cowie B, Cunningham C, de Araujo A, Diap G, Dore G, Doyle J, Elsayed M, Fajardo E, Gane E, Getehun A, Goldberg D, Got T, Hickman M, Hill A, Hutchinson S, Jones C, Kamili S, Khan A, Lee A, Lee TY, Malani J, Morris TM, Nayagam S, Njouom R, Ocama P, Pedrana A, Peeling R, Reddy A, Roberts T, Sacks J, Sarin S, Shimakawa Y, Silva M, Skala P, Taylor-Robinson S, Thompson A, Thursz M, Tonganibeia A, Wallace J, Ward J, Wolff F, Vickerman P, Yau J (2019) Accelerating the elimination of viral hepatitis: a Lancet Gastroenterology & Hepatology Commission. Lancet Gastroenterol Hepatol. https://doi.org/10.1016/S2468-1253(18)30270-X

Cousins S (2024) Egypt's hepatitis success story. Lancet 403:1011–1012. https://doi.org/10.1016/S0140-6736(24)00531-2

de waal R, Lessells R, Hauser A, Kouyos R, Davies M-A, Egger M, Wandeler G, IeDeA-Southern Africa (2018) HIV drug resistance in sub-Saharan Africa: public health questions and the potential role of real-world data and mathematical modelling. J Virus Erad

Dia N, Niang MN, Diadhiou SA, Goudiaby DG, Faye A, Kiori D, Bâ M, Michel R, Diop OM (2013) Spread of Influenza A(H1N1) oseltamivir-resistant viruses in Africa in 2008 confirmed by multiple introductions in Senegal. BMC Infect Dis 13. https://doi.org/10.1186/1471-2334-13-106

Domingo E, Holland JJ (1997) RNA virus mutations and fitness for survival. Ann Rev Microbiol 51:151–178. https://doi.org/10.1146/annurev.micro.51.1.151

Easterbrook PJ, Luhmann N, Bajis S, Min MS, Newman M, Lesi O, Doherty MC (2024) WHO 2024 hepatitis B guidelines: an opportunity to transform care. Lancet Gastroenterol Hepatol 9: 493–495. https://doi.org/10.1016/S2468-1253(24)00089-X

El Behery M, Elghwab AI, Tabll A, El-Sayed, Hamdi E-S, Abdelrazek MA (2025) Review article: Egyptian efforts to control hepatitis C virus in Egypt. AJBAS 6:253–262. https://doi.org/10.21608/ajbas.2025.362040.1251

FAO (2025) Food and agricultural organization of the United Nations. Antimicrobial Resistance [WWW Document]. https://www.fao.org/antimicrobial-resistance/background/what-is-it/en/?utm_source=chatgpt.com. Accessed 20 Aug 2025

Ghoshal A, Mallick J, Sarkar, Suranjana, Ghosh S, Ghosh B, Sarkar, Subhasis (2023) Efflux pumps in antimicrobial resistance: mechanism, regulation and therapeutic implications. J Adv Zool 44: 2575–2580

Gumede SB, Wensing AMJ, Lalla-Edward ST, de Wit JBF, Francois Venter WD, Tempelman HA, Hermans LE (2023) Predictors of treatment adherence and virological failure among people living with HIV receiving antiretroviral therapy in a South African rural community: a sub-study of the ITREMA randomised clinical trial. AIDS Behav 27:3863–3885. https://doi.org/10.1007/s10461-023-04103-2

Herrington CS, Coates PJ, Duprex WP (2015) Viruses and disease: Emerging concepts for prevention, diagnosis and treatment. J Pathol 235:149–152. https://doi.org/10.1002/path.4476

Hoenen T, Groseth A (2022) Virus–host cell interactions. Cells. https://doi.org/10.3390/cells11050804

Hussain M, Galvin HD, Haw TY, Nutsford AN, Husain M (2017) Drug resistance in influenza a virus: the epidemiology and management. Infect Drug Resist. https://doi.org/10.2147/IDR.S105473

Karthika C, Sureshkumar R, Zehravi M, Akter R, Ali F, Ramproshad S, Mondal B, Tagde P, Ahmed Z, Khan FS, Rahman MH, Cavalu S (2022) Multidrug resistance of cancer cells and the vital role of P-glycoprotein. Life. https://doi.org/10.3390/life12060897

Kawasaki J, Suzuki T, Hamada M (2025) Hidden challenges in evaluating spillover risk of zoonotic viruses using machine learning models. Commun Med 5. https://doi.org/10.1038/s43856-025-00903-w

Loosli T, Han N, Hauser A, Josi J, Ingle SM, van Sighem A, Wittkop L, Vehreschild J, Ceccherini-Silberstein F, Maartens G, Gill MJ, Sabin CA, Johnson LF, Lessells R, Günthard HF, Egger M, Kouyos RD (2025) Predicted dolutegravir resistance in people living with HIV in South Africa during 2020–2035: a modelling study. Lancet Glob Health 13:e698–e706. https://doi.org/10.1016/S2214-109X(24)00553-9

Lumley SF, Kimono B, Mugisha J, Makanga R, Mbonye MK, Ojambo K, Waddilove E, Kent C, Ssengendo B, Ndungutse R, McNaughton AL, Muzaale FN, Seeley J, Quick J, Ocama P, Newton R, Matthews PC (2025) Eligibility for hepatitis B virus (HBV) treatment and prevalence of drug resistance in a Ugandan population cohort. https://doi.org/10.1101/2025.04.06.25325341

Maepa MB, Ely A, Kramvis A, Bloom K, Naidoo K, Simani OE, Maponga TG, Arbuthnot P (2022) Hepatitis B virus research in South Africa. Viruses. https://doi.org/10.3390/v14091939

Mahomed K, Wallis CL, Dunn L, Maharaj S, Maartens G, Meintjes G (2020) Case report: emergence of dolutegravir resistance in a patient on second-line antiretroviral therapy. South Afr J HIV Med 21. https://doi.org/10.4102/SAJHIVMED.V21I1.1062

Malinga S, Khan A, Archary M (2023) Breaking the unbreakable: A paediatric case of dolutegravir resistance from KwaZulu-Natal. South Afr J HIV Med 24. https://doi.org/10.4102/sajhivmed.v24i1.1458

Mathew A, Ismael N, Meeds H, Vubil A, Zicai AF, Mabunda N, Blackard JT (2023) Hepatitis B virus genotypes and drug resistance mutations circulating in blood donors in Beira, Mozambique. PLoS One 18. https://doi.org/10.1371/journal.pone.0281855

McColl DJ, Chen X (2010) Strand transfer inhibitors of HIV-1 integrase: Bringing IN a new era of antiretroviral therapy. Antivir Res. https://doi.org/10.1016/j.antiviral.2009.11.004

Meijer A, Rebelo-De-Andrade H, Correia V, Besselaar T, Drager-Dayal R, Fry A, Gregory V, Gubareva L, Kageyama T, Lackenby A, Lo J, Odagiri T, Pereyaslov D, Siqueira MM, Takashita E, Tashiro M, Wang D, Wong S, Zhang W, Daniels RS, Hurt AC (2014) Global update on the susceptibility of human influenza viruses to neuraminidase inhibitors, 2012–2013. Antivir Res 110:31–41. https://doi.org/10.1016/j.antiviral.2014.07.001

Melku M, Gesesew HA, Ward PR (2022) Magnitude and predictors of HIV-Drug resistance in Africa: A protocol for systematic review and meta-analysis. PLoS One. https://doi.org/10.1371/journal.pone.0267159

Mokaya J, McNaughton AL, Hadley MJ, Beloukas A, Geretti AM, Goedhals D, Matthews PC (2018) A systematic review of hepatitis B virus (HBV) drug and vaccine escape mutations in Africa: a call for urgent action. PLoS Negl Trop Dis 12. https://doi.org/10.1371/journal.pntd.0006629

Mokaya J, Maponga TG, McNaughton AL, Van Schalkwyk M, Hugo S, Singer JB, Sreenu VB, Bonsall D, de Cesare M, Andersson M, Gabriel S, Taljaard J, Barnes E, Preiser W, Van Rensburg C, Matthews PC (2020) Evidence of tenofovir resistance in chronic hepatitis B virus (HBV) infection: an observational case series of South African adults. J Clin Virol 129. https://doi.org/10.1016/j.jcv.2020.104548

Molla A, Korneyeva M, Gao Q, Vasavanonda S, Schipper PJ, Mo HM, Markowitz M, Chernyavskiy T, Niu P, Lyons N, Hsu A, Granneman GR, Ho DD, Boucher CA, Leonard JM, Norbeck DW, Kempf DJ (1996) Ordered accumulation of mutations in HIV protease confers resistance to ritonavir. Nat Med 2:760–766. https://doi.org/10.1038/nm0796-760

Nagyová A, Subr Z (2007) Infectious full-length clones of plant viruses and their use for construction of viral vectors. Acta Virol 51:223–237

Naidoo K, Lessells RJ, Dorward J, Moosa MYS, Sookrajh Y, Moodley P, Drain PK, Garrett N (2025) Rapid emergence of dolutegravir resistance on second-line dolutegravir-based ART. South Afr J HIV Med 26. https://doi.org/10.4102/sajhivmed.v26i1.1701

Ndihokubwayo JB, Yahaya AA, Desta AT, Ki-Zerbo G, Odei EA, Keita B, Pana AP, Nkhoma W (2013) Antimicrobial resistance in the African Region: Issues, challenges and actions proposed. African Health Monitor 16:27–30

NICD (2024) National Institute for Communicable Diseases. National HIV Drug Resistance Surveillance Among Adults with Viral Non-Suppression in South Africa [WWW Document]. https://www.nicd.ac.za/national-hiv-drug-resistance-surveillance-among-adults-with-viral-non-suppression-in-south-africa/#:~:text=The%20prevalence%20of%20INSTI%20resistance,the%20need%20for%20continued%20monitoring. Accessed 23 Aug 2025

NICD (n.d.) Influenza Surveillance in South Africa:2024

Nooruzzaman M, Johnson KEE, Rani R, Finkelsztein EJ, Caserta LC, Kodiyanplakkal RP, Wang W, Hsu J, Salpietro MT, Banakis S, Albert J, Westblade LF, Zanettini C, Marchionni L, Soave R, Ghedin E, Diel DG, Salvatore M (2024) Emergence of transmissible SARS-CoV-2 variants with decreased sensitivity to antivirals in immunocompromised patients with persistent infections. Nat Commun 15. https://doi.org/10.1038/s41467-024-51924-3

Nsonga E, Goma M, Ng'ambi WF, Zyambo C (2024) Predicting HIV drug resistance among persons living with HIV/AIDS in Sub-Saharan Africa using population-based HIV impact assessment surveys: 2015–2019. https://doi.org/10.1101/2024.04.11.24305688

Ogbodu OM, Mrara B, Sewani-Rusike C (2025) Interventions to mitigate drug shortages in public health systems in sub-Saharan Africa: a scoping review protocol. BMJ Open 15. https://doi.org/10.1136/bmjopen-2025-101349

Oh DY, Milde J, Ham Y, Calderón JPR, Wedde M, Dürrwald R, Duwe SC (2023) Preparing for the next influenza season: monitoring the emergence and spread of antiviral resistance. Infect Drug Resist 16:949–959. https://doi.org/10.2147/IDR.S389263

Okomo-Adhiambo M, Nguyen HT, Sleeman K, Sheu TG, Deyde VM, Garten RJ, Xu X, Shaw MW, Klimov AI, Gubareva LV (2010) Host cell selection of influenza neuraminidase variants: implications for drug resistance monitoring in A(H1N1) viruses. Antivir Res 85:381–388. https://doi.org/10.1016/j.antiviral.2009.11.005

Patel MC, Nguyen HT, Pascua PNQ, Gao R, Steel J, Kondor RJ, Gubareva LV (2024) Multicountry spread of influenza A(H1N1)pdm09 viruses with reduced oseltamivir inhibition, May 2023–February 2024. Emerg Infect Dis 30:1410–1411. https://doi.org/10.3201/eid3007.240480

Peltzer K, Friend-Du Preez N, Ramlagan S, Anderson J (2010) Antiretroviral treatment adherence among HIV patients in KwaZulu-Natal, South Africa. BMC Public Health 10

Phinius BB, Anderson M, Gobe I, Mokomane M, Choga WT, Phakedi B, Ratsoma T, Mpebe G, Makhema J, Shapiro R, Lockman S, Musonda R, Moyo S, Gaseitsiwe S (2024) High prevalence of hepatitis B virus drug resistance mutations to lamivudine among people with HIV/HBV coinfection in rural and peri-urban communities in Botswana. Viruses 16. https://doi.org/10.3390/v16040592

Pipitò L, Bono E, Tolomeo M, Cascio A (2025) Advances in the management of MPOX infection: therapeutic and vaccination perspectives. Curr Treat Options Infect Dis 17:12. https://doi.org/10.1007/s40506-025-00289-2

Preston BD, Poiesz BJ, Loeb LA, 1988. Fidelity of HIV-1 Reverse Transcriptase, New Series

Ramadan RA, Mohammed AS, Fakhr AE (2018) Molecular characterization of NS5A resistance associated substitutions after failure of Sofosbuvir/Daclatasvir combination therapy in chronic hepatitis C genotype 4a infected Egyptian patients compared to direct-acting antiviral agent (DAA)-naïve sequences key words: hepatitis C virus; NS5A inhibitors; virologic relapse; resistant variants. Egypt J Med Microbiol

Rutstein SE, Chen JS, Nelson JAE, Phiri S, Miller WC, Hosseinipour MC (2019) High rates of transmitted NNRTI resistance among persons with acute HIV infection in Malawi: Implications for first-line dolutegravir scale-up. AIDS Res Ther 16. https://doi.org/10.1186/s12981-019-0220-8

Salam MA, Al-Amin MY, Salam MT, Pawar JS, Akhter N, Rabaan AA, Alqumber MAA (2023) Antimicrobial resistance: a growing serious threat for global public health. Healthcare (Switzerland). https://doi.org/10.3390/healthcare11131946

Sanjuán R, Illingworth CJR, Geoghegan JL, Iranzo J, Zwart MP, Ciota AT, Moratorio G, Gago-Zachert S, Duffy S, Vijaykrishna D (2021) Five challenges in the field of viral diversity and evolution. Front Virol 1. https://doi.org/10.3389/fviro.2021.684949

Sankatsing SUC, Beijnen JH, Schinkel AH, Lange JMA, Prins JM (2004) P glycoprotein in human immunodeficiency virus type 1 infection and therapy. Antimicrob Agents Chemother. https://doi.org/10.1128/AAC.48.4.1073-1081.2004

Shafer RW (2002) Genotypic testing for human immunodeficiency virus type 1 drug resistance. Clin Microbiol Rev. https://doi.org/10.1128/CMR.15.2.247-277.2002

Smyk JM, Szydłowska N, Szulc W, Majewska A (2022) Evolution of influenza viruses—drug resistance, treatment options, and prospects. Int J Mol Sci. https://doi.org/10.3390/ijms232012244

Spearman C (2024) Demystifying the management of Hepatitis B—the WHO 2024 Guidelines on the management of Hepatitis B. South African J Gastroenterol Hepatol 1:19–21. https://doi.org/10.36303/sajgh.0497

Srivastava S, Laxmi, Sharma K, Sridhar SB, Talath S, Shareef J, Mehta R, Satapathy P, Sah R (2024) Clade Ib: a new emerging threat in the Mpox outbreak. Front Pharmacol. https://doi.org/10.3389/fphar.2024.1504154

Stadeli KM, Richman DD (2013) Rates of emergence of HIV drug resistance in resource-limited settings: a systematic review. Antivir Ther. https://doi.org/10.3851/IMP2437

Umutesi G, Shumbusho F, Kateera F, Serumondo J, Kabahizi J, Musabeyezu E, Ngwije A, Gupta N, Nsanzimana S (2019) Rwanda launches a 5-year national hepatitis C elimination plan: a landmark in sub-Saharan Africa. J Hepatol. https://doi.org/10.1016/j.jhep.2019.03.011

UNAIDS, 2030. Global HIV Target Setting for 2030—Global Task Team on 2030 Targets Recommendations—Live document as of 28 March 2025

Vere Hodge A, Field HJ (2011) General mechanisms of antiviral resistance. In: Genetics and evolution of infectious diseases. Elsevier Inc., pp 339–362. https://doi.org/10.1016/B978-0-12-384890-1.00013-3

Wadell G (1983) Cultivation of viruses. In: Textbook of medical virology. Elsevier, pp 38–44. https://doi.org/10.1016/B978-0-407-00253-1.50010-4

Waked I, Esmat G, Elsharkawy A, El-Serafy M, Abdel-Razek W, Ghalab R, Elshishiney G, Salah A, Abdel Megid S, Kabil K, El-Sayed MH, Dabbous H, El Shazly Y, Abo Sliman M, Abou Hashem K, Abdel Gawad S, El Nahas N, El Sobky A, El Sonbaty S, El Tabakh H, Emad E, Gemeah H, Hashem A, Hassany M, Hefnawy N, Hemida AN, Khadary A, Labib K, Mahmoud F, Mamoun S, Marei T, Mekky S, Meshref A, Othman A, Ragab O, Ramadan E, Rehan A, Saad T, Saeed R, Sharshar M, Shawky H, Shawky M, Shehata W, Soror H, Taha M, Talha M, Tealaab A, Zein M, Hashish A, Cordie A, Omar Y, Kamal E, Ammar I, Abd Alla M, El Akel W, Doss W, Zaid H (2020) Screening and treatment program to eliminate hepatitis C in Egypt. N Engl J Med 382:1166

Wang D (2020) 5 challenges in understanding the role of the virome in health and disease. PLoS Pathog 16. https://doi.org/10.1371/journal.ppat.1008318

Wellcome (2024) What is antimicrobial resistance—and how do we prevent it? [WWW Document]. https://wellcome.org/news/what-antimicrobial-resistance-and-how-do-we-prevent-it?utm_source=chatgpt.com. Accessed 20 Aug 2025

Wester CW, Bussmann H, Koethe J, Moffat C, Vermund S, Essex M, Marlink RG (2009) Adult combination antiretroviral therapy in sub-Saharan Africa: lessons from Botswana and future challenges. HIV Ther 3:501

WHO (2016) Consolidated guidelines on the use of antiretroviral drugs for treating and preventing HIV infection, 2nd edn. Recommendations for a Public Health Approach

WHO (2017) HIV drug resistance report 2017. Geneva: World Health Organization; 2017. Licence: CC BY-NC-SA 3.0 IGO

WHO (2018) Progress report on access to hepatitis C treatment: focus on overcoming barriers in low- and middle-income countries, March 2018. Geneva, Switzerland: World Health Organization; 2018 (WHO/CDS/HIV/18.4). Licence: CC BY-NC-SA 3.0 IGO

WHO (2019) WHO recommends dolutegravir as preferred HIV treatment option in all populations [WWW Document]. https://www.who.int/news/item/22-07-2019-who-recommends-dolutegravir-as-preferred-hiv-treatment-option-in-all-populations#:~:text=%C2%A9-,WHO%20recommends%20dolutegravir%20as%20preferred%20HIV%20treatment%20option%20in%20all,initial%20studies%20may%20have%20suggested. Accessed 23 Aug 2025

WHO (2021) HIV drug resistance strategy, 2021 update. Geneva: World Health Organization; 2021. Licence: CC BY-NC-SA 3.0 IGO

WHO (2023) Antimicrobial resistance [WWW Document]. https://www.who.int/news-room/fact-sheets/detail/antimicrobial-resistance. Accessed 20 Aug 2025

WHO (2025a) Fact sheet: HIV drug resistance [WWW Document]. https://www.who.int/news-room/fact-sheets/detail/hiv-drug-resistance#:~:text=Increased%20use%20of%20HIV%20medicines,the%20replication%20of%20the%20virus. Accessed 23 Aug 2025

WHO (2025b) Respiratory virus surveillance in the WHO African region. Epidemiological week 32, August 4 to 10 2025

WHO Africa (2019) WHO unveils plan to tackle rising HIV drug resistance in Africa [WWW Document]. https://www.afro.who.int/news/who-unveils-plan-tackle-rising-hiv-drug-resistance-africa#:~:text=This%20resistance%20occurs%20at%20the,routine%20monitoring%20and%20evaluation%20activities. Accessed 23 Aug 2025

Wilhelmson S, Månsson F, Lindman JL, Biai A, Esbjörnsson J, Norrgren H, Jansson M, Medstrand P (2018) Prevalence of HIV-1 pretreatment drug resistance among treatment naïve pregnant women in Bissau, Guinea Bissau. PLoS One 13. https://doi.org/10.1371/journal.pone.0206406

Wolter N, Buys A, Walaza S, Moyes J, Makhasi M, Kleynhans J, Yun J, Du Plessis M, Moosa F, Kekana D, Mnguni A, Maake L, De Gouveia L, Cohen C, Von Gottberg A (2025) Influenza surveillance in South Africa, weeks 1 to 52, 2024. Public Health Bulletin of South Africa 3

World Bank (2017) Drug-resistant infections a threat to our economic future

World Bank (2024) Addressing the grand pandemic of antimicrobial resistance

Wu Y, Peng Y (2024) Ten computational challenges in human virome studies. Virol Sin. https://doi.org/10.1016/j.virs.2024.04.008

Yeo JY, Goh GR, Tran-To Su C, Ken-En Gan S (2020) The determination of HIV-1 RT mutation rate, its possible allosteric effects, and its implications on drug resistance. Viruses. https://doi.org/10.3390/v12030297

Zambon MC (2013) Surveillance for antiviral resistance. Influenza Other Respir Viruses 7:37–43. https://doi.org/10.1111/irv.12050

Zaniewski E, Skrivankova VW, Brazier E, Avihingsanon A, Cardoso SW, Cesar C, Chenal H, Crabtree-Ramírez BE, Ditangco RA, Ebasone PV, Eley B, Euvrard JG, Fatti G, Huwa JM, Lelo P, Machado DM, Messou EK, Minga AK, Muleebwa J, Mundhe S, Murenzi G, Muyindike WR, Nsonde DM, Obatsa SM, Odhiambo J, Prozesky HW, Rungmaitree S, Semeere AS, Seydi M, Sipambo N, Sudjaritruk T, Technau KG, Tiendrebeogo T, Twizere C, Ballif M (2024) Transition to dolutegravir-based ART in 35 low- and middle-income countries: a global survey of HIV care clinics. AIDS 38:2073–2085. https://doi.org/10.1097/QAD.0000000000004007

Zhang JC, Xie F, Yu XH, Deng ZY, Wang Y, Liang P, Sun L, Zhang FX (2014) Expression levels of P-glycoprotein in peripheral blood CD8+ T lymphocytes from HIV-1-infected patients on antiretroviral therapy. Int J Mol Med 33:431–440. https://doi.org/10.3892/ijmm.2013.1584

Chapter 12
Wastewater-Based Monitoring as an Early Warning for Viral Infections in Africa—Challenges and Prospects

Akebe Luther King Abia and Etando Ayukafangha

12.1 Overview of Wastewater-Based Epidemiology

Wastewater surveillance, also known as wastewater-based epidemiology (WBE), is a robust public health tool that facilitates the tracking of infections within communities. This method offers an economical and non-invasive means for the early identification and monitoring of disease outbreaks. This approach is founded on the idea that pathogens, particularly those responsible for gastrointestinal or respiratory diseases, may be expelled by infected individuals, including asymptomatic individuals, through bodily fluids and faeces for extended or brief periods, eventually making their way to centralised waste treatment facilities via the sewer system (Hamouda et al. 2021). Consequently, wastewater can function as a composite sample from a large community, facilitating the identification of pathogen presence before individuals pursue clinical attention. Thus, applying an appropriate sampling strategy, it is possible to obtain a broad picture of the diseases circulating within a given community connected to the same sewer system, including those not reported earlier by the healthcare facilities (Murakami et al. 2024).

Historically, WBE was employed to monitor Poliovirus, yielding significant insights that aided polio eradication initiatives in multiple regions (Howe 1949; Melnick 1947; Metcalf et al. 1995; Paul 1941; Paul et al. 1940). In Africa, wastewater surveillance significantly contributed to polio monitoring, particularly in nations like Nigeria (Bokinni 2025; Kilaru et al. 2023; Muluh et al. 2016) and

A. L. K. Abia (✉)
Total Environment Research (TEN-R) Group, College of Health Sciences, University of KwaZulu-Natal, Durban, South Africa

Environmental Research Foundation, Westville, South Africa

E. Ayukafangha
Antimicrobial Research Unit, College of Health Sciences, University of KwaZulu-Natal, Durban, South Africa

J. A. Shenge, A. L. K. Abia (eds.), *Viral Diseases and One Health in Africa*,
https://doi.org/10.1007/978-3-032-09613-5_12

Egypt (Shabana et al. 2024), where the identification of Poliovirus in sewage offered an early indication of covert transmission and informed vaccin priority areas. Egypt instituted comprehensive environmental surveillance initiatives that augmented acute flaccid paralysis (AFP) monitoring, facilitating the detection of ongoing viral transmission in high-risk populations. Nigeria's environmental monitoring identified vaccine-derived polioviruses, facilitating focused vaccination initiatives that expedited eradication efforts (Muluh et al. 2016).

Despite its valuable role in disease monitoring, WBE was not highly used as an epidemiological tool. However, the COVID-19 epidemic rekindled global interest in this approach, creating a paradigm shift in disease monitoring through WBE as an early warning tool. Numerous African nations, including South Africa, Senegal, and Kenya, have piloted the surveillance of the Severe Acute Respiratory Syndrome Coronavirus 2 (SARS-CoV-2) in wastewater as part of their comprehensive epidemiological plans. The South African Medical Research Council (SAMRC) implemented a wastewater surveillance program that effectively monitored SARS-CoV-2 variants in the country, confirming clinical findings across two waves after the initial pandemic (Street et al. 2024). Similarly, the Institut Pasteur in Senegal partnered with the Ministry of Health to establish wastewater-based surveillance capabilities in Dakar, showcasing the viability of this method in West Africa (Institut Pasteur 2020). Likewise, Kenya's Ministry of Health facilitated wastewater-based epidemiology (WBE) initiatives in Nairobi that correlated virus quantities in wastewater with local case patterns, offering early alerts for possible outbreaks (Campisano 2025).

The scalability and real-time characteristics of wastewater data have shown their capacity to enhance traditional surveillance systems, particularly in resource-constrained environments or where individual testing access is restricted. In some areas of sub-Saharan Africa, wastewater-WBE is a crucial instrument for evaluating viral transmission dynamics in communities with inadequate healthcare infrastructure, where testing and clinical case reporting may be sporadic or inefficient. This will be particularly crucial in informal settlements and peri-urban regions where healthcare access may be limited, as wastewater monitoring could be used to inform targeted interventions and resource distribution. Moreover, as novel viral dangers arise, WBE in Africa might be swiftly modified for the surveillance of other infections of public health significance.

12.2 Viral Shedding, Entry into, and Survival in Wastewater

Viral shedding refers to the expulsion of viruses from the body of an infected individual with or without symptoms. In some cases, shedding occurs even in healthy individuals (Park et al. 2021). Understanding these mechanisms is essential for managing viral disease spread and potential outbreaks, particularly in regions

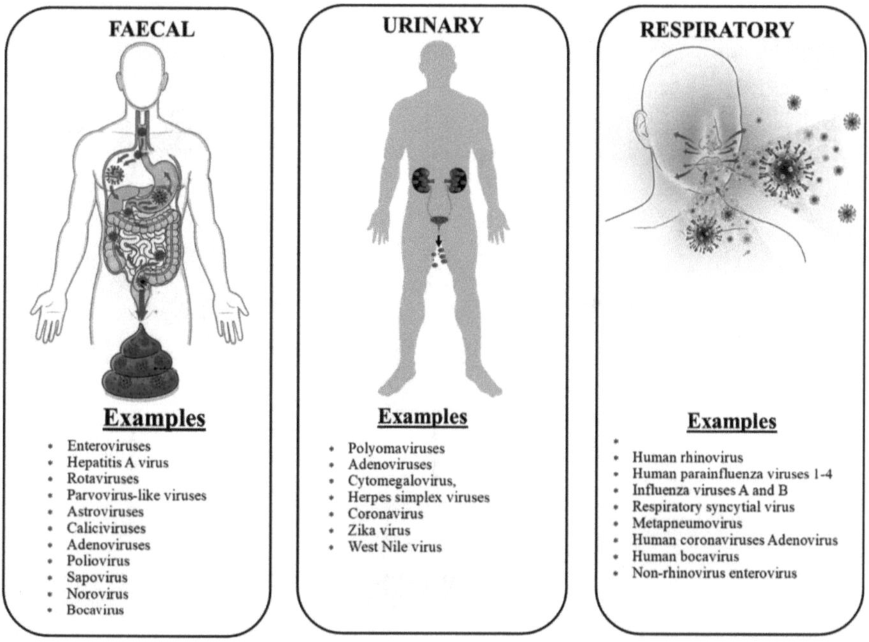

Fig. 12.1 Viral shedding in humans

with inadequate or complete absence of sanitation facilities. Viruses can be excreted from an individual into the environment through three main routes, including through faeces, urine and respiratory aerosols (Fig. 12.1).

Viruses that are excreted through the faecal route are mostly enteric, such as rotavirus, norovirus, adenovirus, and hepatitis A and E (Bosch 1998; Fong and Lipp 2005). However, research indicates that some other viruses involved in extra-intestinal infections, such as SARS-CoV-2, are also shed through the faeces of sick and healthy individuals (Chen et al. 2020; Gupta et al. 2020; Quilliam et al. 2020; Zhang et al. 2020). This is especially pertinent in sub-Saharan Africa, where open defecation and pit latrines remain common in many rural populations, heightening environmental contamination hazards.

Many viruses have been implicated in urinary tract infections in humans, and these can be passed out through the urine of infected persons. Some of them include the human adenoviruses (HAdVs), herpes simplex virus (HSV) (Hanaoka et al. 2019), human polyomavirus (BKV) and cytomegalovirus (Park et al. 2021). Other viruses not necessarily associated with UTIs, but that are still excreted through urine, include the Zika virus and West Nile virus (Park et al. 2021). Studies revealed that SARS-CoV (Xu et al. 2005) can be excreted through urine (Jones et al. 2020).

Air shedding of viruses mostly occurs when infected people sneeze or cough. Several viruses, such as measles, rhinovirus, hantavirus, influenza, mumps, varicella-zoster virus, viral meningitis, and the coronaviruses, have been shown to be airborne with mutation potentials in the atmosphere (Omilabu and Salu 2023).

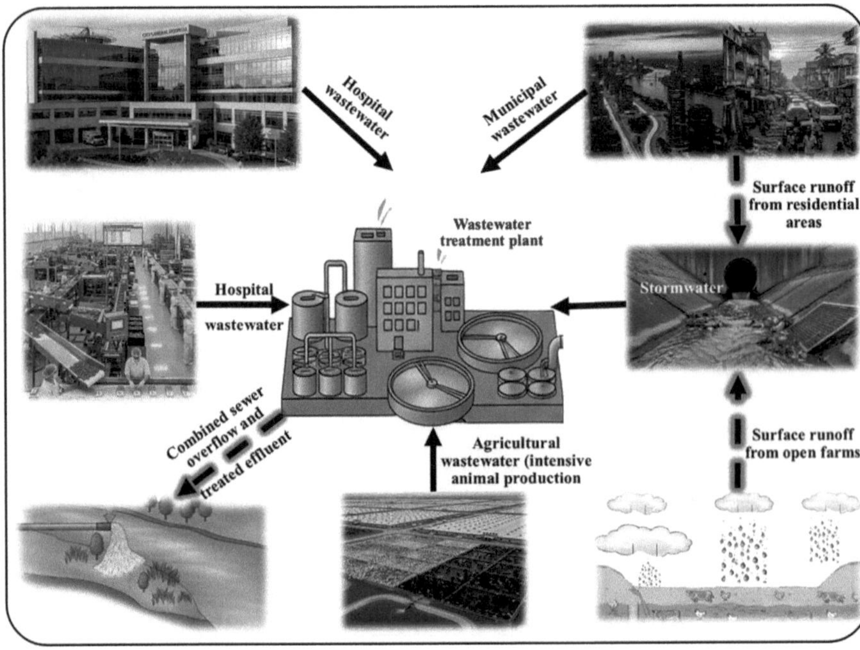

Fig. 12.2 Routes of viral entry into wastewater treatment systems

Airborne viruses can survive in the air for long periods, depending on the prevailing atmospheric conditions such as temperature and relative humidity (Pyankov et al. 2018). Although these viruses are predominantly spread through droplets, their genetic material may settle on surfaces and be washed into wastewater through cleaning and surface sanitation, for example. Several studies have reported on the presence of numerous respiratory viruses in wastewater treatment plants (WWTPs) in developed and developing countries (Ahmed et al. 2023; Raya et al. 2024; Rector et al. 2024).

It should be noted that although the studies indicated in the paragraphs above have focused on viruses implicated in human infections, many other viruses originating from animals can also be shed through the same mechanisms; some of these viruses are zoonotic, therefore, represent a potential health threat to humans (Adriaenssens et al. 2018; Karatas et al. 2025).

Once released from their hosts, these viruses can enter WWTPs through different routes (Fig. 12.2). Therefore, WWTPs could receive viruses through domestic wastewater (Zhang et al. 2016), hospital wastewater (Yuan and Pian 2023), agricultural wastewater (Derbyshire 1976), and industrial wastewater, especially from food processing facilities (Miranda and Schaffner 2019). In Africa, surface runoff carrying viruses (Salemane et al. 2024) may also enter stormwater and reach WWTPs, especially in areas with combined sewer systems. This route is particularly important because of poor sanitation conditions and open defaecation, making this route a substantial, yet less considered route of viral entry into WWTPs.

The survival of viruses outside their natural hosts depends on the interplay of several factors, which could be biological (viral structure, presence/absence of other microbial species, organic matter), physical (prevailing temperature and UV intensity), and chemical (pH, salts, antivirals) (Mehle et al. 2018). Considering coronaviruses, for example, (i) elevated temperatures reduce the overall environmental persistence of the virus; (ii) organic matter in the surrounding matrix may enhance the survivability of coronaviruses (iii) chlorination remains the most efficient and cost-effective disinfection strategy; (iv) membrane bioreactors within wastewater treatment facilities harbor competitive microbial communities capable of inactivating coronaviruses; (v) ultraviolet irradiation constitutes an additional effective approach for viral inactivation (Paul et al. 2021). Thus, wastewater, especially within a WWTP, presents an ideal environment for the survival of numerous microorganisms, including viruses, especially due to its rich nutrient content, tremendous organic matter content and favourable temperature conditions. However, the overall consensus of these studies is that WWTPs are a good proxy for the determination of viral infections within a given community.

12.3 Detection of Viruses in Wastewater

12.3.1 Viral Concentration in Wastewater Samples

The detection of viral RNA and particles in wastewater has gained traction worldwide for monitoring public health risks, including SARS-CoV-2, polio, Ebola and other enteric viruses. Although various analytical methodologies exist, they generally all involve viral concentration, extraction of the viral nucleic material, and molecular detection. In Africa, samples may be from WWTPs, open drainage systems, or pit latrines.

Despite their presence in wastewater, viruses do not usually occur in large enough concentrations to allow for direct extraction of their nucleic materials for downstream applications. Thus, once the samples are collected, viral concentration must be performed using different methods such as polyethylene glycol (PEG) precipitation, aluminium hydroxide ($AlCl_3$) flocculation, adsorption-precipitation or $AlCl_3$ flocculation, adsorption-elution, ultracentrifugation and ultrafiltration (Akter et al. 2024; Sapula et al. 2021).

(a) Different variations of the PEG precipitation exist, but the underlying principle is that PEG, the main polymer, sterically keeps proteins, including viral particles, out of the solvent phase while preferentially trapping the solvent. This enables the proteins to be concentrated to the point of precipitation (Torii et al. 2022). This approach was used in a Kenyan study that identified rotaviruses in different water sources, including wastewater (Kiulia et al. 2010). Similarly, a South African study used the same approach to concentrate viruses in wastewater collected over one year to monitor the emergence of new norovirus variants (Mabasa et al. 2018).

(b) The aluminium hydroxide adsorption-precipitation method involves changing the pH of the wastewater (usually between 3.5 and 6.0) using aluminium chloride, causing aluminium hydroxide to precipitate and produce positively charged flocs. Viral particles, which are typically negatively charged at neutral pH, are drawn to and absorbed by these flocs (Farmer-Diaz et al. 2025). The floc can then be precipitated into a pellet, and the viruses extracted using commercial kits. This method was used in Egypt in a study aimed at determining the number of rotavirus genome copies in water and wastewater (El-Senousy et al. 2023).
(c) The viral adsorption-elution method is based on the adsorption principle, whereby molecules or particles adhere to the surface of a solid material. In this approach, a positively charged filter or membrane is employed to attract and bind the negatively charged viral particles present in the water sample (Akter et al. 2024). Large volumes of water, often several litres, are passed through the filter, enabling the viruses to attach to its surface. This process concentrates the viral particles from a substantial water volume into a considerably smaller and more manageable volume. Following adsorption, the bound viruses are eluted by passing a small volume of an elution buffer through the filter. The buffer, typically of high pH, disrupts the electrostatic interactions between the viruses and the filter surface, thereby releasing the viral particles into the solution (Akter et al. 2024). In Africa, this method has been used in South Africa (Chigor and Okoh 2012) and Tunisia (Othman et al. 2023).
(d) Ultracentrifugation concentrates viruses from liquid matrices by applying extremely high centrifugal forces, often several thousand times greater than the force of gravity, resulting in their sedimentation and accumulation of viral particles as a pellet at the base of the centrifuge tube. This method enables the effective separation of particles based on their biophysical properties, including size, morphology, and density. Ultracentrifugation was used in Ethiopia to concentrate the COVID-19 virus in wastewater, although there was a prior low centrifugation step to remove heavier particles (Ali et al. 2022).
(e) Ultrafiltration (UF) uses semipermeable membranes to separate viral particles from wastewater based on particle size. The membranes typically have pore sizes of about 10–100 nm or molecular weight cut-offs (MWCO) between 10 and 100 kDa, to retain viral particles while allowing water and smaller solutes to pass through (Bleotu et al. 2024). Two main operational configurations that are frequently used include dead-end ultrafiltration (DEUF), in which viruses are trapped on or within the membrane matrix as a result of the liquid sample flowing perpendicular to the membrane surface. An elution or backflushing procedure is then used to retrieve the trapped particles. Unlike DEUF, tangential flow filtration (TFF) allows for the processing of significantly higher quantities because the sample flows parallel to the membrane surface, reducing particle buildup and membrane fouling (Cai et al. 2015; Gibson and Schwab 2011). Some examples of African studies that used UF include South Africa (Ganesh et al. 2014), Tunisia (Othman et al. 2023) and Kenya (Zhou et al. 2020). A summary of the various concentration methods is provided in Table 12.1.

Table 12.1 Comparison of viral concentration methods from wastewater

Method	Principle	Typical sample volume	Recovery (typical/relative)	Advantages	Disadvantages	Typical cost/equipment
Polyethylene glycol (PEG) precipitation	PEG + salt causes viruses to precipitate from clarified concentrate	50 mL—several L (usually applied to pre-concentrated or clarified sample)	Moderate (variable by virus and matrix)	Low cost; widely used; works for many non-enveloped viruses; scalable	Co-concentrates inhibitors and solids; requires cold incubation and centrifugation; recovery variable; long protocol time	Low (centrifuge, PEG reagent)
Aluminium chloride ($AlCl_3$) flocculation	Al^{3+} (or $AlCl_3$) added, pH adjusted → $Al(OH)_3$ flocs adsorb viruses → pellet collected and eluted	100 mL—several L	Low–moderate (matrix dependent)	Very low reagent cost; simple; adapted to low-resource settings	Recovery can be inconsistent, pH sensitive, and can co-concentrate solids/inhibitors	Very low (basic lab equipment, pH meter)
Adsorptio-elution (membrane filtration)	Pass large volume through electropositive/electronegative membrane → viruses adsorb → elute with buffer	0.5–50 L (large volumes feasible)	Moderate-high (depends on membrane, pretreatment)	Handles large volumes; established for enteric viruses; can be combined with secondary concentration	Membrane clogging with turbid wastewaters; elution efficiency variable; membranes cost	Low-moderate (filters, pumps)
Ultracentrifugation	High-g centrifugation pellets viruses directly from the (cleared) sample	≤50–250 mL (limited by rotor tube size)	High for small volumes	Effective pelleting of particles; no chemical reagents needed; high recovery for many viruses	Low throughput; expensive instrument; not practical for many litres	Very high (ultracentrifuge + rotors)
Ultrafiltration	Size- and/or mass-based retention with membranes/hollow fibre filters	50 mL—tens to hundreds of litres	High	Scalable; rapid processing; good recovery for enveloped and non-enveloped viruses	Membrane fouling with turbid wastewater; equipment cost	Moderate–high (filtration rigs, pumps, membranes)

12.3.2 *Isolation of Nucleic Materials and Viral Detection*

Several commercial kits, such as Qiagen RNeasy and Zymo Research, or manual TRIzol-based techniques have been used to extract viral RNA. Effective RNA extraction is crucial for precise detection. So, several researchers have tested and compared most of these kits for their ability to effectively extract viral nucleic materials from different sample types, including wastewater, for downstream applications (Hongjaisee et al. 2022; O'Brien et al. 2021; Perumal et al. 2021; Saeidi et al. 2017). Once extracted, the detection is based on molecular biology methodologies, either individually or combined. Several methods have been used worldwide; these methods have been reviewed extensively (Corpuz et al. 2020). The following paragraphs provide a brief overview of African studies that employed some of these methods.

Reverse Transcription Quantitative Polymerase Chain Reaction (RT-qPCR) is the gold standard for the detection and quantification of viral RNA targeting specific genes. This approach was used for the identification and quantification of viral particles during the COVID-1 pandemic, specifically targeting genes such as N, E, and RdRp for SARS-CoV-2. This methodology was utilised by the South African Medical Research Council (SAMRC) in a countrywide COVID-19 wastewater surveillance initiative in 2021.

Loop-mediated Isothermal Amplification (LAMP) serves as a rapid, less equipment-intensive alternative to RT-qPCR. It is appropriate for resource-constrained environments. South African researchers investigated Reverse transcription loop-mediated isothermal amplification (RT-LAMP) for the detection of SARS-CoV-2 in wastewater and concluded that the method was a cost-effective, user-friendly and time-efficient alternative for detecting SARS-CoV-2 in Wastewater (Amoah et al. 2021).

Next-Generation Sequencing (NGS) is intended for variation monitoring, extensive viral identification, or comprehensive metagenomic surveillance. The National Institute for Communicable Diseases (NICD) of South Africa and many other African studies have used it to detect variations in wastewater (Table 12.2).

Biosensors are currently in their trial phases in Africa and show promise for decentralised testing. Although still in its infancy, a review of the literature revealed a strong focus on electrochemical biosensor research in South Africa, including for regional issues like HIV/AIDs and tuberculosis.

A summary of methods employed in Africa for the detection of viral infections is presented in Table 12.2.

12.4 Prospects of WBE in Africa

Wastewater surveillance has gained significant ground in Africa, especially after the COVID-19 pandemic, and has concentrated on viral targets of significant public health importance, including SARS-CoV-2, Poliovirus, hepatitis viruses, and enteric

Table 12.2 Examples of studies on the detection of viruses in wastewater and some of the methods they used

Technique	Virus target	Countries	Sample type	References
RT-qPCR	Rotaviruses	South Africa	Influent, final effluent, receiving water body	Omatola et al. (2024)
	Human adenovirus, rotavirus and hepatitis A virus	South Africa	Final effluent	Adefisoye et al. (2016)
	Poliovirus	Kenya	River, latrine waste, wastewater	Zhou et al. (2020)
	SARS-CoV-2	Zambia	Raw influent	Shempela et al. (2024)
	Rotavirus A and norovirus (GI and GII)	Botswana	Raw and treated sewage, and surface water	Tubatsi and Kebaabetswe (2022)
	SARS-CoV-2	South Africa	Untreated wastewater	Johnson et al. (2021)
	Enteroviruses and SARS-CoV-2	Tunisia	Different stages of the treatment process	Ibrahim et al. (2023)
RT-LAMP	SARS-CoV-2	South Africa	Untreated wastewater samples	Amoah et al. (2021)
Next-generation sequencing (NGS)—Whole genome sequencing	SARS-CoV-2	Zambia	Raw influent	Shempela et al. (2024)
	Noroviruses	South Africa	Raw sewage and final effluent	Mabasa et al. (2022)
	SARS-CoV-2	South Africa	Sewage (raw or treated, not mentioned)	Yousif et al. (2023)
	Whole viral communities	South Africa	Raw and treated sewage	Osunmakinde et al. (2021)

viruses such as rotavirus and norovirus. These initiatives are essential for mitigating disease burden on the continent, particularly given Africa's socioeconomic and political landscape. With adequate investment in this approach, WBE can significantly revolutionise the continent's public health sector, given its current inadequate disease surveillance due to weak health systems. By learning from the most recent COVID-19 pandemic, WBE can provide real-time epidemic preparedness data throughout the continent in many ways.

(i) Firstly, using WBE to determine the viral load in a community can provide better information necessary for instituting and implementing public health interventions. Quantifying viral concentrations in wastewater can help in quantifying infection prevalence, monitoring temporal patterns, and offering early warnings of developing outbreaks. This information could facilitate prompt mitigative measures (Keshaviah et al. 2023). In African contexts, combining these findings with clinical reports from the community health facilities and hospitals can enhance the precision of outbreak predictions in regions with deficient clinical reporting systems. This approach was particularly helpful during the COVID-19 pandemic. It facilitated the identification of the causative virus in the absence of positive clinical cases, making it instrumental for cost-effective, population-wide monitoring, which is critical for the resource-limited African status.

(ii) Secondly, WBE can help mitigate the deficiencies in disease testing and monitoring. A chronic deficiency in testing capabilities plagues most African countries due to the absence or poor nature of available infrastructure. At the onset of the COVID-19 pandemic, restricted testing capabilities were observed in nations such as Senegal, Uganda, Nigeria, and the Democratic Republic of the Congo (Bosonkie et al. 2023). This challenge, although almost global, was more prominent in Africa. In such a case, WBE could provide valuable information on areas where testing could be focused by determining the viral load in different communities. For example, the South African Medical Research Council (SAMRC) launched a national wastewater surveillance program in South Africa, which identified surges in SARS-CoV-2 RNA in wastewater up to two weeks before the rise in clinical cases. This enabled local health authorities in some provinces to implement focused public health communications and enhance hospital readiness (SAMRC 2021).

(iii) Thirdly, WBE could be used to establish disease progression or trends within a community. Variations in viral RNA concentrations, rather than absolute numbers, serve as the most dependable markers of infection trends. In most cases, the need for individual case testing drops as the outbreak reduces. Here, WBE could be very instrumental in observing trends in the community without the need for intensive testing of individuals. Determining the trend is also important, especially following the emergence of new variants of the disease, as was the case with COVID-19. In Singapore, for example, scientists observed that new variants of Omicron appeared in WWTPs at the same time as the first cases were reported in the country (Singer et al. 2023). Therefore, Africa could benefit from this approach and monitor the spread of viral infections within communities. This would also allow public health officials to determine where there is a high likelihood of exposure to a viral pathogen, thus establishing communities at a greater risk of potential outbreaks (Aghaei et al. 2024).

(iv) Finally, WBE data could be used to generate a disease map for an entire country without the need to test every individual, which is practically not possible. Using data from WBE surveys, health officials can generate a database of the disease burden, spread and trends within the country, allowing them to identify potential hotspots for future outbreaks. This could prompt actions like the dispatch of mobile clinics to specific areas, especially in places like Africa, where access to health facilities could be challenging due to road infrastructure.

12.5 Challenges to Implementing WBE in Africa

It can be said without doubt that WBE is one of the most promising tools for disease epidemiology in modern times, based on the remarkable wealth of information that has been generated using the approach globally. However, despite its potential to monitor viral infections, the approach is faced with several challenges, especially in developing nations like those in Africa.

(i) The most significant of these problems within the African context is the unavoidable truth that most countries within the continent still lack centralised sewage collection systems; where they exist, they are not functional or function sub-optimally (Abia et al. 2023). While most urban areas may possess advanced sanitation infrastructure, rural regions without sewage treatment facilities could hinder the process of wastewater sampling. With a very low percentage of households connected to centralised systems, this influences both sample frequency and data representativeness, as a significant amount of data is lost due to the presence of alternative sanitary facilities like pit latrines and septic tanks. In some more rural or informal settlements or slums, where open defecation is still practised, it will not be possible to accurately determine the viral load or burden without individual sampling within the community, which in itself will not be feasible technically and financially.

(ii) Another major challenge is the lack of standardised methods for the evaluation of wastewater for epidemiological purposes. As observed in Table 12.2, for example, different studies sample different points within the WWTP. However, a better representation of the community would be the raw influent before it goes through any processes in the plant. Furthermore, there is a lack of information regarding the optimal timing for sampling, the frequency of sampling, and the quantity of the sample that should be collected. Moreover, comparison of analysis methods showed that some concentration methods, for example, performed better than others. However, most studies are financially limited and cannot afford some of these methods. Standardisation of sampling and testing protocols for WBE of viruses is essential for the reliability of surveillance data. Without such standardisation, it would be challenging to compare results across borders.

(iii) Viral detection in wastewater is rapidly advancing, with high-throughput sequencing techniques being at the forefront of this advancement. The limited availability of PCR and advanced molecular testing technologies in most African nations hampers the accurate detection of viruses in wastewater. However, although these technologies are gradually gaining ground in Africa, they are still limited by the cost of instrumentation and consumables, which makes the cost per sample usually unaffordable for routine monitoring. This, therefore, forces most countries to outsource this service to some developed countries, which imposes further financial stress and limits the number of samples that can be analysed at any given time.

(iv) Sequencing techniques generate a tremendous amount of data that requires skilled bioinformaticians to handle. While such skills are gradually being introduced into schools, a lot still needs to be done to allow the continent to meet Western levels. In some cases, the cost of attendance for these courses often deters many people from applying due to their financial backgrounds.

(v) The preceding challenges mentioned above have a ripple effect on the WBE data reporting and converting such data into action. Inappropriate reporting could either overestimate the viral disease burden, resulting in the wasteful allocation of funds for interventions in areas that do not require them. Conversely, underreporting may lead to insufficient fund allocation, resulting in potential outbreaks. This is exacerbated by the lack of sufficient integration among sectors. In numerous African countries, most sectors function in silos. However, for effective WBE of viral infections in Africa, data from wastewater surveillance must be integrated with that across various sectors, including water, health, and environment.

(vi) Apart from its wide use during the COVID-19 pandemic, WBE is still not a topic of national priority in many African countries. Most countries that have developed national action plans focus on human health and, to some extent, animal health. WBE is still regarded as an environmental health issue, instead of an epidemiological tool for the benefit of human health. This results in reduced funding allocation for WBE. Thus, the approach remains more of a research agenda where academicians focus more on generating data for publication purposes than to inform national priorities.

(vii) Many people in some parts of Africa are displaced due to armed conflicts. Such significant movement of populations, especially refugees and migrants, exacerbates the challenges of wastewater surveillance initiatives. If such displaced populations are in camps, such camps could also be considered as communities. However, where they are dispersed, it becomes challenging to collect representative samples in such cases.

12.6 Recommendations

(i) Wastewater-based epidemiology should not be regarded as a one-size-fits-all, as evident by the fact that most African countries do not have centralised sewer systems. As such, African countries must develop country-specific approaches defined by the country's realities. For example, new sampling approaches should be designed to include collection from surface water, pit latrines, and septic systems. This should be followed by the standardisation of methods, at least at the national and continental level, where countries have similar infrastructural characteristics. It should, however, be noted that seasonal precipitation and flooding in various regions of Africa may dilute virus concentrations in wastewater, leading to erroneous or inconsistent findings, and thus, must be considered when using alternative sampling approaches.

(ii) In addressing the lack of instrumentation and skills for WBE of viral infections in Africa, initiatives such as the African CDC's Pathogen Genomics Initiative have begun efforts to establish continental frameworks. This should be supported by other institutions such as the WHO. Furthermore, the initiative should also be reinforced with training in environmental virology, a skill which is currently highly deficient on the continent. Additionally, public awareness should be raised about the possibility of wastewater surveillance.
(iii) Integrating wastewater data with clinical and other existing surveillance systems would enhance disease monitoring by combining wastewater surveillance with clinical testing and health records, hence providing more comprehensive and relevant public health insights.
(iv) Political commitment and support from governments should be evident. African governments must see WBE as a national priority, necessary to safeguard the health of their populations. In so doing, there will be sufficient funding allocation for viral disease surveillance through wastewater.

12.7 Conclusions

Wastewater surveillance has proven to be a cost-effective, early-warning, and population-wide instrument for monitoring viral outbreaks in Africa. Despite numerous constraints impeding this approach, the growing implementation of WBE in Africa is gradually but greatly enhancing the continent's pandemic preparedness and response capabilities. Continuous research and global cooperation, as exemplified by the Africa CDC, may assist in surmounting certain obstacles. For better output from this technique, it is imperative to augment investment in infrastructure, human resources, and policy formulation, alongside fostering regional collaboration to standardise processes and facilitate data sharing.

References

Abia ALK, Baloyi T, Traore AN, Potgieter N (2023) The African wastewater resistome: identifying knowledge gaps to inform future research directions. Antibiotics. https://doi.org/10.3390/antibiotics12050805

Adefisoye MA, Nwodo UU, Green E, Okoh AI (2016) Quantitative PCR detection and characterisation of human adenovirus, rotavirus and hepatitis a virus in discharged effluents of two wastewater treatment facilities in the Eastern Cape, South Africa. Food Environ Virol 8:262–274. https://doi.org/10.1007/s12560-016-9246-4

Adriaenssens EM, Farkas K, Harrison C, Jones DL, Allison HE, McCarthy AJ (2018) Viromic analysis of wastewater input to a river catchment reveals a diverse assemblage of RNA viruses. mSystems 3. https://doi.org/10.1128/msystems.00025-18

Aghaei M, Khoshnamvand N, Janjani H, Dehghani MH, Karri RR (2024) Exposure to environmental pollutants: a mini-review on the application of wastewater-based epidemiology approach. J Environ Health Sci Eng. https://doi.org/10.1007/s40201-024-00895-0

Ahmed W, Bivins A, Stephens M, Metcalfe S, Smith WJM, Sirikanchana K, Kitajima M, Simpson SL (2023) Occurrence of multiple respiratory viruses in wastewater in Queensland, Australia: potential for community disease surveillance. Sci Total Environ 864. https://doi.org/10.1016/j.scitotenv.2022.161023

Akter J, Smith WJM, Liu Y, Kim I, Simpson SL, Thai P, Korajkic A, Ahmed W (2024) Comparison of adsorption-extraction (AE) workflows for improved measurements of viral and bacterial nucleic acid in untreated wastewater. Sci Total Environ 908. https://doi.org/10.1016/j.scitotenv.2023.167966

Ali S, Gudina EK, Gize A, Aliy A, Adankie BT, Tsegaye W, Hundie GB, Muleta MB, Chibssa TR, Belaineh R, Negessu D, Shegu D, Froeschl G, Wieser A (2022) Community wastewater-based surveillance can be a cost-effective approach to track COVID-19 outbreak in low-resource settings: feasibility assessment for Ethiopia context. Int J Environ Res Public Health 19. https://doi.org/10.3390/ijerph19148515

Amoah ID, Mthethwa NP, Pillay L, Deepnarain N, Pillay K, Awolusi OO, Kumari S, Bux F (2021) RT-LAMP: a cheaper, simpler and faster alternative for the detection of SARS-CoV-2 in wastewater. Food Environ Virol 13:447–456. https://doi.org/10.1007/s12560-021-09489-7

Bleotu C, Matei L, Dragu LD, Necula LG, Pitica IM, Chivu-Economescu M, Diaconu CC (2024) Viruses in wastewater—a concern for public health and the environment. Microorganisms. https://doi.org/10.3390/microorganisms12071430

Bokinni Y (2025) Nigeria's polio battleground. Nat Afr. https://doi.org/10.1038/d44148-025-00153-x

Bosch A (1998) Human enteric viruses in the water environment: a minireview. Int Microbiol 1: 191–196. https://doi.org/10.2436/im.v1i3.39

Bosonkie M, Egbende L, Namale A, Fawole OI, Seck I, Kizito S, Kaba D, Kiwanuka SN, Diallo I, Bello S, Kabwama SN, Kashiya Y, Monje F, Dairo MD, Bondo B, Namuhani N, Leye MMM, Adebowale AS, Bassoum O, Bamgboye EA, Fall M, Salawu M, Afolabi R, Ndejjo R, Wanyenze RK, Mapatano MA (2023) Improving testing capacity for COVID-19: experiences and lessons from Senegal, Uganda, Nigeria, and the Democratic Republic of Congo. Front Public Health 11. https://doi.org/10.3389/fpubh.2023.1202966

Cai L, Yang Y, Jiao N, Zhang R (2015) Evaluation of tangential flow filtration for the concentration and separation of bacteria and viruses in contrasting marine environments. PLoS One 10. https://doi.org/10.1371/journal.pone.0136741

Campisano D (2025) How Kenya built a wastewater-based surveillance system: 6 questions answered [WWW Document]. https://www.aphlblog.org/how-kenya-built-a-wastewater-based-surveillance-system-6-questions-answered/. Accessed 8.2.25

Chen Y, Chen L, Deng Q, Zhang G, Wu K, Ni L, Yang Y, Liu B, Wang W, Wei C, Yang J, Ye G, Cheng Z (2020) The presence of SARS-CoV-2 RNA in the feces of COVID-19 patients. J Med Virol 92:833–840. https://doi.org/10.1002/jmv.25825

Chigor VN, Okoh AI (2012) Quantitative RT-PCR detection of hepatitis a virus, rotaviruses and enteroviruses in the Buffalo River and source water dams in the Eastern Cape Province of South Africa. Int J Environ Res Public Health 9:4017–4032. https://doi.org/10.3390/ijerph9114017

Corpuz MVA, Buonerba A, Vigliotta G, Zarra T, Ballesteros F, Campiglia P, Belgiorno V, Korshin G, Naddeo V (2020) Viruses in wastewater: occurrence, abundance and detection methods. Sci Total Environ 745. https://doi.org/10.1016/j.scitotenv.2020.140910

Derbyshire JB (1976) Fate of animal viruses in effluent from liquid farm wastes. J Milk Food Technol 39:214

El-Senousy WM, Rashed MK, Kamel MA, Hasan SF (2023) Human rotavirus genome copies and infectious units in water and wastewater in Egypt. Egypt J Chem 66:1801–1814. https://doi.org/10.21608/ejchem.2023.225241.8344

Farmer-Diaz K, Matthew-Bernard M, Cheetham S, Mitchell K, Macpherson CNL, Ramos-Nino ME (2025) Optimized aluminum hydroxide adsorption–precipitation for improved viral detection in wastewater. Int J Environ Res Public Health 22. https://doi.org/10.3390/ijerph22020148

Fong T-T, Lipp EK (2005) Enteric viruses of humans and animals in aquatic environments: health risks, detection, and potential water quality assessment tools. Microbiol Mol Biol Rev 69:357–371. https://doi.org/10.1128/MMBR.69.2.357-371.2005

Ganesh A, Lin J, Singh M (2014) Detecting virus-like particles from the Umgeni River, South Africa. Clean (Weinh) 42:393–407. https://doi.org/10.1002/clen.201200564

Gibson KE, Schwab KJ (2011) Tangential-flow ultrafiltration with integrated inhibition detection for recovery of surrogates and human pathogens from large-volume source water and finished drinking water. Appl Environ Microbiol 77:385–391. https://doi.org/10.1128/AEM.01164-10

Gupta S, Parker J, Smits S, Underwood J, Dolwani S (2020) Persistent viral shedding of SARS-CoV-2 in faeces – a rapid review. Color Dis 22:611–620. https://doi.org/10.1111/codi.15138

Hamouda M, Mustafa F, Maraqa M, Rizvi T, Aly Hassan A (2021) Wastewater surveillance for SARS-CoV-2: lessons learnt from recent studies to define future applications. Sci Total Environ. https://doi.org/10.1016/j.scitotenv.2020.143493

Hanaoka N, Ito S, Konagaya M, Nojiri N, Yasuda M, Fujimoto T, Deguchi T (2019) Infectious human adenoviruses are shed in urine even after disappearance of urethral symptoms. PLoS One 14. https://doi.org/10.1371/journal.pone.0212434

Hongjaisee S, Jabjainai Y, Sakset S, Preechasuth K, Ngo-Giang-huong N, Khamduang W (2022) Comparison of simple RNA extraction methods for molecular diagnosis of Hepatitis C virus in plasma. Diagnostics 12. https://doi.org/10.3390/diagnostics12071599

Howe HA (1949) Epidemiology of poliomyelitis in the light of modern research. Am J Med 6:537–550. https://doi.org/10.1016/0002-9343(49)90127-8

Ibrahim C, Hammami S, Khelifi N, Hassen A (2023) Detection of enteroviruses and SARS-CoV-2 in Tunisian wastewater. Food Environ Virol 15:224–235. https://doi.org/10.1007/s12560-023-09557-0

Institut Pasteur (2020) Program analyzing the spread of the SARS-CoV-2 virus in high and low incidence areas of COVID-19 in Senegal [WWW Document]. https://www.pasteur.fr/en/institut-pasteur/institut-pasteur-world/news/program-analyzing-spread-sars-cov-2-virus-high-and-low-incidence-areas-covid-19-senegal. Accessed 8.2.25

Johnson R, Muller CJF, Ghoor S, Louw J, Archer E, Surujlal-Naicker S, Berkowitz N, Volschenk M, Bröcker LHL, Wolfaardt G, van der Walt M, Mutshembele AM, Malema S, Gelderblom HC, Mdhluli M, Gray G, Mathee A, Street RA (2021) Qualitative and quantitative detection of SARS-CoV-2 RNA in untreated wastewater in Western Cape Province, South Africa. S Afr Med J 111:198–202. https://doi.org/10.7196/SAMJ.2021.V111I3.15154

Jones DL, Baluja MQ, Graham DW, Corbishley A, McDonald JE, Malham SK, Hillary LS, Connor TR, Gaze WH, Moura IB, Wilcox MH, Farkas K (2020) Shedding of SARS-CoV-2 in feces and urine and its potential role in person-to-person transmission and the environment-based spread of COVID-19. Sci Total Environ 749. https://doi.org/10.1016/j.scitotenv.2020.141364

Karatas M, Bloemen M, Swinnen J, Roukaerts I, Van Gucht S, Van Ranst M, Wollants E, Matthijnssens J (2025) Untapped potential of wastewater for animal and potentially zoonotic virus surveillance: pilot study to detect non-human animal viruses in urban settings. Environ Int 199. https://doi.org/10.1016/j.envint.2025.109500

Keshaviah A, Diamond MB, Wade MJ, Scarpino SV, Ahmed W, Amman F, Aruna O, Badilla-Aguilar A, Bar-Or I, Bergthaler A, Bines JE, Bivins AW, Boehm AB, Brault JM, Burnet JB, Chapman JR, Chaudhuri A, de Roda Husman AM, Delatolla R, Dennehy JJ, Diamond MB, Donato C, Duizer E, Egwuenu A, Erster O, Fatta-Kassinos D, Gaggero A, Gilpin DF, Gilpin BJ, Graber TE, Green CA, Handley A, Hewitt J, Holm RH, Insam H, Johnson MC, Johnson R, Jones DL, Julian TR, Jyothi A, Kohn T, Kuhn KG, La Rosa G, Lesenfants M, Manuel DG, D'Aoust PM, Markt R, McGrath JW, Medema G, Moe CL, Murni IK, Naser H, Naughton CC, Ogorzaly L, Oktaria V, Ort C, Karaolia P, Patel EH, Paterson S, Rahman M, Rivera-Navarro P, Robinson A, Santa-Maria MC, Schmitt H, Smith T, Stadler LB, Stassijns J, Stenico A, Street RA, Suffredini E, Susswein Z, Trujillo M, Wolfe MK, Yakubu H, Zanoli Sato MI (2023) Wastewater monitoring can anchor global disease surveillance systems. Lancet Glob Health. https://doi.org/10.1016/S2214-109X(23)00170-5

Kilaru P, Hill D, Anderson K, Collins MB, Green H, Kmush BL, Larsen DA (2023) Wastewater surveillance for infectious disease: a systematic review. Am J Epidemiol. https://doi.org/10.1093/aje/kwac175

Kiulia NM, Netshikweta R, Page NA, Van Zyl WB, Kiraithe MM, Nyachieo A, Mwenda JM, Taylor MB (2010) The detection of enteric viruses in selected urban and rural river water and sewage in Kenya, with special reference to rotaviruses. J Appl Microbiol 109:818–828. https://doi.org/10.1111/j.1365-2672.2010.04710.x

Mabasa VV, Meno KD, Taylor MB, Mans J (2018) Environmental surveillance for noroviruses in selected South African wastewaters 2015–2016: emergence of the novel GII.17. Food Environ Virol 10:16–28. https://doi.org/10.1007/s12560-017-9316-2

Mabasa VV, van Zyl WB, Ismail A, Allam M, Taylor MB, Mans J (2022) Multiple novel human norovirus recombinants identified in wastewater in Pretoria, South Africa by Next-Generation Sequencing. Viruses 14. https://doi.org/10.3390/v14122732

Mehle N, Gutiérrez-Aguirre I, Kutnjak D, Ravnikar M (2018) Water-mediated transmission of plant, animal, and human viruses. Adv Virus Res 101:85–128. https://doi.org/10.1016/bs.aivir.2018.02.004

Melnick JL (1947) Poliomyelitis virus in urban sewage in epidemic and in nonepidemic times. Am J Epidemiol 45:240–253. https://doi.org/10.1093/oxfordjournals.aje.a119132

Metcalf TG, Melnick JL, Estes MK (1995) From detection of virus in sewage and water by isolation to identification by molecular biology—a trip of over 50 years. Ann Rev Microbiol 49:461–487. https://doi.org/10.1146/annurev.mi.49.100195.002333

Miranda RC, Schaffner DW (2019) Virus risk in the food supply chain. Curr Opin Food Sci. https://doi.org/10.1016/j.cofs.2018.12.002

Muluh TJ, Hamisu AW, Craig K, Mkanda P, Andrew E, Adeniji J, Akande A, Musa A, Ayodeji I, Nicksy G, Banda R, Tegegne SG, Nsubuga P, Oyetunji A, Diop O, Vaz RG, Muhammad AJG (2016) Contribution of environmental surveillance toward interruption of poliovirus transmission in Nigeria, 2012–2015. J Infect Dis 213:S131–S135. https://doi.org/10.1093/infdis/jiv767

Murakami M, Ando H, Yamaguchi R, Kitajima M (2024) Evaluating survey techniques in wastewater-based epidemiology for accurate COVID-19 incidence estimation. Sci Total Environ 954:176702. https://doi.org/10.1016/j.scitotenv.2024.176702

O'Brien M, Rundell ZC, Nemec MD, Langan LM, Back JA, Lugo JN (2021) A comparison of four commercially available RNA extraction kits for wastewater surveillance of SARS-CoV-2 in a college population. Sci Total Environ 801. https://doi.org/10.1016/j.scitotenv.2021.149595

Omatola CA, Olasehinde TA, Olaniran AO (2024) Relative abundance and the fate of human rotavirus in wastewater during treatment processes: identification of potential infectious rotavirus in the final effluents and receiving aquatic milieu in Durban area, South Africa. Environ Monit Assess 196. https://doi.org/10.1007/s10661-024-12888-5

Omilabu SA, Salu OB (2023) Medically important airborne viruses. In: Aeromicrobiology. Elsevier, pp 205–241. https://doi.org/10.1016/B978-0-323-96122-6.00010-4

Osunmakinde CO, Selvarajan R, Mamba B, Msagati TAM (2021) Viral communities distribution and diversity in a wastewater treatment plants using high-throughput sequencing analysis. Pol J Environ Stud 30:3189–3201. https://doi.org/10.15244/pjoes/127888

Othman I, Helmi A, Slama I, Hamdi R, Mastouri M, Aouni M (2023) Evaluation of three viral concentration methods for detection and quantification of SARS-CoV-2 in wastewater. J Water Health 21:354–360. https://doi.org/10.2166/wh.2023.264

Park S, Kim ET, Huh J-S (2021) Virus in the urine of healthy people and patients with infectious diseases. Urogenit Tract Infect 16:44–48. https://doi.org/10.14777/uti.2021.16.2.44

Paul JR (1941) The virus of poliomyelitis in stools and sewage. JAMA: The Journal of the American Medical Association 116:493. https://doi.org/10.1001/jama.1941.02820060041009

Paul JR, Trask JD, Gard S (1940) II. Poliomyelitis virus in urban sewage. J Exp Med 71:765–777. https://doi.org/10.1084/jem.71.6.765

Paul D, Kolar P, Hall SG (2021) A review of the impact of environmental factors on the fate and transport of coronaviruses in aqueous environments. NPJ Clean Water. https://doi.org/10.1038/s41545-020-00096-w

Perumal N, Jain RK, Sharma A, Chaurasia D (2021) Performance comparison of commercial RNA extraction kits for the diagnosis of SARS-CoV-2. J Clin Sci Res 10:157–159. https://doi.org/10.4103/jcsr.jcsr_90_20

Pyankov OV, Bodnev SA, Pyankova OG, Agranovski IE (2018) Survival of aerosolized coronavirus in the ambient air. J Aerosol Sci 115:158–163. https://doi.org/10.1016/j.jaerosci.2017.09.009

Quilliam RS, Weidmann M, Moresco V, Purshouse H, O'Hara Z, Oliver DM (2020) COVID-19: the environmental implications of shedding SARS-CoV-2 in human faeces. Environ Int. https://doi.org/10.1016/j.envint.2020.105790

Raya S, Malla B, Shrestha S, Sthapit N, Kattel H, Sharma ST, Tuladhar R, Maharjan R, Takeda T, Kitajima M, Tandukar S, Haramoto E (2024) Quantification of multiple respiratory viruses in wastewater in the Kathmandu Valley, Nepal: potential implications of wastewater-based epidemiology for community disease surveillance in developing countries. Sci Total Environ 920. https://doi.org/10.1016/j.scitotenv.2024.170845

Rector A, Bloemen M, Thijssen M, Pussig B, Beuselinck K, Van Ranst M, Wollants E (2024) Respiratory viruses in wastewater compared with clinical samples, Leuven, Belgium. Emerg Infect Dis 30:141–145. https://doi.org/10.3201/eid3001.231011

Saeidi N, Gu X, Goh SG, Xin CLY, Gin KYH (2017) Evaluating the efficacy of commercial kits for viral DNA/RNA extraction. Water Pract Technol 12:80–86. https://doi.org/10.2166/wpt.2017.015

Salemane K, Coetzee LZ, Pocock G, Genthe B, Taylor MB, Mans J (2024) Water-based epidemiological investigation of Hepatitis E virus in South Africa. Food Environ Virol 16:338–350. https://doi.org/10.1007/s12560-024-09596-1

SAMRC (2021) SAMRC wastewater surveillance dashboard. An early warning system for COVID-19 infections [WWW Document]. https://www.samrc.ac.za/wbe/. Accessed 8.10.25

Sapula SA, Whittall JJ, Pandopulos AJ, Gerber C, Venter H (2021) An optimized and robust PEG precipitation method for detection of SARS-CoV-2 in wastewater. Sci Total Environ 785. https://doi.org/10.1016/j.scitotenv.2021.147270

Shabana MR, Zaghloul AY, El Shaarawy TH, Elleboudy NS, Aboshanab KM (2024) Monitoring the VDPV2 outbreak in Egypt during 2020–2021 highlights the crucial role of environmental surveillance and boosting immunization in combating poliovirus. BMC Infect Dis 24. https://doi.org/10.1186/s12879-024-09731-0

Shempela DM, Muleya W, Mudenda S, Daka V, Sikalima J, Kamayani M, Sandala D, Chipango C, Muzala K, Musonda K, Chizimu JY, Mulenga C, Kapona O, Kwenda G, Kasanga M, Njuguna M, Cham F, Simwaka B, Morrison L, Muma JB, Saasa N, Sichinga K, Simulundu E, Chilengi R (2024) Wastewater surveillance of SARS-CoV-2 in Zambia: an early warning tool. Int J Mol Sci 25. https://doi.org/10.3390/ijms25168839

Singer AC, Thompson JR, Filho CRM, Street R, Li X, Castiglioni S, Thomas KV (2023) A world of wastewater-based epidemiology: viewpoint. Nat Water 1:408–415. https://doi.org/10.1038/s44221-023-00083-8

Street R, Mathee A, Reddy T, Mahlangeni NT, Mangwana N, Nkambule S, Webster C, Dias S, Sharma JR, Ramharack P, Louw J, Surujlal-Naicker S, Berkowitz N, Mdhluli M, Gray G, Muller C, Johnson R (2024) One year of wastewater surveillance in South Africa supporting COVID-19 clinical findings across two waves of infection. Microorganisms 12. https://doi.org/10.3390/microorganisms12112230

Torii S, Oishi W, Zhu Y, Thakali O, Malla B, Yu Z, Zhao B, Arakawa C, Kitajima M, Hata A, Ihara M, Kyuwa S, Sano D, Haramoto E, Katayama H (2022) Comparison of five polyethylene glycol precipitation procedures for the RT-qPCR based recovery of murine hepatitis virus, bacteriophage phi6, and pepper mild mottle virus as a surrogate for SARS-CoV-2 from wastewater. Sci Total Environ 807. https://doi.org/10.1016/j.scitotenv.2021.150722

Tubatsi G, Kebaabetswe LP (2022) Detection of enteric viruses from wastewater and river water in Botswana. Food Environ Virol 14:157–169. https://doi.org/10.1007/s12560-022-09513-4

Xu D, Zhang Z, Jin L, Chu F, Mao Y, Wang H, Liu M, Wang M, Zhang L, Gao GF, Wang FS (2005) Persistent shedding of viable SARS-CoV in urine and stool of SARS patients during the convalescent phase. Eur J Clin Microbiol Infect Dis 24:165–171. https://doi.org/10.1007/s10096-005-1299-5

Yousif M, Rachida S, Taukobong S, Ndlovu N, Iwu-Jaja C, Howard W, Moonsamy S, Mhlambi N, Gwala S, Levy JI, Andersen KG, Scheepers C, von Gottberg A, Wolter N, Bhiman JN, Amoako DG, Ismail A, Suchard M, McCarthy K (2023) SARS-CoV-2 genomic surveillance in wastewater as a model for monitoring evolution of endemic viruses. Nat Commun 14. https://doi.org/10.1038/s41467-023-41369-5

Yuan T, Pian Y (2023) Hospital wastewater as hotspots for pathogenic microorganisms spread into aquatic environment: a review. Front Environ Sci. https://doi.org/10.3389/fenvs.2022.1091734

Zhang CM, Xu LM, Xu PC, Wang XC (2016) Elimination of viruses from domestic wastewater: requirements and technologies. World J Microbiol Biotechnol. https://doi.org/10.1007/s11274-016-2018-3

Zhang T, Cui X, Zhao X, Wang J, Zheng J, Zheng G, Guo W, Cai C, He S, Xu Y (2020) Detectable SARS-CoV-2 viral RNA in feces of three children during recovery period of COVID-19 pneumonia. J Med Virol 92:909–914. https://doi.org/10.1002/jmv.25795

Zhou NA, Fagnant-Sperati CS, Komen E, Mwangi B, Mukubi J, Nyangao J, Hassan J, Chepkurui A, Maina C, van Zyl WB, Matsapola PN, Wolfaardt M, Ngwana FB, Jeffries-Miles S, Coulliette-Salmond A, Peñaranda S, Shirai JH, Kossik AL, Beck NK, Wilmouth R, Boyle DS, Burns CC, Taylor MB, Borus P, Meschke JS (2020) Feasibility of the bag-mediated filtration system for environmental surveillance of poliovirus in Kenya. Food Environ Virol 12:35–47. https://doi.org/10.1007/s12560-019-09412-1

Chapter 13
Use of Genomics for the Detection of Viral Infections—Is Africa Well-Equipped?

Selvarajan Ramganesh, Ramar Ramesh, Nfor Gilbert Karngong, and Akebe Luther King Abia

13.1 Introduction

Viruses have coexisted with humans for centuries, adapting to diverse environments and continuing to pose challenges to global health (Taylor 2015). Their existence, initially obscure, was revealed through advances in microbiology—beginning with the invention of the microscope. The foundation of virology was established with studies on the tobacco mosaic virus (TMV) by Stanley (Rossmann 2013). From these early discoveries, a range of techniques for studying and identifying viruses emerged, including X-ray fiber diffraction analysis by Bernal and Fankuchen and the elucidation of viral icosahedral structures by Watson and Crick (Taylor 2015). Among these, nucleic acid amplification methods have undergone rapid evolution, progressing from the identification of single viruses to the simultaneous detection of multiple viruses in complex samples. These technological advancements have greatly expanded research into human, animal, and plant viruses. However, such

S. Ramganesh (✉)
Department of Environmental Science, College of Agricultural Sciences (CAS), University of South Africa-Florida Campus, Roodepoort, South Africa

Department of Biochemistry, J.J. College of Arts and Science (Autonomous), Pudukkottai, Tamil Nadu, India

R. Ramesh
Department of Biochemistry, J.J. College of Arts and Science (Autonomous), Pudukkottai, Tamil Nadu, India

N. G. Karngong
Catholic University of Central Africa, Yaounde, Cameroon

A. L. K. Abia (✉)
Total Environmental Research (TEN-R) Group, College of Health Sciences, University of KwaZulu-Natal, Durban, South Africa

Environmental Research Foundation, Westville, South Africa

J. A. Shenge, A. L. K. Abia (eds.), *Viral Diseases and One Health in Africa*,
https://doi.org/10.1007/978-3-032-09613-5_13

progress has not been uniformly distributed; many low- and middle-income countries still rely on basic, often time-consuming and labor-intensive diagnostic methods. This technological limitation continues to hinder effective viral surveillance, timely outbreak response, and comprehensive research in regions that usually bear the highest burden of viral diseases.

13.2 Genomics—Its Enormous Benefits

Genomics has emerged as an indispensable tool for identifying and understanding new and unknown viral infectious pathogens that can cause widespread devastation and transcend geographical boundaries (Tegally et al. 2022). The advent of genomic technologies has significantly transformed our ability to monitor, characterize, and respond to these viral threats. Through detailed analysis of viral genomes, researchers can unravel the mechanisms of viral evolution, transmission dynamics, and emergence of new variants, providing insights that were previously unattainable.

Next-generation sequencing (NGS) and whole-genome sequencing (WGS) represent groundbreaking advancements in the field of genomics. NGS technologies enable the rapid sequencing of DNA and RNA, allowing researchers to decode the entire genetic blueprint of viruses within a matter of days. This fast turnaround accelerates outbreak investigations, informs vaccine and therapeutic development, and enhances the detection of novel or emerging pathogens. WGS, in particular, offers a comprehensive view of a virus's genetic architecture, facilitating in-depth studies of its evolutionary history, transmission patterns, and mutation rates. These approaches are not only pivotal for understanding the biology of known viruses but are also crucial in identifying and monitoring new viral threats as they arise. Despite these advancements, the uptake of genomic diagnostics in Africa has historically lagged behind other regions, mainly due to limited infrastructure, a shortage of skilled personnel, and inadequate investment in research and technology. Before the COVID-19 pandemic, many African countries lacked robust genomic sequencing capabilities, often relying on laboratories outside the continent for sequencing and analysis (Morgan 2023). This dependence has impeded timely surveillance, local capacity-building, and independent research initiatives.

Africa, however, has long been a hotspot for significant viral outbreaks, including Ebola virus disease, Marburg virus disease, Crimean-Congo haemorrhagic fever, Rift Valley fever, Yellow fever, Lassa fever, and, most recently, COVID-19 (Chauhan et al. 2020; Gear 1989). The emergence and re-emergence of these viruses underscore the urgent need for improved local capacity in genomics and bioinformatics. Strengthening genomics infrastructure within Africa would not only accelerate the detection and monitoring of infectious disease outbreaks but also enable tailored, context-specific responses that are essential for effective public health management. This chapter aims to highlight key African studies that have leveraged NGS and WGS technologies in viral research. By highlighting their successes, challenges, outcomes, and limitations, the chapter aims to provide a comprehensive overview of the current landscape. The insights gained will provide policymakers with valuable guidance, underscoring the strategic importance of investing in advanced research tools. Such investments are critical to enhancing Africa's preparedness and resilience in the face of ongoing and future viral disease threats.

13.3 Africa in the Genomic Research Landscape

Since the introduction of genomic research, each decade demonstrates a clear and progressive increase in the number of African countries actively participating in genomics research, as well as a notable intensification of research activity and funding (Fig. 13.1). In the 1990s, genomic research capacity was primarily limited to a small number of countries with minimal investment and limited infrastructure. Most countries had either no activity or were reliant on external collaborations for genomics initiatives. By the 2000s, more countries began to establish the foundations for genomic research, with moderate growth in infrastructure, capacity-building, and early regional collaborations. The 2010s mark a turning point, characterized by significant expansion in research networks, increased domestic and international funding, and the emergence of pan-African initiatives such as H3Africa. This period saw an increase in countries investing in sequencing facilities, bioinformatics training, and locally driven research projects, resulting in greater

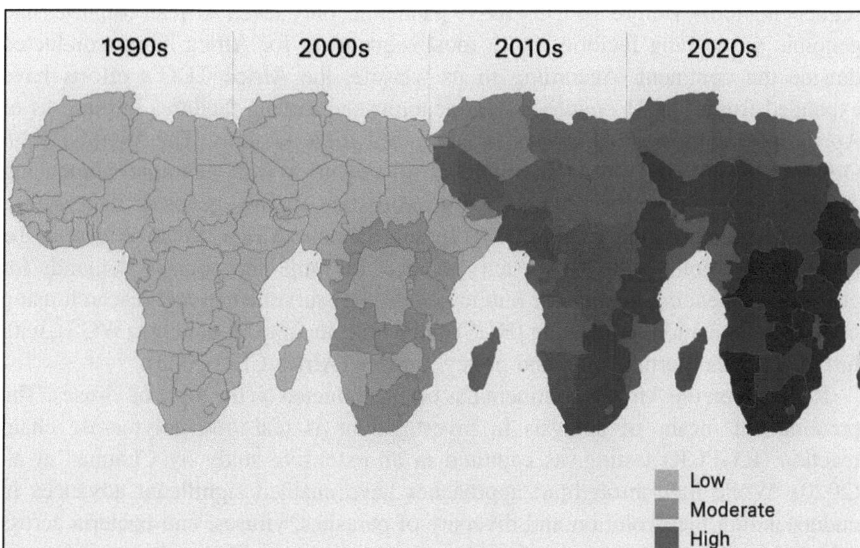

Fig. 13.1 The figure illustrates the evolution of genomic research and funding intensity across Africa from the 1990s to the 2020s. (*Low*: Limited or emerging genomic research activity and funding; *Moderate*: Established research centers and increased investment; *High*: Extensive genomic research activity with significant funding and multiple flagship projects)

scientific output and the development of continent-wide expertise. In the 2020s, the pace and intensity of genomic research across Africa accelerated rapidly, driven in part by the urgent need for local surveillance and response during the COVID-19 pandemic. Many countries established advanced sequencing centers, increased funding for genomics projects, and launched collaborative networks to monitor and study a wide array of viral and other infectious diseases. The result is a dramatic transformation from isolated efforts in a handful of countries to a continent-wide landscape characterized by widespread and high-level genomic research activity and investment. This expansion highlights Africa's increasing ability to conduct advanced genomics research independently, inform public health policy, and respond promptly to emerging disease threats.

Africa has risen to the challenge with ambitious targets and institutions established in the private sector to mitigate that disadvantage, aiming to enable swift action by local governments to prevent future epidemics. In-house genomic sequencing capacity can significantly reduce the time for a public health response to viral illnesses for governments. For instance, in-country sequencing times are shorter than off-continent sequencing times by as much as 64 days, resulting in a two-month reduction in the time for a public health response (Kwon 2022). This responsibility has largely been taken up by the African Centres for Disease Control and Prevention (Africa CDC), a public-sector initiative established in 2017. That same year, the Africa CDC initiated pathogenic microbial genomic sequencing, although the COVID-19 pandemic rapidly expanded its activities (Africa CDC 2023). The organization's goal is to ensure that all African countries have access to genome sequencing tools. Before the COVID-19 pandemic, only seven African countries had genomic sequencing facilities, with most sequencing for Africa being conducted outside the continent. According to its website, the Africa CDC's efforts have expanded from 7 to 31 countries with genomic sequencing facilities in place as of April 2023, with ongoing efforts to strengthen these systems. The World Health Organization (WHO) puts that figure at 40 countries with genomic sequencing capacity as of September 2022, with 46 countries sharing genomic data with a public database (Africa CDC, 2023). In sub-Saharan Africa, South Africa is the leader in genomics with the capacity to meet the time and country demands for genomic sequencing quality for public health viral surveillance and research using both next-generation sequencing (NGS) and whole genome sequencing (WGS), with full government participation and policy in place (Africa CDC 2023).

Research on the African continent has been conducted on the topic of viruses. The predominant means of analysis in investigations is real-time polymerase chain reaction (RT-PCR) testing, as captured in an extensive study by Chauhan et al. (2020). While high-throughput approaches have enabled significant advances in understanding the evolution and diversity of parasites, viruses, and bacteria across Africa, it is important to note that not all sequencing work has been performed locally; in many cases, samples have been analyzed in laboratories outside the continent. Additionally, high-throughput sequencing has been applied to plant viral research in at least 20 African countries. Notably, two countries in East Africa, along with South Africa, have accounted for the majority of research output in this area (Ibaba and Gubba 2020). This reflects both the growing capacity for genomics in Africa and the persistent challenges of infrastructure and local expertise, which have limited the continent-wide adoption and application of advanced sequencing technologies.

13.4 High-Throughput Sequencing Viral Studies in Africa

Across the African continent, several countries have begun adopting high-throughput gene sequencing methods to enhance viral research and surveillance (Table 13.1).

Table 13.1 Summary of high-throughput sequencing viral research in selected African countries

Country	Key viral genomics studies and milestones	Sequencing facility/ location	Notable outcomes and policy actions
Algeria	COVID-19 genome evolution (via GISAID data); S. aureus WGS for AMR (analysis done in UK)	No local WGS (samples analyzed abroad)	Early use of WGS; limited local sequencing infrastructure
South Africa	NGS for plant viruses (Closteroviridae); H5N1 bird flu outbreak traced using WGS (Stellenbosch University)	Stellenbosch University, others	Demonstrated capacity for in-country sequencing and outbreak tracing
Senegal	NGS for acute febrile illness, identification of multiple viruses (analysis at broad institute, USA); WGS of COVID-19; plasmodium falciparum population genomics	Limited local (some analysis abroad)	Characterized local SARS-CoV-2 clade; expanded pathogen discovery via metagenomics
Nigeria	First SARS-CoV-2 genome sequenced in Africa; Lassa fever virus evolution studies; deployment of portable sequencing tools	NRL, NIMR, CPHL, ACEGID, UDUTH	Multiple local sequencing labs; National Genomics Surveillance Consortium (2024)
DR Congo	Post-2018 Ebola outbreak, implementation of genomic surveillance system	Local labs supported by government	Policy-driven adoption of high-throughput sequencing for outbreak response

Abbreviations: *WGS* Whole-Genome Sequencing, *NGS* Next-Generation Sequencing, *AMR* Antimicrobial Resistance, *ACEGID* African Centre of Excellence for Genomics of Infectious Disease, *NRL* National Reference Laboratory, *NIMR* Nigerian Institute of Medical Research, *CPHL* Central Public Health Laboratory, *UDUTH* Usmanu Danfodiyo University Teaching Hospital, *NCDC* Nigeria Centre for Disease Control

13.4.1 Algeria

A study on the evolution of COVID-19 in North Africa (Sudan, Egypt, Algeria, Morocco, Libya, and Tunisia) analyzed whole-genome sequences (WGS) of viral strains recorded in the GISAID database; however, genomic sequencing was not conducted locally for this study (Menasria and Aguilera 2022). In another instance, other than viral surveillance, WGS was utilized to genetically characterize antimicrobial resistance in *Staphylococcus aureus* isolated from two Algerian hospitals. While the samples were collected in Algeria, the sequencing analysis itself was performed at a partner university in the UK (Namoune et al. 2023).

13.4.2 South Africa

South Africa has demonstrated robust viral genomics research capacity. One study applied next-generation sequencing (NGS) to analyze two variants of the Closteroviridae virus family, which affect grapevines and grapefruit, and determined the sequencing depth required for effective detection (Visser et al. 2016). Outbreaks of H5N1 High Pathogenicity Avian Influenza in South Africa in 2023 were caused by two distinct sub-genotypes of Clade 2.3.4.4b Viruses (Abolnik et al. 2024). Genomic sequencing was conducted at the University of Stellenbosch in South Africa in 2023 to assess viral bird flu strains in wild birds and farm chickens. This work aimed to trace the source of the outbreak, as well as its epidemiology and evolution, in comparison with clades from other parts of the world and Africa.

13.4.3 Senegal

NGS has been instrumental in identifying non-malarial causes of acute febrile illness in Senegal, revealing the presence of eight viruses associated with febrile disease, including flaviviruses, coronaviruses, herpesviruses, and picornaviruses, as well as bacteria and fungi (Orf et al. 2024). Another study identified five different viruses in hospital blood samples, while also investigating bacterial vectors through 16S analysis (Levine et al. 2024). Although these metagenomic analyses were performed at the Broad Institute in the USA, all samples originated from Senegal. Local WGS studies on COVID-19 have also characterized a unique Senegalese clade derived from the Brazilian P.1 lineage, with more than 1100 single nucleotide polymorphisms identified (Ndiaye et al. 2023) An investigation utilized WGS combined with population genetic methods to examine evolutionary forces shaping diversity in the parasite population in Senegal to isolates of *Plasmodium falciparum*, the malaria-causing parasite, recognizing the implications of understanding gene selection for drug targeting (Chang et al. 2012).

13.4.4 Nigeria

Nigeria has five genomic sequencing facilities as recognized by the World Health Organization (WHO): the National Reference Laboratory (NRL), Nigerian Institute of Medical Research (NIMR), Central Public Health Laboratory (CPHL), Lagos, the African Centre of Excellence for the Genomics of Infectious Disease (ACEGID) and Usmanu Danfodiyo University Teaching Hospital (UDUTH), 4 of which are government-owned, showing an active government policy and effort at the national level to utilize (Nigeria Expands Genomic Sequencing Intervention beyond COVID-19 | WHO | Regional Office for Africa 2022). A PCR laboratory in the country identified the country's first case of Ebola virus disease in a returnee from another African nation in 2014. That same lab sequenced the first SARS-CoV-2 genome in Africa and made it publicly available. The lab carries out viral research using genomic sequencing. It has even partnered with the Sabeti Lab at the Broadway Institute to do research which traced the evolution of the Lassa fever virus, revealing its "ancient origins" and uncovering seven different lineages through sequencing (Broad Institute 2024; Gire et al. 2012; Siddle et al. 2018). The Nigeria Centre for Disease Control and Prevention (NCDC) used portable genomic sequencing tools in 2018 to identify a Lassa fever outbreak, thereby facilitating an effective public health response (NCDC 2019). In May 2024, the NCDC established a National Genomics Surveillance Consortium, demonstrating the government's commitment to genomic sequencing for safeguarding public health and positioning Nigeria as a "genomic sequencing hub in the global south" (Ileyemi and James 2024). Nigeria also has a government establishment that handles viral research in animals, the National Veterinary Research Institute; however, it does not list genomic diagnostics as part of its diagnostic tools. However, genomic testing facilities in Nigeria are insufficient for effective healthcare; although the government is involved in genomic sequencing, there is no policy specifically promoting neonatal genomic screening in Nigeria.

13.4.5 Democratic Republic of Congo

Following its tenth Ebola virus disease outbreak in Nord Kivu in 2018, the Democratic Republic of Congo established a genomic surveillance system using high-throughput sequencing, reflecting government support for genomics in public health (Kinganda-Lusamaki et al. 2021). Table 13.1 summarises some of the research that used high-throughput sequencing in Africa over time.

13.5 Challenges to Implementing Genomics Research in Africa

Despite the promise of genomics for revolutionizing healthcare, infectious disease surveillance, and agricultural biotechnology in Africa, the continent continues to face numerous barriers that hinder the widespread adoption and sustainability of genomics research (Adebamowo et al. 2018). Implementing genomics research in Africa faces numerous systemic and infrastructural challenges. Securing timely and sustained funding is a significant barrier, as many projects are delayed or halted due to bureaucratic hurdles, limited domestic investment, or dependence on short-term international grants. This financial instability hinders both ongoing research and the ability to maintain or upgrade laboratory infrastructure. Furthermore, the continent suffers from a shortage of local experts and technical staff trained in genomics and bioinformatics. Inadequate capacity-building programs and limited professional development opportunities often compel African scientists to seek training abroad, which can result in resource constraints and a brain drain. Many research centers lack access to advanced sequencing platforms, reliable internet, or even cold-chain storage facilities. Furthermore, frequent power outages and poor connectivity further disrupt operations and international collaboration. Additional obstacles include limited access to research facilities, particularly in rural or underserved regions, and the absence of centralized genomic data repositories, which impedes data sharing and long-term studies. Computing and bioinformatics infrastructure is often insufficient for handling large genomic datasets, leading to analysis bottlenecks and underutilization of sequencing outputs. Moreover, the development of harmonized ethical, legal, and policy frameworks for genomics research remains slow, raising concerns over privacy, informed consent, and benefit-sharing. Language barriers, low public awareness of genomics, administrative hurdles, and difficulties importing necessary reagents further complicate the research landscape.

13.6 Advantages for Genomic Sequencing Infrastructure and Capacity Building in Africa

Building genomic sequencing infrastructure and capacity in Africa provides crucial advantages for public health and research. Local facilities and skilled personnel enable rapid detection of both new and known viruses, allowing for timely outbreak response and more effective disease control. This strengthens the continent's health systems, reduces reliance on external laboratories, and helps mitigate loss of life during epidemics. Additionally, owning and managing genomic data empowers African researchers to set local research agendas, ensures data sovereignty, and promotes scientific independence. Capacity building fosters expertise, facilitates training for future scientists, and supports regional and international collaborations.

Ultimately, investing in genomics equips Africa to address its unique health challenges while contributing to the global scientific community.

13.7 Recommendations

African governments are strongly encouraged to integrate genomic sequencing infrastructure into national health policies to ensure efficient and effective public health response systems that prioritize saving lives. Investment in both technology and workforce development is essential, as building local expertise and maintaining modern facilities will empower countries to detect, monitor, and respond rapidly to disease outbreaks and emerging health threats.

Given the continent's limited financial resources, it is also recommended that governments actively pursue regional collaboration. By partnering with neighboring countries and leveraging existing regional hubs—such as those supported by the Africa CDC African nations can maximize the use of available resources while gradually developing their in-country capabilities. These strategic partnerships will help bridge current gaps in infrastructure and expertise, ensuring broader access to genomic tools and ultimately strengthening Africa's capacity to safeguard public health.

References

Abolnik C, Roberts LC, Strydom C, Snyman A, Roberts DG (2024) Outbreaks of H5N1 high pathogenicity avian influenza in South Africa in 2023 were caused by two distinct sub-genotypes of clade 2.3.4.4b viruses. Viruses 16(6). https://doi.org/10.3390/v16060896

Adebamowo SN, Francis V, Tambo E, Diallo SH, Landouré G, Nembaware V, Dareng E, Muhamed B, Odutola M, Akeredolu T, Nerima B, Ozumba PJ, Mbhele S, Ghanash A, Wachinou AP, Ngomi N (2018) Implementation of genomics research in Africa: challenges and recommendations. Glob Health Action 11(1). https://doi.org/10.1080/16549716.2017.1419033

Africa CDC (2023) A six-year journey: advancing pathogen genomics in Africa –. Retrieved June 26, 2024, from https://africacdc.org/news-item/a-six-year-journey-advancing-pathogen-genomics-in-africa/

Broad Institute (2024) A new viral surveillance system in West Africa is showing the world how to prevent the next pandemic. Retrieved June 29, 2024, from https://www.broadinstitute.org/news/new-viral-surveillance-system-west-africa-showing-world-how-prevent-next-pandemic

Chang HH, Park DJ, Galinsky KJ, Schaffner SF, Ndiaye D, Ndir O, Mboup S, Wiegand RC, Volkman SK, Sabeti PC, Wirth DF, Neafsey DE, Hartl DL (2012) Genomic sequencing of Plasmodium falciparum malaria parasites from Senegal reveals the demographic history of the population. Mol Biol Evol 29(11):3427–3439. https://doi.org/10.1093/MOLBEV/MSS161

Chauhan RP, Dessie ZG, Noreddin A, El Zowalaty ME (2020) Systematic review of important viral diseases in Africa in light of the 'One Health' concept. Pathogens 9(4). https://doi.org/10.3390/PATHOGENS9040301

Gear JHS (1989) Clinical aspects of African viral hemorrhagic fevers. Rev Infect Dis 11(Suppl 4): s777–s782. https://doi.org/10.1093/CLINIDS/11.SUPPLEMENT_4.S777

Gire SK, Stremlau M, Andersen KG, Schaffner SF, Bjornson Z, Rubins K, Hensley L, McCormick JB, Lander ES, Garry RF, Happi C, Sabeti PC (2012) Emerging disease or diagnosis? Science 338(6108):750–752. https://doi.org/10.1126/SCIENCE.1225893

Ibaba JD, Gubba A (2020) High-throughput sequencing application in the diagnosis and discovery of plant-infecting viruses in Africa, a decade later. Plants 9(10). https://doi.org/10.3390/plants9101376

Ileyemi M, James L (2024) Health security: Nigerian agency inaugurates national genomics consortium. Retrieved June 29, 2024, from https://www.premiumtimesng.com/news/top-news/699245-health-security-nigerian-agency-inaugurates-national-genomics-consortium.html

Kinganda-Lusamaki E, Black A, Mukadi DB, Hadfield J, Mbala-Kingebeni P, Pratt CB, Aziza A, Diagne MM, White B, Bisento N, Nsunda B, Akonga M, Faye M, Faye O, Edidi-Atani F, Matondo-Kuamfumu M, Mambu-Mbika F, Bulabula J, Di Paola N et al (2021) Integration of genomic sequencing into the response to the Ebola virus outbreak in Nord Kivu, Democratic Republic of the Congo. Nat Med 27(4):710–716. https://doi.org/10.1038/S41591-021-01302-Z

Kwon D (2022) 100,000 coronavirus genomes reveal COVID's evolution in Africa. Nature. https://doi.org/10.1038/D41586-022-03070-3

Levine ZC, Sene A, Mkandawire W, Deme AB, Ndiaye T, Sy M, Gaye A, Diedhiou Y, Mbaye AM, Ndiaye IM, Gomis J, Ndiop M, Sene D, Faye Paye M, MacInnis BL, Schaffner SF, Park DJ, Badiane AS, Colubri A et al (2024) Investigating the etiologies of non-malarial febrile illness in Senegal using metagenomic sequencing. Nat Commun 15(1):1–13. https://doi.org/10.1038/s41467-024-44800-7

Menasria T, Aguilera M (2022) Genomic diversity of SARS-CoV-2 in Algeria and north African countries: what we know so far and what we expect? Microorganisms 10(2). https://doi.org/10.3390/MICROORGANISMS10020467/S1

Morgan PJ (2023) World of Genomics: Nigeria. Retrieved June 29, 2024, from https://frontlinegenomics.com/world-of-genomics-nigeria/

Namoune R, Djebbar A, Mekler R, McHugh M, Bekara MEA, Decano A, Holden MTG, Sebaihia M (2023) Whole genome sequencing and molecular epidemiology of clinical isolates of Staphylococcus aureus from Algeria. Microorganisms 11(8):2047. https://doi.org/10.3390/MICROORGANISMS11082047

Ndiaye AJS, Beye M, Lo G, Kacel I, Sow A, Leye N, Padane A, Mboup A, Diop-Ndiaye H, Sokhna C, Kane CT, Colson P, Fenollar F, Mboup S, Fournier PE (2023) Genomic epidemiology of SARS-CoV-2 in urban settings in Senegal. Viruses 15(6). https://doi.org/10.3390/V15061233/S1

Nigeria Centre for Disease Control and Prevention (2019) Retrieved June 29, 2024, from https://ncdc.gov.ng/news/161/innovative-genomics-tool-directs-public-health-response-early-in-outbreak

Nigeria expands genomic sequencing intervention beyond COVID-19 | WHO | Regional Office for Africa (2022) Retrieved June 29, 2024, from https://www.afro.who.int/countries/nigeria/news/nigeria-expands-genomic-sequencing-intervention-beyond-covid-19

Orf GS, Ahouidi AD, Mata M, Diedhiou C, Mboup A, Padane A, Manga NM, Dela-del Lawson AT, Averhoff F, Berg MG, Cloherty GA, Mboup S (2024) Next-generation sequencing survey of acute febrile illness in Senegal (2020–2022). Front Microbiol 15. https://doi.org/10.3389/fmicb.2024.1362714

Rossmann MG (2013) Structure of viruses: a short history. Q Rev Biophys 46(2):133–180. https://doi.org/10.1017/S0033583513000012

Siddle KJ, Eromon P, Barnes KG, Mehta S, Oguzie JU, Odia I, Schaffner SF, Winnicki SM, Shah RR, Qu J, Wohl S, Brehio P, Iruolagbe C, Aiyepada J, Uyigue E, Akhilomen P, Okonofua G, Ye S, Kayode T et al (2018) Genomic analysis of Lassa virus during an increase in cases in Nigeria in 2018. N Engl J Med 379(18):1745–1753. https://doi.org/10.1056/NEJMOA1804498

Taylor MW (2015) Viruses and man: a history of interactions. Springer, pp 1–430. https://doi.org/10.1007/978-3-319-07758-1/COVER

Tegally H, San JE, Cotten M, Moir M, Tegomoh B, Mboowa G, Martin DP, Baxter C, Lambisia AW, Diallo A, Amoako DG, Diagne MM, Sisay A, Zekri ARN, Gueye AS, Sangare AK, Ouedraogo AS, Sow A, Musa AO et al (2022) The evolving SARS-CoV-2 epidemic in Africa: insights from rapidly expanding genomic surveillance. Science (NY) *378*(6615). https://doi.org/10.1126/SCIENCE.ABQ5358

Visser M, Bester R, Burger JT, Maree HJ (2016) Next-generation sequencing for virus detection: covering all the bases. Virol J 13(1):1–6. https://doi.org/10.1186/S12985-016-0539-X/FIGURES/2

Chapter 14
Burden of Viral Diseases on the Psychosocial Well-Being of Africans

Nyitor A. Shenge

14.1 Introduction: What Are Viral Diseases?

Viral diseases are caused by organisms that are particles, lack independent or autoreplicatory cellular machinery, and contain nucleic acid as a genetic material. In simpler terms, viral diseases are any infections you get from a virus, which is a tiny organism that uses your cells to reproduce itself. A virus is a type of germ (pathogen) so small that it can only be seen under a microscope. All viruses carry a small piece of genetic information (DNA or RNA) inside a protective coating (capsid). A virus can be likened to an envelope carrying instructions. Conversely, human cells are akin to an entire factory which contains instructions and all the equipment needed to execute them. These instructions allow the body to build proteins and make more cells based on these instructions.

Viral infections usually cause respiratory and digestive illnesses, but viruses can infect most other body parts. Types of viral infections include respiratory infections (affecting the nose, throat, airways, and lungs), digestive system infections (affecting the stomach, intestines, or liver), and viral hemorrhagic fevers (affecting blood clotting and weakening blood vessels, which can lead to potentially life-threatening bleeding). Others are sexually transmitted infections (STIs), exanthematous (rash-causing) infections, neurological infections and congenital infections. Since viruses do not have cells, they also do not have all the necessary components to replicate themselves. Therefore, if they want to replicate themselves, they have to intrude into our cells and use our machinery to do it (replicate). This phenomenon (viruses replicating) makes you sick with a viral infection. Infections with viruses and bacteria can present similar symptoms such as fever, cough and rashes. Therefore, the only way to know what kind of infection you have is to present yourself for assessment by a healthcare provider.

N. A. Shenge (✉)
Department of Psychology, University of Ibadan, Ibadan, Nigeria

J. A. Shenge, A. L. K. Abia (eds.), *Viral Diseases and One Health in Africa*,
https://doi.org/10.1007/978-3-032-09613-5_14

14.2 Viral Diseases as Threats to Public Health

Viral diseases constitute major threats to public health due primarily to the significant health challenges that they pose. They are among modern medicine's most important human health concerns, causing many acute infections, chronic diseases, and virus-associated malignancies. A wide variety of viruses affect millions of people worldwide each year. These include human immunodeficiency virus (HIV), hepatitis C, influenza, rotavirus, chikungunya, and dengue, which affect millions of people each year worldwide. Globally, and especially in Africa, there are threats of viral emergence and pandemics with which humanity and, notably, Africans regularly contend (Dunn and Connor 2012). Reports of the emergence of novel strains of H1N1 flu and previously unrecognised pathogens, such as severe acute respiratory syndrome (SARS) coronavirus and SFTS bunyavirus, further present challenges to global public health.

Remarkably, the health of humans, animals and plants is threatened by these emerging and re-emerging pathogens, most of which have devised means of adapting easily to the environment, including possessing resistant mutations in their genomes. The emergence of new viruses, including but not limited to haemorrhagic fever viruses such as Ebola, Marburg and Lassa fever viruses, and respiratory pathogens such as avian and human influenza, SARS-CoV, MERS viruses, most from zoonotic reservoirs, constitute a rising global challenge, which may result in significantly high morbidity and mortality in human population in the nearest future.

Similarly, vector-borne zoonotic viral diseases, including Rift Valley fever, yellow fever, dengue, chikungunya and West Nile, transmitted by arthropod vectors from many animal reservoirs occur frequently in the tropics, exhibiting previously unseen patterns of infection and spread. These patterns are facilitated by many intrinsic factors, such as mutated sites in the viral genome; they are also driven by external factors, including urbanisation, displacement, human migration and climate change. Transmission of emerging viruses is not restricted; therefore, they can easily cross boundaries and pose a serious threat to the human population in new geographical areas. Here, we outline the features of common emergent viral agents, factors that facilitate their emergence, effects, control and sustained management in the environment.

Viral infections are challenging to treat. A few medications can be used, but treatment usually involves supportive care (i.e. support for the immune system, rest, and a nutritious diet). Stress, pain, and fatigue compromise the immune function, predisposing the person to a viral infection. In this regard, therapeutic massage to support parasympathetic dominance is beneficial.

14.3 The Sporadic Nature of Viral Diseases

Viral diseases are highly sporadic. This refers to their unpredictable and scattered occurrence, where outbreaks may appear in isolated areas rather than widespread epidemics. Factors accounting for isolated rather than widespread epidemics include environmental changes, human activities, and the inherent nature of viruses. Environmental changes encompass human activities, such as agriculture and deforestation, and they can alter ecosystems and bring humans into contact with previously inaccessible viruses or their hosts. As mentioned above, the African continent is highly vulnerable due to the weak or near absence of environmental regulatory laws, among other factors.

By their nature, viruses can adapt to new hosts, resulting in the emergence of new infections in human populations. Changes in host population, demographics, migration patterns, and even individual behaviours can shape the spread of viruses. Ecological factors can play out in the form of climate change, urbanisation, and other environmental factors that can also influence the distribution and transmission of viruses. In Africa, as in other parts of the globe, sporadic viral diseases occur in different ways. For instance, some haemorrhagic fevers, like those caused by the Junin virus, are often found in specific areas due to the presence of rodent hosts. New viral infections such as AIDS similarly appear in human populations. These can have sporadic outbreaks before becoming widespread. Outbreaks of viral diseases in domestic animals, such as vesicular stomatitis virus in cattle, can also be sporadic. Consequences of sporadic outbreaks may include economic losses and public health threats. The sporadic nature of viral diseases suggests the need for ongoing research to understand their origins, transmission, and control.

14.4 Ecological and Socioeconomic Implications of Viral Diseases

Viral diseases are known to disrupt people's efforts to function normally, as they lead to changes in national behavioural patterns and have shut down usual day-to-day functioning, particularly in collectivist societies. These lead to economic and other losses. During COVID-19, social-physical distancing was, for instance, found to affect the psychological well-being of people, especially in collectivist settings such as Africa. It disrupted normal functioning and contrasted the tendency to acclimatise to social identities, social groups, and social participation (Ejoke et al. 2023). With more than 70% of the total COVID-19 cases in Africa originating from South Africa, Egypt, Nigeria, Ghana, and Algeria alone, it is significant to understand the impact of the pandemic on the psychological well-being of Africans. This was made worse by the practice of social-physical distancing.

Restricting people through social distancing alters their daily routine and livelihood, and such changes may cause people to experience deprivation of personal freedom and loneliness, and become devoid of purpose (Ejoke and Khumalo 2020; Mbiti 1990; Venkatesh and Edirappuli 2020). The loss of freedom, therefore, is significant for people. This is particularly so in collectivist societies, which cherish values such as reciprocity and harmony on which economic livelihoods and sustainability largely depend.

14.5 Viral Diseases as Burdens on the Psychological Well-Being of Africans

Psychological well-being is key to survival behaviours, productive ties with others, and living a purposeful and meaningful life, yet little attention is given to it, especially in Africa. Psychological well-being refers to the development of an individual's real potential, attained by achieving a state of harmony and affected by both challenging and rewarding life events (Ryff 1989, 1995). Ryff (1995) identifies six core dimensions of psychological well-being: positive relationships with others, personal mastery, autonomy, a feeling of purpose and meaning in life, and personal growth and development. Each of these dimensions points to a different challenge people find in their efforts to function positively (Keyes et al. 2002; Ryff and Keyes 1995).

Insights from Ryff's research on development during life provide a better understanding of what quality of life entails and how individuals strive to attain it (Ryff and Keyes 1995). Theoretically, the derived dimensions of positive psychological health encompass self-acceptance, positive relations with others, autonomy, environmental mastery, purpose in life, and personal growth (Ryff 1989a).

Psychological well-being is key to a wide range of human survival behaviours, productive interpersonal relationships, purposeful living, and continued growth. However, little attention has been given to the well-being of Africans during COVID-19. This is despite the empirical evidence that social-physical distancing in a collectivist setting such as Africa affects the psychological well-being of the people; it disrupts normal functioning.

Evidence shows that social-physical distancing for a long time strains people's psychological well-being (Ejoke and Khumalo 2020). Therefore, there is a need for relevant authorities to consider activities or practices that assure people's happiness. During COVID-19, psychological well-being was not satisfactorily achieved across Africa. A well-lived life among Africans, characterised by their collective nature in everyday life, is judged by communal living and interpersonal relationships. As such, restricting people through social distancing alters their daily routine and livelihood. There is a clear indication that while the use of social-physical distancing could lead to reduced disease spread, it does have a negative impact on the psychological well-being of the African people. This reduced psychological well-being stems from the fact that social-physical distancing is in contrast with the natural inclination of Africans to connect with others in search of social support, especially in difficult situations.

In addition to the economic and physical burdens that viral diseases place on Africans, some government decisions and policies regarding viral disease outbreaks, including lockdowns, social distancing, self-isolation, and other movement restrictions, lead to reduced social and psychological well-being among the general population and health workers.

14.6 Suggestions for Ameliorating the Situation

The emergence of viral diseases almost always brings to the forefront the urgent need to prepare for the consequences of associated epidemics and pandemics. The outcome of such outbreaks also affects people's physical and mental health. Primary attention is given to physical health, including therapies and treatment of pneumonic symptoms. Consequently, the profound importance of psychological health, orchestrated by the viral infection, isolation, restricted social activities, and trouble sleeping, culminating in stress, anxiety, and episodes of depressive reactions, is ignored. Being infected by a virus and being stressed by the infection have consequences. Therefore, interventions and medications for ameliorating viral infections should also provide improved psychological health. In this regard, scholars have raised concerns about the need for policymakers to balance physical and psychological health (Galea et al. 2020; Holmes et al. 2020; Van Bavel et al. 2020).

Africans are known to be collective in their everyday life, whereby communal living and interpersonal relationships are traditional values and beliefs for judging a well-lived life. Communal connectedness and interpersonal engagement are predominant in Africa. Therefore, social connectedness for Africans is key. Past studies have shown that communal living, frequent social interactions, and spending more time talking with others contribute to greater well-being (Bernstein et al. 2018). Similarly, Margolis and Lyubomirsky (2020) argued that people who engage in more social interactions rather than control activities report higher levels of positive emotion and social connectedness. Recognising that maintaining psychological well-being is vital for people's daily living, it is suggested that an effective applicable policy and a better well-being intervention during a viral outbreak should come to the fore with a clear understanding of what constitutes sound psychological well-being. Identifying factors that negatively impact psychological well-being during viral outbreak interventions and eliminating or minimising them is necessary.

In evaluating the psychological well-being of individuals and groups, authorities should factor in both objective and subjective parameters of psychological well-being. Based on empirical evidence available in the relevant extant literature, special provisions should be made for disadvantaged populations when intervening in viral disease outbreaks. As was observed during the COVID-19 pandemic, there is a need for relevant authorities always to make concerted efforts to preserve the social identities of people when managing viral outbreaks. This is because social identities are essential ingredients that people need to satisfy their basic psychological needs, like belongingness, self-esteem esteem, the need for control, and meaningful existence. This further brings to the fore the importance of social identities, connectedness, and happiness.

Attention should be given to what Ryff (1989a) believes constitutes vital elements of well-being. These include happiness, life satisfaction, and positive affect. During pandemics, authorities, particularly those in Africa, should prioritise health (mental and physical) and interventions that aim to enhance the quality of human living. It is therefore recommended that policymakers consciously try to strike a balance between fighting viral infections and the psychological well-being of the people.

References

Bernstein MJ, Zawadzki MJ, Juth V, Benfield JA, Smyth JM (2018) Social interactions in daily life: within-person associations between momentary social experiences and psychological and physical health indicators. J Soc Pers Relat 35(3):371–394

Dunn EF, Connor JH (2012) HijAkt: the PI3K/Akt pathway in virus replication and pathogenesis. In: Shenolikar S (ed) Progress in molecular biology and translational science, vol 106. Academic, pp 223–250. ISSN 1877-1173. https://doi.org/10.1016/B978-0-12-396456-4.00002-X

Ejoke UP, Khumalo IP (2020) Psychological perspective of experienced happiness during COVID-19 pandemic in South Africa. Gender Behav 18(4):16839–16856

Ejoke UP, Ehigie OB, Shenge NA, Madukwe AU, Obosi AC, Ucho (2023) Social-physical distancing and psychological well-being of Africans during COVID-19 pandemic: a conceptual view. Afr J Dev Stud 13(3):121–144

Galea S, Merchant RM, Lurie N (2020) The mental health consequences of COVID-19 and physical distancing: the need for prevention and early intervention. JAMA Intern Med *180*(6):817–818

Holmes EA, O'Connor RC, Perry VH, Tracey I, Wessely S, Arseneault L et al (2020) Multidisciplinary research priorities for the COVID-19 pandemic: a call for action for mental health science. Lancet Psychiatry *7*(6):547–560

Keyes CL, Shmotkin D, Ryff CD (2002) Optimising well-being: the empirical encounter of two traditions. J Pers Soc Psychol 82(6):1007

Margolis S, Lyubomirsky S (2020) Experimental manipulation of extraverted and introverted behavior and its effects on well-being. J Exp Psychol Gen 149(4):719–731. https://doi.org/10.1037/xge0000668

Mbiti JS (1990) African religions and philosophy, 2nd edn. Heinemann Educational Publishers, Oxford

Ryff CD (1989) Happiness is everything, or is it? Explorations on meaning of psychological well-being. J Pers Soc Psychol 57:1069–1081

Ryff CD (1989a) Beyond Ponce de Leon and life satisfaction: new directions in quest of Successful Ageing. Int J Behav Dev 12:35–55

Ryff CD (1995) Psychological well-being in adult life. Curr Dir Psychol Sci 4(4):99–104

Ryff CD, Keyes CLM (1995) The structure of psychological well-being revisited. J Pers Soc Psychol 69:719–727

Van Bavel JJ, Baicker K, Boggio PS, Capraro V, Cichocka A, Cikara M et al (2020) Using social and behavioural science to support COVID-19 pandemic response. Nat Hum Behav 4(5): 460–471. https://doi.org/10.1038/s41562-020-0884-z

Venkatesh A, Edirappuli S (2020) Social distancing in covid-19: what are the mental health implications? BMJ 369

Chapter 15
The Politics in Public Health—Political Dimensions to Leadership in a Public Health Emergency Like COVID-19

Celestina Obiekea

15.1 Introduction

Africa has faced numerous severe public health crises over the last three decades, including the Human Immunodeficiency Virus/Acquired Immune Deficiency Syndrome (HIV/AIDS) pandemic, the Ebola virus Disease outbreak, persistent Yellow Fever, Cholera and Meningitis outbreaks, the COVID-19 pandemic and most recently the Mpox outbreaks. While some of these diseases are of bacterial origin, a greater proportion of these public health emergencies are due to viruses.

Viruses, by their very nature, possess some unique characteristics (ability to survive outside hosts and in the environment, high mutation rates, ability to infect a wide range of hosts, obligate intraparasitism, and reservoirs in animal populations) that make them able to persist and thrive across human, animal and environmental health interfaces, making them one of the most popular contributors to the interconnectedness of these three interfaces in what is referred to as the "One Health Approach".

As the world continues to become more interconnected into what is now referred to as a "Global Village", and with increasing urbanisation and changes in environmental dynamics, the factors (such as weather, vector and/or host availability and selection pressure) that determine the transmission and spread of these diseases are also changing.

The interconnectedness of the world, as well as the interconnectedness of the various sectors in a One-Health Approach and the likelihood that public health emergencies will often disrupt other non-public health aspects of society, such as the economy, trade and travel, as witnessed with the COVID-19 pandemic underscores the importance of critically understanding the role that politics and political

C. Obiekea (✉)
Abuja, Nigeria

J. A. Shenge, A. L. K. Abia (eds.), *Viral Diseases and One Health in Africa*,
https://doi.org/10.1007/978-3-032-09613-5_15

leadership plays in ensuring that public health emergencies are well coordinated and delivered for the best outcomes for health and non-health benefits.

The COVID-19 pandemic was not merely a public health emergency but a litmus test for political leadership across the globe. In Africa, where health systems are often under-resourced and constrained, the crisis laid bare the critical role of political leaders in navigating complex and nuanced challenges. From enforcing lockdowns to managing vaccine distribution, African leaders faced unparalleled pressures to balance public health imperatives with economic stability, social cohesion, and political survival.

Africa's diversity, culturally, politically, and economically, means that no one single leadership model fits all countries. While some countries rely on decentralised governance structures to deliver health services, others depend on highly centralised systems. This variability underscores the need for nuanced analyses of how leadership operates in practice during public health crises.

Compounding these structural differences are historical and contemporary challenges, including colonial legacies, weak health infrastructures, and limited access to global health resources, yet African leaders have also demonstrated resilience and ingenuity, adapting strategies to local contexts and leveraging regional collaborations to combat the pandemic.

This chapter aims to:

1. Educate readers on the political dimensions of leadership in public health emergencies.
2. Highlight compelling case studies that highlight both successes and failures.
3. Offer actionable policy recommendations to strengthen leadership structures.

The author does not aim to fully exhaust the role of politics in public health emergencies but rather to get a conversation started on the foundations of an area of discourse that is gaining more traction due to the COVID-19 pandemic.

15.2 Definition of Terms

Public Health "This is the science and art of preventing disease, prolonging life, and promoting health through the organised efforts and informed choices of society, organisations, public and private communities, and individuals" (Winslow 1920; Gatseva and Argirova 2011). It includes activities such as disease surveillance, health education, and the implementation of health policies.

Politics This refers to the activities associated with the governance of a country or other area, especially the debate or conflict among individuals or parties having or hoping to achieve power (Aiyede 2023). In public health, politics involves the decisions made by governments and other influential bodies that affect public health policies, resource allocation, and response strategies.

Leadership is the ability to guide and influence individuals or groups toward a common goal (Yukl 2012). In public health emergencies, leadership involves setting direction, making critical decisions, mobilising resources, and effectively coordinating efforts to address the crisis.

Public Health Emergency This is the incidence or imminence of a disease or health condition brought on by bioterrorism, a pandemic or epidemic, or new and highly contagious pathogens that have a high potential to have a significant negative influence on public health. A prompt and thorough answer is necessary (Madhav et al. 2017).

One Health This approach acknowledges the connection between human, animal, and environmental health (Zhou and Zheng 2024). It emphasises the need for interdisciplinary collaboration to address complex health challenges.

15.3 How Public Health Emergencies Disrupt Communities and Economies

Public health emergencies are not just medical crises; they ripple through every aspect of society, upending livelihoods, straining social fabric, and destabilising economies. The COVID-19 pandemic, in particular, illuminated the multifaceted disruptions that health crises can bring, from eroding trust in institutions to widening socioeconomic inequalities.

Public health emergencies place a lot of strain on communities beyond causing personal strain to individuals. They often disrupt socio-economic activities, exacerbating inequalities and eventually contributing to an overall interruption of community, country and international development goals.

During the response to the COVID-19 pandemic (and other public health emergencies), communities with limited access to healthcare, rural populations, informal settlements, and displaced persons faced disproportionately severe impacts. Gender disparities also intensified, with women bearing the brunt of caregiving responsibilities while facing heightened risks of domestic violence and economic exclusion. Fear of infection, isolation, and grief compounded psychological stress across communities and limited access to mental health services, especially in low-resource settings, left many struggling to cope.

In African communities where a significant portion of the population relies on informal work, lockdowns and movement restrictions devastated livelihoods; street vendors, market traders, and daily wage earners faced sudden income losses with limited access to government relief. Businesses, particularly Small and Medium Enterprises (SMEs), were forced to shut down or reduce operations, resulting in widespread job losses; youth unemployment, already high in many African nations, surged further during the pandemic, creating long-term economic scarring.

Many African nations borrowed heavily to finance emergency responses, exacerbating existing debt crises and diverting resources to address immediate crises that strained health systems, disrupting routine care for chronic diseases, maternal health, and immunisation programs.

15.4 Some Public Health Emergencies in Africa Over the Last Three Decades

Over the last 30 years, Africa has faced multiple public health emergencies, many of which have been of viral origin. These crises have posed significant challenges due to the continent's varying healthcare infrastructure, economic limitations, and political contexts.

The HIV/AIDS pandemic from the 1980s till the present still heavily affects countries like South Africa, Nigeria, Uganda, and Kenya. Many African countries have launched and are still maintaining elaborate response programmes to the pandemic. Perhaps, before the most recent COVID-19 pandemic, no other public health emergency fully encapsulated politics' effect on countries' responses to public health emergencies. For instance, due to political denialism, South Africa's early response delayed attempts at prevention and effective treatment. The country's response improved as soon as the political denialism was removed, and the country became a leader in providing Antiretroviral Therapy (ART) on the continent (Nattrass 2008).

The greatest and deadliest Ebola outbreak so far in history occurred between 2014 and 2016, mainly impacting Guinea, Liberia, and Sierra Leone. The outbreak also had sporadic cases in other countries, including Mali, Nigeria, Senegal, the United States, and Europe, due to international travel (WHO 2023).

Other viruses such as Lassa Fever virus, Yellow Fever virus, Marburg virus, Crimean Congo virus, Mpox virus continue to cause ongoing outbreaks in several African countries such as Nigeria, Sierra Leone, DRC, Liberia and Angola; most of these countries experience annual outbreaks (that are almost predictable) requiring leadership in the countries to take more contemporary approaches to improving disease surveillance and response measures as well as public awareness efforts.

Most recently, the COVID-19 pandemic caused by the Severe Acute Respiratory Syndrome Coronavirus 2 (SARS-CoV-2) affected all African countries and highlighted the need for regional leadership and collaboration, nuanced approaches tailored to individual countries' context. Indeed, the COVID-19 pandemic and countries' response to it have highlighted more than ever the role politics and political actors can play in managing public health emergencies.

15.5 Importance of Political Leadership During Health Emergencies: COVID-19 as a Case Study

Effective political leadership during public health emergencies is multidimensional, requiring coordination across various levels of governance. In Africa, where diverse political systems intersect with complex public health needs, political leadership plays a pivotal role in determining the trajectory of a crisis. The responses to HIV/AIDS, Ebola, and COVID-19 underscore the spectrum of political actions that can either mitigate or exacerbate public health challenges.

Let us examine some of the critical roles that political leadership play in managing public health emergencies.

15.5.1 Decision-Making Authority and the Power to Formulate Health Regulations and Policies

During all the phases of the management of public health emergencies (before, during and after), political leaders hold critical decision-making authority and the power to formulate and enforce health regulations and policies. In Africa, where diverse health challenges require adaptable strategies, the capacity of leaders to exercise these powers effectively often determines the outcomes of such emergencies.

The power to formulate and enforce health regulations and/or policies enables political leaders to address the immediate demands of public health emergencies while also building long-term resilience. Effective policymaking involves collaboration with public health experts, scientists, and international organisations to ensure evidence-based decisions. In Uganda, President Yoweri Museveni's administration was lauded for its early adoption of the "Test and Treat" strategy during the HIV/AIDS epidemic, which significantly improved access to antiretroviral therapy and reduced transmission rates (Parkhurst 2002). This policy was rooted in close partnerships with health organisations and community leaders, exemplifying the importance of inclusive decision-making.

Political leaders, particularly heads of state and health ministers, wield significant influence during public health emergencies. Their authority allows them to declare emergencies, allocate budgets, and direct national responses. For example, during the 2014–2016 Ebola outbreak in Liberia, President Ellen Johnson Sirleaf invoked emergency powers to implement curfews, restrict movement, and establish treatment centres. Though initially controversial, these decisive actions proved essential in controlling the outbreak and preventing its escalation (Abramowitz 2017).

Governors and local government officials play pivotal roles at sub-national levels in implementing national directives and tailoring responses to local contexts. In Nigeria's fight against COVID-19, state governors imposed localised lockdowns and set up isolation centres, demonstrating how decentralised decision-making can enhance responsiveness and adaptability (Nkengasong and Mankoula 2020).

15.5.2 Resource Allocation

Resource allocation is one of the most critical powers wielded by political leaders during public health emergencies. It involves directing financial, human, and logistical resources to address immediate and long-term needs (Hanson et al. 2022). In Africa, where health systems are often underfunded and stretched, effective resource allocation can significantly influence the trajectory of public health emergencies. Like other government agencies, National Public Health Institutes (NPHIs) are funded through national budgetary allocations subject to national budgetary cycles, processes and approvals. Often, the leadership of public health institutes have to lobby political leaders and get them to see the importance of ensuring sufficient budget allocations to manage public health emergencies (including prevention, control and sustainability measures). Health ministers, who are often political appointees, most times have to be convinced that allocating resources to the management of public health emergencies and public health security in general (Ihekweazu and Ihekweazu 2024) is beneficial and cost-effective, and this lack of urgency can often have dire consequences. Budgets are also often reprioritised to fund emergency responses, including the procurement of medical supplies, construction of treatment facilities, and deployment of healthcare workers. During the 2014–2016 Ebola outbreak in Sierra Leone, President Ernest Bai Koroma redirected national funds toward response efforts and sought international aid to bolster the country's overwhelmed healthcare system (Richards 2016).

Political leaders also have the authority to mobilise and deploy human resources, including healthcare workers, law enforcement, and volunteers, to manage public health emergencies. This was evident during the Ebola outbreak in Liberia, where President Ellen Johnson Sirleaf directed the training and deployment of thousands of healthcare workers to affected areas. Similarly, local and community leaders in Nigeria were key in mobilising traditional healers and religious leaders to support polio eradication efforts, effectively addressing vaccine hesitancy and improving coverage (Jegede 2007).

During the COVID-19 pandemic, several African countries faced strikes by healthcare workers protesting unsafe working conditions and insufficient compensation. This undermined the response activities in some of the affected countries and highlighted the need for political leaders to prioritise the welfare of frontline responders to sustain effective crisis management.

In addition to directing and controlling domestic resources, political leaders often negotiate and secure international aid during public health emergencies. The African Union's efforts to establish the African Vaccine Acquisition Task Team (AVATT) during COVID-19 exemplified the power of collective political leadership in mobilising resources for the continent. National leaders also collaborated with global institutions like the World Health Organization and the Global Fund to secure funding, vaccines, and technical expertise (Nkengasong et al. 2021).

15.5.3 Inter-Agency Coordination

Inter-agency coordination is a cornerstone of effective public health emergency management, and political leaders often play a pivotal role in facilitating collaboration among diverse stakeholders. This coordination involves harmonising efforts across government agencies at the national and sub-national levels, health institutions, private entities, and international organisations to ensure a cohesive response. Political leaders frequently establish centralised coordination mechanisms during public health crises to streamline responses. These structures enable the integration of various agencies and ensure a unified strategy. In Nigeria, during the reaction to the COVID-19 pandemic, President Muhammadu Buhari directed the setting up of the Presidential Task Force (PTF) that brought together all health and non-health government agencies, development partners and private sector to coordinate the country's response to the pandemic efficiently. At the regional level, the Africa CDC collaborated with national governments to standardise testing protocols, manage vaccine procurement, and establish the African Medical Supplies Platform (Nkengasong et al. 2021).

Conversely, a lack of coordination can undermine response efforts. During the early phases of the COVID-19 pandemic, conflicting directives between national governments and local authorities in some African countries created confusion, delaying the implementation of critical measures such as lockdowns and testing (Nkengasong and Mankoula 2020). These instances highlight the importance of clear leadership and coordination to avoid fragmented responses.

In transboundary health emergencies, political leaders must coordinate efforts across national borders to address shared challenges. The West African Ebola outbreak exemplified the importance of regional solidarity, with leaders of affected countries collaborating through platforms such as the Mano River Union. Similarly, during COVID-19, the African Union's leadership in creating the African Vaccine Acquisition Task Team (AVATT) underscored the role of political leaders in mobilising collective action to secure vaccines for the continent (Nkengasong et al. 2021).

15.5.4 Public Communication and Trust-Building

The authority to make decisions and formulate policies also carries the responsibility of maintaining public trust, and transparent communication, inclusivity, and accountability are essential to ensure compliance with health regulations. Public health emergencies are often accompanied by a surge in misinformation, which can undermine response efforts, and political leaders have the power to counter misinformation by providing evidence-based information and partnering with credible voices, such as health experts and community leaders. Leaders who engage with communities, as seen in Liberia's Ebola response, foster greater public cooperation and resilience. On the other hand, opaque decision-making processes can lead to resistance and misinformation, as evidenced by vaccine hesitancy in some African countries during the COVID-19 pandemic (Nkengasong et al. 2021).

Poor communication or the spread of misinformation by political leaders can erode public trust. During the COVID-19 pandemic, Tanzanian President John Magufuli dismissed the severity of the virus during the early phase of the country's response and discouraged testing, promoting unverified remedies instead. This approach sowed confusion and undermined the credibility of health authorities and international guidelines (Yaya et al. 2021).

Trust-building is a long-term process but becomes especially critical during emergencies. It also involves acknowledging and addressing the structural inequalities that exacerbate health crises. Leaders who engage marginalised communities and ensure equitable access to healthcare resources are more likely to sustain public confidence. During COVID-19, countries like Ghana demonstrated trust-building by offering free testing and subsidised treatment, signalling a commitment to equitable care (Nkengasong et al. 2021).

When political leaders fail to communicate effectively or prioritise political agendas over public health, trust in leadership can erode, leading to noncompliance and heightened vulnerability. In some African countries, inconsistent messaging during COVID-19 and reports of corruption in managing pandemic funds led to widespread scepticism about government directives. This erosion of trust hampered vaccination campaigns and other preventive measures, prolonging the pandemic's impact (Yaya et al. 2021).

15.6 Political Leadership during the COVID-19 Response in Africa: Country-Specific Deep Dives and Case Scenarios

The COVID-19 pandemic presented a litmus test for political leadership across Africa. Leaders faced the dual challenge of safeguarding public health while mitigating economic and social upheaval. This section examines the political dimensions of leadership in South Africa, Nigeria, and Rwanda, showcasing how their unique political contexts influenced their responses to the pandemic.

15.6.1 South Africa: Managing a Decentralised Health System amid Political Tension

South Africa is a constitutional democracy with a three-tier system of government and an independent judiciary. The political structure is based on the Constitution of South Africa (1996), which provides for a unitary state with decentralised governance across national, provincial, and local levels.

During the early stages of the pandemic, the national government, led by President Cyril Ramaphosa, centralised decision-making under the Disaster Management Act (2002) (Republic of South Africa, 2002). This gave the National Coronavirus Command Council (NCCC) control over pandemic policies, including lockdown regulations and economic restrictions. However, this approach undermined provincial autonomy, as provincial governments had limited decision-making power (Heywood 2020). Provinces such as the Western Cape, governed by the opposition Democratic Alliance (DA), pushed back against the centralised response. The Western Cape government criticised blanket lockdown measures imposed by the national government, arguing that provincial variations in infection rates required a more localised approach (Pillay 2021).

President Cyril Ramaphosa declared a national state of disaster early in the pandemic, enabling swift implementation of lockdown measures to curb the virus's spread and provide time to bolster healthcare capacities. In South Africa and many countries, while the public health authorities may make recommendations on what type and level of non-medical or non-pharmaceutical measures are required to contain outbreaks, it is ultimately the political leaders who hold the power to announce such stringent measures and ensure their implementation in full.

The rollout of COVID-19 vaccines in South Africa was delayed due to political and logistical challenges. The national government initially opted for a centralised procurement strategy, which the provincial governments criticised as slow and inefficient (Madhi et al. 2021). This resulted in some provincial governments attempting to procure vaccines independently, leading to further clashes with national authorities (Pillay 2021).

Overall, South Africa's COVID-19 response was heavily influenced by political tensions between different levels of government. Coordination between the national and provincial governments was critical in managing resource allocation and healthcare delivery, and the constant battle for political autonomy between the national and provincial governments often hampered the response efforts.

15.6.2 Nigeria: Federal Coordination and Innovative State-Level Responses

Nigeria operates a federated political system with political power shared between the three arms of government (federal, state and local). This federal system created a mosaic of responses to the pandemic, with varying levels of effectiveness across the states.

Health matters are on Nigeria's concurrent legislative list, meaning that both federal and state governments have responsibilities when it comes to the administration of health matters. While issues relating to policy development, coordination and standardisation are generally left to the federal government, it is usually understood that the state (and sometimes local governments) are responsible for ensuring that these policies are implemented and necessary resources are allocated to realise this implementation. This dichotomy of responsibilities often creates challenges for effective response to public health emergencies in the country, especially as there is frequently limited clarity on who is responsible for what, what boundaries exist for all parties and what situations could trigger emergency approaches.

The Federal Government, led by President Muhammadu Buhari, established the Presidential Task Force (PTF) on COVID-19 to coordinate nationwide inter-ministerial efforts and mitigate the impact of the pandemic on Nigerians (Bolu et al. 2022). The PTF was led by the Secretary to the government of the federation and comprised heads of key ministries and agencies and international development partners such as the World Health Organization (WHO). In responding to the pandemic, the federal and state governments exercised their powers to implement strict whole-of-society approaches such as travel bans and lockdowns.

Along parallel lines, state governments also created coordination structures led by the Commissioners of Health and, in some instances, the state Governors themselves. For example, Lagos State instituted its command centre, which sometimes implemented measures that were way ahead of the federal government's. Similarly, Kaduna State implemented its state-level lockdown.

Challenges brought about by this dichotomy of responsibilities included communication gaps between federal and state governments, occasionally hampering the uniformity of interventions, disagreement between federal and state governments on the true extent of infections (for instance, the Kogi state governor at the time till the end of his tenure refused NCDC and national surveillance officers entry into the state, claiming that the state had no COVID-19 cases). Other challenges included the general lack of trust in government.

In addition to the operations of the executive arm of government (at both federal and state levels), the legislative arms of government (Senate and House of Representatives at the federal and state houses of representatives at the state level) also ammended existing laws that empowered respective agencies to carry out their duties fully and better. For instance, the senate passed a resolution as early as March 2020, urging the Federal Government to increase funding to the Nigeria Centre for Disease Control (NCDC) to respond efficiently to the pandemic, introduced and expedited passage of the Economic Stimulus Bill. The National Assembly also amended the existing Medical Schemes Act to enhance the regulatory framework for healthcare delivery during the crisis (Dan-Azumi and Abubakar 2020).

Considering Nigeria's federated political context, these legislative actions aimed to ensure a cohesive and practical approach to managing the pandemic across the federal and state levels.

15.6.3 Rwanda: Centralised Leadership and Strict Censorship

Rwanda's political landscape is characterised by a strong centralised government, strict political control, and a developmental state model. Under President Paul Kagame, Rwanda's centralised political system allowed for a rapid and coordinated pandemic response. Before the pandemic, Rwanda was widely regarded as one of Africa's most stable and efficiently governed countries and one of its most politically restrictive (Reyntjens 2021).

When COVID-19 emerged, Rwanda's political system was critical in shaping its response. The government adopted a centralised, science-driven, and enforcement-heavy approach that effectively contained the virus and reflected Rwanda's broader political framework. The state-controlled media ensured that public messaging was clear and consistent, helping curb misinformation and increase compliance (Mukarubuga 2021).

Rwanda implemented some of the most stringent lockdown measures on the continent early in the pandemic. The government used drones to disseminate public health messages and monitor compliance with social distancing measures. It worked closely with local leaders and community health workers to ensure the widespread dissemination of accurate information.

The government of Rwanda also enacted several pieces of legislation in response to the pandemic. Some of these legislations include Presidential orders on state of emergency (which declared a nationwide state of emergency, granting extraordinary powers to the government to manage the pandemic), tax relief and restructuring (which allowed temporary tax exemptions for businesses affected by lockdowns as well as directed commercial banks to restructure loans for affected borrowers), laws on Use of Digital Contact Tracing and Surveillance for COVID-19 (which legalised the use of mobile tracking and digital monitoring for COVID-19 containment and required telecommunication providers to share data with health authorities). Others include laws that amended the penal code to introduce fines and imprisonment for anyone violating the COVID-19 health regulations and establishing the COVID-19 Economic Recovery Fund (CERF).

Rwanda's response demonstrated the power of centralised leadership in ensuring swift and cohesive action. However, concerns about the suppression of dissent during the pandemic, heavy-handed law enforcement, human rights violations, limited transparency and accountability, and a lack of inclusivity highlighted the challenges of over-centralised governance during public health crises and the delicate balance between public health enforcement and civil liberties.

15.7 Lessons for Future Public Health Emergencies

The COVID-19 pandemic highlighted both the vulnerabilities and strengths of African political leadership. As the continent prepares for future public health crises, the focus must be on building resilient institutions, fostering inclusive leadership, and leveraging local and regional collaboration. By learning from past experiences and investing in proactive measures, Africa can emerge stronger and better prepared to tackle the challenges of tomorrow. Specifically, there should be a focus on:

- Political leaders must be equipped with the skills to respond effectively to complex emergencies. Programs focusing on evidence-based decision-making, crisis communication, and ethical leadership are critical.
- Regional institutions like the Africa CDC can spearhead leadership development initiatives tailored to African contexts.
- Leaders must communicate openly about challenges and decisions during crises to foster public trust.
- Decentralisation of health governance and empowering subnational governments to act swiftly in emergencies can reduce bureaucratic delays. Countries with decentralised systems, like Nigeria, highlight the importance of local decision-making capabilities.
- Traditional and religious leaders play a crucial role in mobilising communities. Involving them early in planning and implementation ensures greater compliance and trust.
- Solutions must be tailored to each country's unique cultural, economic, and political realities.
- Inclusive leadership that reflects the diversity of the population fosters equitable responses.
- As seen in Nigeria, decentralised approaches demonstrate the value of flexibility and adaptability.

15.8 Conclusion

The COVID-19 pandemic has underscored the critical role of political leadership in managing public health emergencies in Africa. The responses of South Africa, Nigeria, and Rwanda to the COVID-19 pandemic highlight the diversity of political leadership styles, clear communication, community engagement, and innovative solutions. Each country faced unique challenges, but common themes emerged, such as the need for adaptable and inclusive leadership to mitigate the impact of public health crises, the role of legislation as a tool for political action and the importance of decisive action. The pandemic has also revealed the importance of building resilient institutions, fostering inclusive leadership, and leveraging local and regional collaboration. By learning from past experiences and investing in proactive measures, Africa can emerge stronger and better prepared to tackle future public health emergencies. Political leaders must be equipped with the skills to respond effectively to complex emergencies, and regional institutions like the Africa CDC can play a pivotal role in spearheading leadership development initiatives tailored to African contexts. Ultimately, the lessons learned from the COVID-19 pandemic can guide the continent in building a more resilient and equitable public health system.

References

Abramowitz S (2017) Ebola: discourses in disease, security, and global health. Routledge

Aiyede ER (2023) Governance and politics of public policy in Africa. In: Public policy and research in Africa. Springer, Cham, p 87

Bolu O, Mustapha B, Ihekweazu C, Muhammad M, Hassan A, Abdulwahab A, Asekun AA, Nsirim R, Okechukwu E, Attah I, Swaminathan M (2022) Effect of Nigeria presidential task force on COVID-19 pandemic, Nigeria. Emerg Infect Dis 28(Suppl 1):S168

Dan-Azumi JD, Abubakar (2020) Role of parliaments in managing pandemics: an evaluation of National Assembly's response to Covid-19. In: A political economy of pandemics and consequences of Covid-19 for Nigeria. Abuja, National Institutes for Legislative and Democratic Studies (NILDS), pp 320–348

Gatseva PD, Argirova M (2011) Public health: the science of promoting health. J Public Health 19: 205–206

Hanson K, Brikci N, Erlangga D, Alebachew A, De Allegri M, Balabanova D, Blecher M, Cashin C, Esperato A, Hipgrave D, Kalisa I (2022) The Lancet Global Health Commission on financing primary health care: putting people at the centre. Lancet Glob Health 10(5):e715–e772

Heywood M (2020) South Africa's COVID-19 response: strengths, weaknesses, and political challenges. Daily Maverick, 15 May. Available at: www.dailymaverick.co.za/article/2020-05-15. Accessed 11 Feb 2025

Ihekweazu C, Ihekweazu V (2024) An imperfect storm. Outside the Box Learning Resources Ltd., Naas, Co, Kildare

Jegede AS (2007) What led to the Nigerian boycott of the polio vaccination campaign? PLoS Med 4(3):e73

Madhav N, Oppenheim B, Gallivan M, Mulembakani P, Rubin E, Wolfe N (2017) Pandemics: risks, impacts, and mitigation. In: Disease control priorities: improving health and reducing poverty, 3rd edn. World Bank Group, Washington, DC

Madhi SA, Gray GE, Adebayo E (2021) COVID-19 vaccine rollout in South Africa: challenges and opportunities. Lancet Glob Health 9(7):e1010–e1020

Mukarubuga A (2021) Economic and social challenges of Rwanda's COVID-19 response. J Afr Public Policy 15(3):90–110

Nattrass N (2008) AIDS and the scientific governance of medicine in post-apartheid South Africa. Afr Aff 107(427):157–176

Nkengasong JN, Mankoula W (2020) Looming threat of COVID-19 infection in Africa: act collectively, and fast. Lancet 395(10227):841–842

Nkengasong JN et al (2021) Africa CDC'S leadership in Africa's COVID-19 vaccine rollout. Nat Med 27(1):20–22

Parkhurst JO (2002) The Ugandan success story? Evidence and claims of HIV-1 prevention. Lancet 360(9326):78–80

Pillay D (2021) Provincial responses to COVID-19: the case of the Western cape. S Afr J Public Health 15(4):120–135

Reyntjens, F. (2021) The politics of pandemic response in Rwanda: between public health and political control. Oxford University Press
Richards P (2016) Ebola: how a people's science helped end an epidemic. Zed Books
Winslow C-EA (1920) The untilled fields of public health. Science 51:23
World Health Organization (2023) Ebola outbreak 2014–2016 overview. Available at: https://www.who.int/news-room/fact-sheets/detail/ebola-virus-disease. Accessed 13 Feb 2025
Yaya S et al (2021) COVID-19 in Africa: lessons from a continent's response. Lancet Glob Health 9(5):e593–e594
Yukl G (2012) Leadership: what is it. Cases in leadership, 3rd edn. Sage, Thousand Oaks, pp 1–42
Zhou X, Zheng J (2024) Building a transdisciplinary science of One Health with a global vision. Glob Health J 8(3):99–102

Index

J. A. Shenge, A. L. K. Abia (eds.), *Viral Diseases and One Health in Africa*,
https://doi.org/10.1007/978-3-032-09613-5

MIX
Papier aus verantwortungsvollen Quellen
Paper from responsible sources
FSC® C105338

If you have any concerns about our products,
you can contact us on
ProductSafety@springernature.com

In case Publisher is established outside the EU,
the EU authorized representative is:
Springer Nature Customer Service Center GmbH
Europaplatz 3, 69115 Heidelberg, Germany

Printed by Libri Plureos GmbH
in Hamburg, Germany